D0148838

FLUID EXCHANGES

Artists and Critics in the AIDS Crisis

AIDS is an acronym that was largely unknown only a decade ago. Today AIDS has meaning for virtually everyone in the western world. But the nature of its meaning varies wildly, from the stark reality faced by people infected by the HIV virus and those who love them to those who encounter AIDS only as a 'plague' hysterically exploited in the media. In between lies a range of expression about AIDS in art, literature, drama, film, and critical theory.

In this volume, an international group of contributors discuss the ways in which the arts and humanities have presented AIDS. They exchange ideas across lines of liberalism and radicalism, art and theory, social realities and political agendas. In the process they raise difficult questions: How does the vocabulary of AIDS shape popular conception about HIV infection? How can we counter the response to AIDS that equates sex with death and health with piety? What is the impact of AIDS on gay identity?

Since AIDS first became known to the general public ten years ago, its medical and political aspects have largely eclipsed the spiritual and cultural dimensions. These essays address that imbalance. They consider the impact of AIDS, not only on the bodies of persons with HIV infection, but on the hearts and minds of us all.

JAMES MILLER is Faculty Professor of Arts, University of Western Ontario, and author of *Measures of Wisdom: The Cosmic Dance in Classical and Christian Antiquity.*

FLUID EXCHANGES:

Artists and Critics in the AIDS Crisis

edited by James Miller

University of Toronto Press
Toronto Buffalo London

© University of Toronto Press 1992
Toronto Buffalo London
Printed in Canada

ISBN 0-8020-5892-2 (cloth)
ISBN 0-8020-6824-3 (paper)

Printed on acid-free paper

Canadian Cataloguing in Publication Data

Main entry under title:

Fluid exchanges: artists and critics in the AIDS crisis
ISBN 0-8020-5892-2 (bound) ISBN 0-8020-6824-3 (pbk.)
1. AIDS (Disease) in art. I. Miller, James L., 1951– .

NX180.A25F58 1992 704.9'496169792 C91-095665-0

This book has been supported by the Canada Council and Ontario Arts Council under their block grant programs, and by a grant from the Visual AIDS Committee.

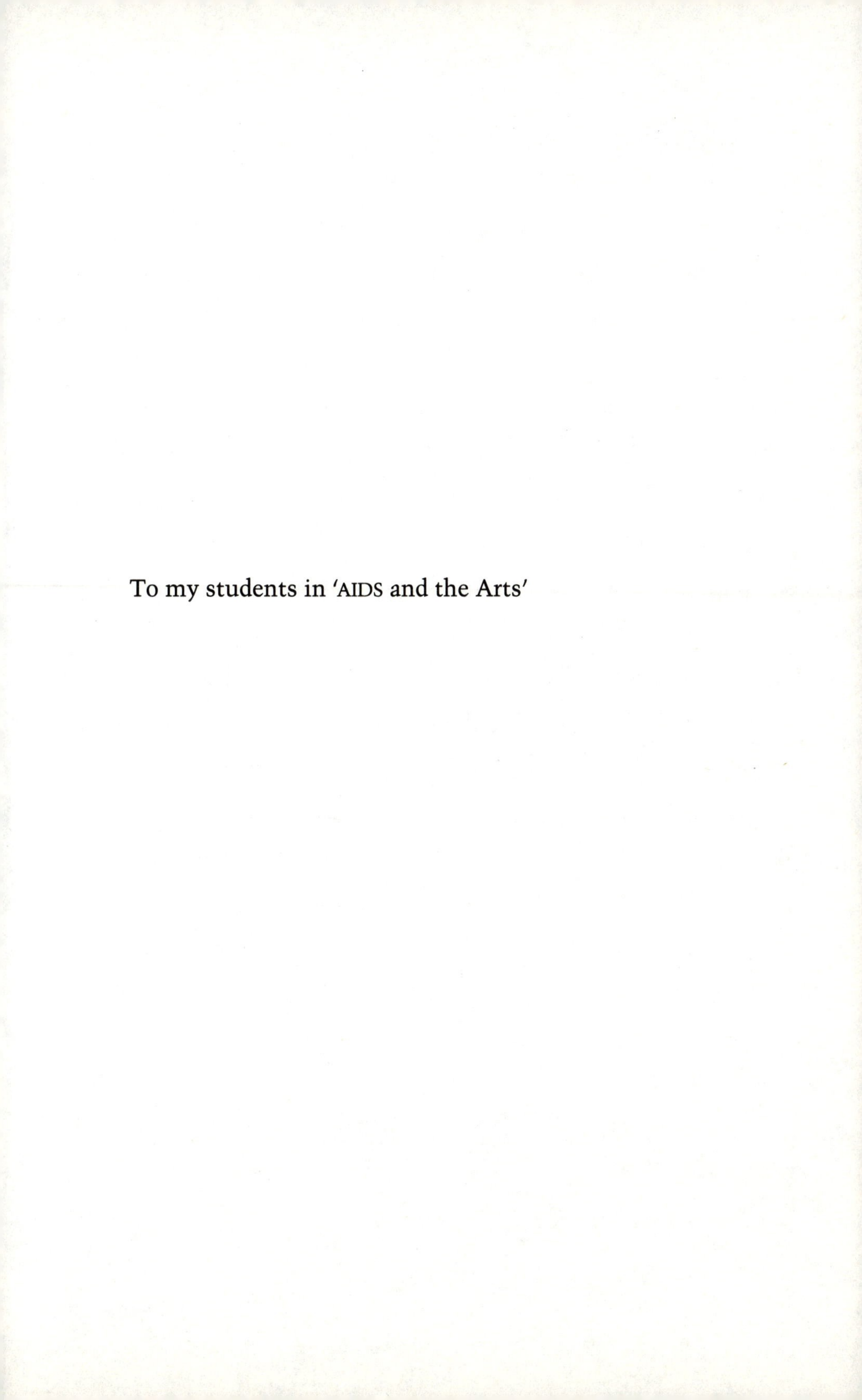

To my students in 'AIDS and the Arts'

Contents

Acknowledgments / xi

Introduction / 3
JAMES MILLER

PHOTOGRAPHY

Visible Lesions: Images of the PWA in America / 23
Appendix: AIDS Archives and Resources for Visual Researchers / 44
JAN ZITA GROVER

Plates for Introduction and Grover and Gagnon essays following page 51

A Convergence of Stakes: Photography, Feminism, and AIDS / 53
MONIKA GAGNON

PAINTING

'The Soul is the Prison of the Body': Fabo on Foucault / 65
DAVID WHITE

Plates for White and Miller essays following page 88

Our Lady of AIDS: The Occult Design of André Durand's *Votive Offering* / 89
JAMES MILLER

FILM AND VIDEO

The Syndrome is the System: A Political Reading of *Longtime Companion* / 111
BART BEATY
Erotic Self-Images in the Gay Male AIDS Melodrama / 122
THOMAS WAUGH
Parma Violets for Wayland Flowers / 135
JOHN GREYSON

MEMORIALS AND PUBLIC ART

The Scythe, the Scales, and the Palette: AIDS and the Rupture of Representational Strategies / 146
MONIQUE BRUNET-WEINMANN

Plates for Brunet-Weinmann, Harris, and O'Malley essays following page 161

On Reading the Obituaries in the *Bay Area Reporter* / 163
DANIEL HARRIS

PREVENTION CAMPAIGNS

The Representation of AIDS in Third World Development Discourse / 169
JEFF O'MALLEY
Portfolio One: Posters from the Visual AIDS Exhibition, London Regional Art and Historical Museums, 11–20 October 1988 / 177

CRISIS AND CRITICISM

Criticism as Activism / 185
Appendix: Le Manifeste de Montréal / 211
JAMES MILLER

Plates for Miller essay following page 214

Portfolio Two: 'The Body & Society' Exhibition: Embassy Cultural House, London, Ontario, September–December 1988 / 215

MEDIA AND MEDIATION

'John': *London Free Press*, 1 April 1988 / 222
DAHLIA REICH

The AIDS-Timmy: Reflections on a Cultural Niche / 228
DAVID KINAHAN
'A Fair Representation of His Feelings': A Reply to David Kinahan / 236
DAHLIA REICH

Plates for Reich, Gordon/Crossman, Patton, and Kroker essays following page 239

'aids kills fags dead ...': Cultural Activism in Grand Bend / 241
Appendix: AIDS and the Human Rights Code / 253
JOHN GORDON AND CLARENCE CROSSMAN
'Fighting spirit remains in 29-year-old victim': *London Free Press*, 8 July 1991 / 255
DAHLIA REICH

LITERATURE

AIDS in the Novel: Getting It Straight / 257
JAMES MILLER
Cell Wars: Military Metaphors and the Crisis of Authority in the AIDS Epidemic / 272
BRIAN PATTON

LEGAL AND POLITICAL DISCOURSE

Law as an 'Art Form' Reflecting AIDS: A Challenge to the Province and Function of Law / 287
MARGARET A. SOMERVILLE
The State, Public Policy, and AIDS Discourse / 305
BARRY D. ADAM

PSYCHOSEXUAL DISCOURSE

Sacrificial Sex / 321
ARTHUR KROKER
The Possibilities of Permutation: Pleasure, Proliferation, and the Politics of Gay Identity in the Age of AIDS / 329
SIMON WATNEY

Notes on Contributors / 369

Photo Credits / 373

Index / 375

Acknowledgments

When David Stimpson first suggested to me that a book could be formed from the papers of the 'Representing AIDS' conference, he also urged me to sound out the idea with Prudence Tracy at the University of Toronto Press. Her encouragement to go ahead with it – come what may – got it off the ground in the spring of 1989.

Come what may, of course, inevitably came: reactionary forces opposed to the radical character of the project slowed down its realization in spite of our urgent sense of its usefulness in the discourse wars sparked by the epidemic. Forced to rethink my counter-discursive tactics, I depended on Prudence's unshaken confidence in the project to guide me through the tricky process of reconceiving it as more than an academic archive. Fortunately, her editorial wisdom prevented me from proceeding with a dull volume of conference proceedings when that was all I thought it would ever be allowed to be. With diplomatic skills worthy of her allegorical namesake, she went to bat for this book more often, I'm sure, than I'll ever know.

Thanks to her dialectical fairmindedness, the manuscript was sent out to readers whose divergent political and cultural viewpoints assured it a thorough going-over from all sides. William Zion challenged its diversity of approaches and provoked me to defend the discord of its marginalized agendas. Peter Millard questioned the value of polemical strategies that came off as tactless attacks, but also criticized the dispassionate tact of arguments that ignored the urgency of the crisis. Paula Treichler pointed out the weak links in the chain of articles (starting with the original draft of my introduction) and called for a clarification of the organization of the contents. John St James exposed much else that needed clarifying or rewording. Their invaluable readings virtually reshaped the book.

If James Etherington, Catherine Finlayson, and Peta Lomberg of London Life had not expanded my vision of cultural activism to include much beyond the classroom and the gallery, the London sections of the book would have been narrowly focused on academic issues. Their continuing support for the local and international projects reflected in this volume is much appreciated by all the London contributors. Thanks to a subvention from the Visual AIDS Committee, whose work has been supported by generous grants from London Life since 1988, the cost of photographing the AIDS posters reproduced in these pages has been sizeably reduced and the price of the paperback edition held within reasonable bounds.

To the resource centre at the AIDS Committee of London, a copy of this book will be gratefully donated by me on behalf of the Visual AIDS Committee. Betty Anne Thomas and the dedicated ACOL staff have never failed to help me out whenever I needed a statistic checked, a poster hunted down, a medical term defined, a newspaper article retrieved, or a community-based hug administered.

My colleagues at Western, Tom Lennon, Madeline Lennon, John Nicholas, Richard Green, and Alice Mansell, offered their personal (which is to say political) support of the 'AIDS and the Arts' program from its beginnings in 1988. Melissa Hardy helped me to face the terrors of nuclear-family meltdown by springing me from the closet of my own cowardice with her characteristic courage. Linda Nicholas kept my spirits up by proving that there really was a beach at the end of it all. John Stracuzza gently outed me to myself, with a little help from *Idomeneo*.

The steady friendship of all these people through the tumultuous days of my coming out – which coincided, not coincidentally, with the long coming-to-be of this anthology – sustained it as well as me.

FLUID EXCHANGES

Artists and Critics in the AIDS Crisis

Introduction

JAMES MILLER

Since 1985, when the first AIDS activist groups proclaimed their radical agendas in the United States, Britain, and Canada, artists and critics have joined forces in increasing numbers to fight the epidemic of fear and bigotry attending the AIDS crisis. Their alliance with the activists continues into the 1990s all along the undefended border between the university and what used to be known as the Real World. Drawn together at international conferences and local gallery openings, at private vigils and public demonstrations, they have found a common project in fighting AIDS discrimination with words and images that challenge the discursive foundations of contemporary social reality. This volume is part of that ongoing critical project.

The engagement of artists and critics in AIDS activism did not come about simply because the Human Immunodeficiency Virus (HIV) had already infected many members of their overlapping communities by the mid-1980s. Nor was it due entirely to the angry momentum of local protest groups rallied to the defence of human rights or civil liberties in the dark years before the epidemic was widely perceived as a threat to the 'general public.' The rapid sophistication of artistic and critical responses to the AIDS crisis no doubt reflects the cosmopolitan character of the specific publics where 'AIDS awareness' as a social cause was born. Its genesis in New York, San Francisco, Toronto, Montreal, and London was favoured by ethnological as well as epidemiological factors: the peculiar self-reflexiveness of these cultural capitals, with their interconnected universities and museums and multitudes of commercial and alternative art galleries, inscribed itself on the tabula rasa of the new illness from the start and promoted its very mysteriousness as a subject for immediate artistic and academic meditation.

Of course other epidemics have affected the production of cultural objects and the construction of cultural history, and often deeply. But never so rapidly or so politically as AIDS: though millions of people in the Third World die of cholera or malaria each year, who has ever marched down Fifth Avenue for the rights of cholera victims or attended a Queen Street exhibition of postmodern malarial art? In the capitals of the First World, AIDS was perceived as a crisis for the arts even before it received its official medical name.

Perhaps what remained of late-sixties liberalism in the academic life of the 1970s had something to do with the conception of AIDS awareness as an activist aesthetic project – if only because the university (or at least some universities) continued to offer ideological support for various disenfranchised groups mobilized during the heyday of the student rebellions. Chief among these were women, blacks, and gays, whose liberationist causes were being championed on the alternative art scene well before the epidemic struck. After its outbreak representatives from all three oppressed constituencies, notably female prostitutes, Haitian immigrants, and male homosexuals, found themselves swiftly and searingly reclassified as 'high-risk groups' in the discriminatory discourse of public health. When early reports of the 'special' vulnerability of women, blacks, and gays to immune deficiency surfaced in the mainstream media, their advocates in the arts (some of whom were male, white, and straight) were quick to express opposition to the dominant political construction of the AIDS crisis in the West, which included, as it still does, the perniciously consoling role of the 'AIDS victim.'

Yet even such a coincidence of ethical sympathies, a continuity of old countercultural allegiances, is not enough to explain the exceptional imaginative vigour and intellectual thrust of their militant strategies on the newly mapped battleground of cultural activism. Nothing invented at the university in recent years has acted as more of a stimulus to the socially reforming zeal of AIDS activism than 'critical theory,' a dynamic and complicated fusion of radical social philosophies and sceptical reading techniques. If academics were in need of a jump-start after the spluttering decline of structuralism, which had failed to provide them with a key to all mythologies, they got more than they bargained for in the crackling 'poststructuralist' channels into which their faculties of arts and social sciences were decisively tapping. Try as they might to contain it within conventional disciplines and course-offerings in the late 1970s, the multilateral explosion of critical theory through the 1980s has rocked the privileged foundations of the university itself. It was a blast to be felt all over the map, including the map of the Real World where the AIDS crisis was being constructed as a global menace to the good life of Western capitalist democracies.

Crucial to the ideology of radical AIDS activism are the twin concepts of social marginalization and inferiorization developed by theorists in the arts and social sciences and expanded by politically active artists influenced by critical theory. Borne on the university currents of feminism, civil libertarianism, and gay liberation, these notions have passed without resistance into the sophisticated counterdiscourse of groups like ACT UP ('AIDS Coalition To Unleash Power') in America, OutRage in Britain, and AIDS ACTION NOW! in Canada. As an institutional forum for utopian social transformations, the university has provided artists and activists with a common ground of liberationist consciousness where they have strengthened each other's resolve to confront the AIDS crisis by calling for a profound rethinking of social order and the operations of political power.

It should come as no surprise, then, that the present volume should have been published by a university press for readers in the Real World who want to do more than read about the AIDS crisis. In dealing with the fantasy world of political agendas, the contributors to the volume have not forgotten the worldly reality of tight money and discriminatory funding. Consequently, with the encouragement of the University of Toronto Press, we have agreed to donate all profits from the sale of this publication to AIDS ACTION NOW! in recognition of its constructive use of the mainstream media to end the scandalous ban on the sale of experimental drugs (such as dextran sulfate, manufactured in Ontario) to persons with AIDS in Canada.

As an application of critical theory to an actual crisis, this work could not be a quiet little anthology of artistic musings and academic meditations on sex, death, and the indomitable human spirit. It is too urgent in its outspokenness, too large in its cultural concerns, to be vaulted up like a time capsule in the silence of a university library. Lob it at anyone who tries to bury it there. With its volatile mixture of postmodern scepticism, radical feminism, gay liberationism, and liberal individualism, this volume is bound to explode on contact with the family values of the New Right and to shake up quite a few other well-organized prejudices and cherished belief systems in the process. Its contents spring from heated discussions among artists and critics mobilized against AIDS by their strong theoretical convictions. Where their convictions differ or clash, no attempt has been made to neutralize or reconcile them from a position of external editorial power. To have done so would have been to falsify the complex evidence of their engagement with the issues and to ignore the stubbornly democratic spirit of their debates.

As a result, this volume is markedly dialectical in character. The diversity of arguments in it, enunciated from various national, political, and sexual standpoints, is meant to provoke constructive debate on the role of the arts in AIDS activism for the 1990s, even as it reflects the engagement of artists and critics with the ethics and politics of AIDS representation in the 1980s.

The urgent need for such engagement was proclaimed in 1987 by British art critic Simon Watney in *Policing Desire*, a provocative study of discriminatory AIDS commentary in the British media. It was also proclaimed in 1987 by American cultural theorist Douglas Crimp in his manifesto-like essay 'AIDS: Cultural Analysis / Cultural Activism.' The latter work introduces an archive of critical articles and activist documents by various authors (including Watney) edited by Crimp under the same title as his essay and published as a thematically unified issue of the New York theory journal *October* (winter 1987). This now legendary issue was reprinted in 1988 by MIT Press as an academic book, which made it look somewhat less radical – or at least less avant-garde – than its electrifying jolts of kulturkritik actually are by comparison with the elegiac biographies, analgesic deathbed dramas, and bourgeois cautionary tales that still dominate the non-medical literature on AIDS.[1]

As an extension of the still relatively small theoretical branch of that literature, this anthology owes much to the ground-breaking work of Watney and Crimp. They are the gay eminences behind it, and though what we have produced is not presented as a 'gay studies book' in the narrowly ghettoized sense, any more than theirs were, the continuities of form and method between their applications of critical theory to the AIDS crisis and ours are obvious enough to require only brief comment.

Watney's community-rousing voice is to be heard all through these pages, in direct quotations, in turns of phrase, in footnotes, and in the final polemical essay, which he contributed as an entrelacement of its psychosexual and sociopolitical themes. Crimp's direct impact on the volume, apart from the frequent references to his key concept of cultural activism and his controversial privileging of activist aesthetic practices, is noticeable chiefly in its anthological structure. Besides critical essays, contemporary artworks, and media clips, this collection, like his, includes a number of archival documents relevant to the politics of AIDS resistance. Where Crimp published the 'Denver Principles' of the American PWA Coalition, for instance, I have reproduced the text of the international 'Manifeste de Montréal.'[2]

Like the *October* anthology, moreover, this volume is emphatically not the work of any one critic or artist. It is a collective effort, which means that in some measure its contributors had to come to terms with their theoretical and professional differences in order to define their common goals as cultural activists. Too often in the past, scholars in the tenured security of the university looked down on the unstable art world as theoretically unsophisticated or anti-intellectual – even when strongly principled artists who were challenging the heterosexist and capitalist ethos of that world were ransacking the academy for critical terms and concepts that they subsequently modified in their often textually abstruse work. On the disputed border between the academy and the art world a vainglorious competition persists between text-based and image-based thinkers – a hangover from the ecphrastic rivalry between philosophical poets and painters of the Renaissance. The *October* anthology in its very form argued that this competition should, and could, be abandoned in the interests of forging a strong alliance between critics and artists to meet the cultural challenges of the epidemic. Such an alliance was forged anew in the production of this volume.

Though its contributors have particularized the activist agenda to suit their own political ideas, intellectual concerns, and artistic visions, most of them have looked to the social philosophy of Michel Foucault for critical guidance and have chosen discourse analysis as the best theoretical starting-point from which to attack the problematics of AIDS representation. That Foucault's social philosophy of 'discipline' and 'disciplines' has been fashionably applied to many critical problems in the arts throughout the 1980s is no reason in itself for this choice, of course. Nor is the darkly ironic circumstance that Foucault himself died of AIDS in, of all years, 1984. Rather, it is his strong theoretical emphasis on the historical inseparableness of knowledge systems and power structures, and on the isolating medical 'gaze' that constructed the systems and structures currently dominating the lives of 'AIDS victims,' that has drawn so many critics and artists into the collective task of disengagement from the powers that be (including university hierarchies) in preparation for defiant engagement with their propagandists and power-brokers over AIDS-related issues.[3]

From time to time in the volume other lines of cultural analysis – from feminist dialectics to deconstructionist wordplay to post-Freudian psychoanalytic theory to gay-liberation erotics – are followed through, tried out, woven into the critical agenda. No single approach would be sufficient to explain or expose all the cultural implications and political subtexts of all the representations of the epidemic. There are just too many of them now, too many (to my non-medical 'gaze' at least) that are poignantly inexplicable or grossly inexcusable to merit academic attention. Nevertheless, in the welter of conflicting representations and responses, Foucauldian scepticism emerges as the dominant intellectual force behind the whole effort, lending the volume a theoretical coherence that I thought at first simply reflected my own bias as a gay sceptic reeling before the old academy. In the course of editing the anthology, however, I have come to see its dependence on Foucault as a testimony to the persistent vitality of his unsettling political wisdom.

In moving on from the *October* anthology, the contributors to the present volume have striven to extend the Foucault-based cultural analysis initiated by Watney and Crimp across a broader range of artistic media and representational contexts than their pioneering essays covered. Where they focused on the contrast between mass-media representations and counterdiscursive artworks – tabloid photos of 'AIDS victims' versus activist art installations, network news coverage of the 'gay plague' versus ACT UP protest videos – we have broadened the critical scope to include public memorial art, private elegiac erotica, religious icons, photography exhibitions, government poster campaigns, mainstream magazine graphics, local newspaper profiles, and gay film as well as video. More prominence has been given to verbal representations of AIDS (as distinct from verbal commentary on AIDS) in this anthology than was granted to literary works by Crimp, whose anthology was largely based in, and somewhat biased by, the concerns of the visual arts. Writings as diverse as pulp novels, chronicle histories, obituary verses, political speeches, autobiographical essays, feature articles, advertising slogans, and video scripts come under analysis, or attack, in our scan of the ever-expanding field of cultural responses to the epidemic.

If this volume may be said to have its own perspective, it is at once more localized and more international than Watney's British-focused media criticism or Crimp's America-centred cultural analysis. Its local focus is (of all places) London, Ontario – a far cry from the Thatcher-bloated London decried in *Policing Desire* or the Reagan-blighted New York acting up in *October* 43. Like English Canada as a whole, London, Ontario has traditionally looked to Britain for cultural models and to America for cultural direction, but in doing so changes what it finds to suit the provincial ethos of its citizens. The same may be said of this volume: it has cosmopolitan connections and aspirations while remaining resolutely provincial at its core.

Accordingly, its two central groups of articles are devoted to the testing out of cultural-activist theory in a hometown context at some geographical and cultural distance from the metropolises hit hardest by the crisis. If cultural activism can be seen to work in a conservative haven like London, Ontario, where even the weeds on our lawns (not to mention the 'devices and desires of our own hearts,' as the local Anglicans say) fall under the cheerful regulation of bourgeois standards of propriety, then chances are other arrière-garde communities with large lawns and low crime rates will question what goes for 'AIDS awareness' in their parts and cease ignoring or denying the need for community-based action to stop the epidemic.

Ironically, by working on hometown activist projects, the London contributors to this volume developed strong bonds of sympathy and cross-cultural solidarity with other local people caught up in the global politics of the epidemic – Zambian villagers who draw their own AIDS posters because the government publicity rots in warehouses in Lusaka; West Berlin curators who struggle against the heterosexism of the 'AIDS-Staat' by organizing defiant exhibitions of homoerotic art; Latin American street kids who gather round their local video machine to enjoy a safer-sex cartoon produced in Toronto; San Franciscan leathermen who wave giant condoms at the crowds lining Market Street for the annual Freedom Day Parade. Our work reached out to theirs, even as theirs extended to ours. It was 'collective' in a much broader sense than we at first imagined. As a result, this volume in more than a vague symbolic sense is also their work: even its strictly 'Canadian content' is socially centrifugal, culturally relativistic, driven by an internationalist impetus that moves well beyond the World Health Organization slogans about 'the global crisis' and 'the world-wide effort to stop it.'

The multi-cultural contents of the volume have been linked and divided into ten sections. The five sections preceding the London sequence ('Photography,' 'Painting,' 'Film and Video,' 'Memorials and Public Art,' and 'Prevention Campaigns') are chiefly concerned with the visual representation of AIDS, while the three sections following it ('Literature,' 'Legal and Political Discourse,' and 'Psychosexual Discourse') focus on verbal representation. The two core sections on London ('Crisis and Criticism' and 'Media and Mediation') analyse a number of complex mixed-media representations in which words and images converge, combine, and compete.

Looking back over the tumultuous first decade of the epidemic, or epidemics as she would insist, San Francisco art critic Jan Zita Grover opens the first section with a decisively clarifying study of the culturally discernible periods in the history of the American AIDS crisis as reflected in photographic images of PWAs (Persons with AIDS). Her provocative analysis of competing stratagems for presenting 'the human face of AIDS' from aesthetic and activist viewpoints in photography exhibitions is followed by Toronto art critic Monika Gagnon's feminist analysis of the prevalent social constructions of the 'abject bodies' of female patients, male homosexuals, and shell-shocked soldiers. Gagnon's concluding discussion of nineteenth-century medical photographs of male hysterics provides a fascinating historical analogue to the kinds of clinically isolating and inferiorizing images of 'AIDS victims' criticized by Grover.

The self-empowering artbooks of Canadian painter Andy Fabo provide the visual focus for the opening essay of section two. Reading them in the light of literary and art history, David White of the University of Western Ontario explores Fabo's (and his own) struggle to sustain the erotic and social agenda of gay liberation through the debilitating paradoxes of the Age of AIDS. His critical gaze, like Fabo's recurrent image of the artist's eye, is turned towards the possibility of regeneration, a rebirth of gay identity coinciding with an astonishing renaissance of figural art. A critical gaze of sheer astonishment – my own – is subsequently cast over a very different kind of painting, an icon of rebirth from the opposite end of the West's weird spectrum of plague fantasies. Humbly entitled *Votive Offering*, it is a mystic exaltation in oils by Canadian-born, British-based artist André Durand. Despite their ideological differences, Durand and Fabo both depict (and venerate in quite unconventional ways) the figure of St Sebastian in his old role as patron saint of the plague-stricken.

In the third section the critical focus shifts from static to moving pictures of the crisis. All three essays in this section explore gay resistance to the dominant heterosexist fantasies about sex and death in the Age of AIDS as represented on film or video. In the first essay, a political reading of Norman René's *Longtime Companion*, Bart Beaty, a member of the AIDS and the Arts seminar at the University of Western Ontario, considers how the reactionary character of realism in mainstream American cinema affects a supposedly progressive representation of gay men as tragic victims of the epidemic. In the second essay Thomas Waugh of Concordia University offers a spirited defence of the melodramatic as a serious and traditional expression of gay sensibility, analysing the emergent gay cinema's tearful and at times cheerful variations on the old soap-opera theme of the decline and fall of the ailing lover. On a lighter (though no less serious) note, Toronto-based filmmaker John Greyson defends the tradition of gay aestheticism as a valid and potent counterdiscourse to the puritanical crisis-mentality of mainstream culture. His apologia for the long-lost Gilded Age introduces his hilarious 'Fake Video Script' on dandyism as activism in a world turned upside down by the Green Monkey. In opposition to artists like Fabo and Durand, Greyson argues that we do not need a renaissance in the arts to end the crisis. We need a resistance movement.

Why not resistance through renaissance? That is the route recommended for mainstream cultural activists (in opposition to radical aesthetes like Greyson) by Montreal art critic Monique Brunet-Weinmann in her essay on the rupturing of representational strategies in response to AIDS. After confronting the charnel-house images in the public art of the AIDS poster, and meditating on the memento-mori theme of a fantasy memorial by Canadian artist Richard Purdy, she concludes by hailing a new renaissance of life-affirming imagery for the 1990s to counter the morbid medievalizing of the 1980s. Memorials to the AIDS dead take many surprising forms, often reinventions of traditional mourning rites and announcements. From his Castro Street vantage point, essayist Daniel Harris looks at one of these reinvented forms – the printed obituary – as it appears, with its blurry photos and verse lamentations, in a San Francisco gay weekly. What he sees on the obit page week after week is a miniature version of the NAMES Project Quilt, as a desperately personal and sentimental space eked out for the triumph of love in the thought-policed confines of the public domain.

In that domain are posted many signs of the medical crisis that are also implicitly signs of cultural crisis, and nowhere is the advertisement of public anxiety more apparent than in the graphic art produced for AIDS prevention campaigns in the developing world. Though such art is ostensibly designed to present and illustrate 'AIDS facts,' often for semi-literate or illiterate target groups, it unerringly touches on deep-rooted fantasies about the erotic body and its political control. These fantasies find visual expression as omens of economic ruin, symptoms of moral decline, icons of sanctified monogamy, and allegories of religious transcendence.

They are by no means confined to the developing world: in fact, they often originate in the chauvinist and imperialist propaganda of the First World developers. So Ruth Wilson, a health-education officer for CUSO (Canadian University Students Overseas), reveals in her comments on the representation of women in a portfolio of Third World AIDS posters at the start of section five. Her practical approach to the plight of the HIV-infected multitudes in the Third World is subsequently complemented by the theoretical approach of Jeff O'Malley, a Canadian officer at the Global Program on AIDS at the World Health Organization in Geneva. Employing the tactics of discourse analysis, O'Malley contrasts the First World discourse of economic developmentalism with its rival, public-health progressivism, by which AIDS is widely constructed in the Third World.

Sections six and seven, on cultural activism in London, Ontario, can be read together as an extended case study of how a small community of artists, academics, and activists met the challenge of modifying and reconciling their highly local perceptions of the epidemic with critical theories and cross-cultural perspectives on AIDS as a global crisis. The 'Crisis and Criticism' section opens with a personal essay about my confrontations with the colliding worlds at the Fifth International Conference on AIDS in Montreal as contrasted with my previous experiences in the socially interactive and integrating spheres of arts activism around AIDS issues in London. The essay also provides an account of the AIDS and the Arts program initiated at the University of Western Ontario and the AIDS-related art exhibitions organized in London galleries in 1988, concluding with the formulation of a six-point agenda for arts activists working at a local level. The section ends with a portfolio of twelve photographs documenting one of the London exhibitions, a three-part series of contemporary artworks addressing the critical issue of 'The Body & Society.' Fabo was one of the twelve artists represented in the shows, which were all mounted at the Embassy Cultural House under the curatorial direction of Jamelie Hassan and her gallery board in conjunction with my AIDS and the Arts seminar at the university. Following Hassan's lead, I have come to regard the 'Body & Society' exhibition as London's answer to the New Museum of Contemporary Art's installation 'Let the Record Show ...' documented and commended by Crimp in his discussion of AIDS activism on the New York art scene.

The five articles in the local 'Media and Mediation' section, which correspond to the cosmopolitan medical critiques in Crimp's anthology, are linked together by a common focus on the social identity and activist initiatives of one person living with AIDS in London, Ontario. He is John Gordon, a social worker who was brought to the city's attention in 1988 by a feature article on his life as a 'young AIDS victim' by the *London Free Press*. The section opens with a reprint of this article, written by *Free Press* journalist Dahlia Reich, as it appeared in the paper along with several slice-of-life photographs by Susan Bradnam. In an essay following it, David Kinahan of the University of Western Ontario compares Reich's well-intentioned representation of Gordon as a young victim with the 'Timmy' role carved out years ago as a profitable niche for handicapped kids in the Canadian cultural landscape. Reich, in turn, speaking from the practical standpoint of a journalist who must work within the social and ethical constraints of the mainstream media, provides an indignant apologia for her feature in direct response to Kinahan's theory-based criticisms. Agreeing wholeheartedly with Reich's reading of what the feature accomplished at the time, Gordon goes on in his own words to fill out the picture of himself as an AIDS activist by describing his efforts to remove a scandalous T-shirt from the shelves of a novelty store in an Ontario resort town. AIDS educator Clarence Crossman subsequently reflects on the significance of Gordon's action in light of the Ontario Charter of Human Rights, which has given gay people and their allies across the province a legal incentive to fight the prejudices exacerbated by the epidemic. The 'Media and Mediation' section concludes with a follow-up report by Reich on Gordon's physical and spiritual condition three years after the original feature on his life with AIDS appeared in the *Free Press*.

Prejudicial fantasies of the plague find expression in AIDS fiction and non-fiction alike, as Brian Patton of the University of Western Ontario and I contend in the 'Literature' section. Greyson's Green Monkey would feel right at home in the fantastic world populated by AIDS villains and CDC heroes in Randy Shilts's best-selling chronicle of the epidemic, which I read as a Dickensian tour-de-force in a satiric essay on why straights die bloated, and gays ethereally slim, in popular AIDS fiction. Whose world are we fighting for in the 'War on AIDS'? The military metaphors so common in medical and biographical accounts of the epidemic are the stimuli for Patton's consideration of the crisis of authority underlying the rhetoric of power in the rival AIDS narratives of the late 1980s.

While the previous two sections pointed towards the largely verbal domain of legal and political discourse shaping (if not fully dictating) majority conceptions of the epidemic, section nine foregrounds the rhetoric of law and politics in so far as these are employed by governments to represent, and at times to override, the interests of HIV-infected people. Margaret Somerville of McGill University offers a critique of most AIDS legislation as purely symbolic action, a ritual gesture of exclusion and solidarity in the face of global disaster. Like the arts, then, the law is not just a means of responding to the AIDS crisis. It is a medium for constructing and in a sense creating the crisis to promote prevailing systems of belief, knowledge, and power. With formidable clarity, speaking not only as a sociologist of marginality but also as a community-based activist who has had to deal with multiple levels of government in furthering the cause of PWA rights, Barry Adam of the University of Windsor goes on to examine the translation of official AIDS discourse into state policy, and to analyse its appalling effects on the lives of the people branded by lawmakers and politicians as deviant, unhealthy, or impure.

The final section of the volume considers the twin discourses of sexuality and psychology as political tools for the representation and repression of people 'at risk' for HIV infection. The two essays in it present a sharp contrast in rhetorical style and theoretical approach to psychosexual discourse in the Age of AIDS. Arthur Kroker of Concordia University speaks in an idiom all his own – an almost poetic synthesis of French psychoanalytic and poststructuralist terminology, American political catch-phrases, and German philosophical allusions – while Simon Watney writes as a radical gay polemicist uncompromising in his attack on psychoanalytic conceptions of 'the Homosexual' and unyielding in his condemnation of 'Assimilationism' as a valid gay community response to the epidemic.

Different as their approaches are, both men speak like prophets in their readings of AIDS as a crisis of sexual identity. Sex itself, or rather what's happening to it in postmodern America, is analysed by Kroker with apocalyptic urgency. No less oracular is Watney's essay on self-empowerment through the radicalization of gay identity, which I first read on an East German train bound for West Berlin at the time the Wall fell: two experiences of liberation indissolubly linked in my memory. The recurrent concerns in the volume – activism versus aestheticism, periodization, the crisis of authority, the control of collective memory, the fantasy of magical self-protection, the politics of safer sex, the transvaluation of mourning rituals, the common mind searching for new meaning in things – all converged for me on that train in Watney's provocative argument. The prophetic note on which the volume ends is intended to provoke more discussion of these issues, more impassioned articulation of where we can go from here in meeting the AIDS crisis with words and images.

The dialectical restlessness of the volume reflects the experience of the artists, academics, and activists who attended a symposium on the cultural dimensions of the AIDS crisis at the University of Western Ontario in October 1988. Most of the authors and artists whose work appears in these pages participated in 'Representing AIDS,' as the symposium was called, either as speakers or discussants.

The setting for 'Representing AIDS' was subversively (if accidentally) symbolic: all fifteen speeches on the program were delivered in the main auditorium of University Hospital as arranged by Western's Office of Continuing Medical Education. Ironically, though not surprisingly, the entire event was ignored by the doctors and nurses of the hospital and by London's large medical community. It was evidently perceived by the practical-minded hospital staff as an oddly disquieting but fortunately temporary intrusion into their technical domain – an offbeat 'cultural affair' – as if cultural affairs did not intrude at every moment onto the sacred ground of scientific objectivity and medical pragmatism. In one way or another, all the speakers on the program challenged the insularity of the medical construction of AIDS. Some exposed its patriarchal and mechanistic presuppositions. Others examined its social consequences. Still others strove to excite political resistance to its potentially dehumanizing influences.

Critical as they all were of unquestioned medical authority, none of the speakers would have driven the doctors out of the city as Socrates had driven the poets out of his republic. Even the most radical artists and theorists at the symposium acknowledged the extraordinary advances of medical science in retroviral research, and considered the daunting epidemiological and economic challenges facing health-care professionals dedicated to ending the crisis. Starting from a common assumption that the medical sciences are enmeshed in the sophisticated culture of images that defines and to some extent determines contemporary life in the West, the speakers turned their critical attention to the various cultural institutions that create or control the representations of AIDS for society at large. The media, the visual arts, the performing arts, public art and advertising, the legal system, the public-health agencies, and the policy-making offices of the state – a wide spectrum of sources engaged in the representation of the epidemic was examined in the light of their aesthetic strategies and controlling discourses.

Debates between mainstream liberals and radical liberationists (there were no vocal conservatives or fundamentalists at the symposium) were sparked by four recurrent issues: whether memorial art or any traditional aesthetic practice had a role to play in AIDS activism; whether the state should censor as 'hate literature' any representation of the epidemic perceived to be discriminatory or insulting to persons with AIDS; whether the formulation of new laws specifically addressing AIDS issues was merely a symbolic action or a practical move in the direction of ending the crisis; and whether critical theory as an interdisciplinary academic enterprise could do anything to further the main cause (often strangely neglected) of ending the epidemic. These issues continue to be raised in the dialectical cross-fire between papers and images in this volume.

If there was one point on which all the speakers at the symposium seemed to agree, it was the urgent need to oppose representations designed to isolate persons with AIDS from the uninfected 'general public.' AIDS education campaigns targeted at this mythical majority (which chiefly consists of white male heterosexual taxpayers) were condemned for fitting the various social groups commonly dualized by the official administrators of the epidemic – gays versus straights, blacks versus whites, foreigners versus nationals, fallen women versus fallible men – into the politically charged categories of the Sick and the Well.

Andy Fabo, in his challenging keynote address at the symposium, tied all these issues together by speaking not only as one who has dealt with AIDS in his work but also as one who deals with AIDS in himself. Placing himself at a critical distance from university debates, he pointed to the inevitable limitations of all academic discourses, even the most professedly radical, when he warned us not to be so mesmerized by theory that we failed to resolve our aesthetic and political disputes into practical action capable of rallying society as a whole to the personal cause, the principal cause, of saving the erotic body from the 'delirium' of the plague.

This timely admonition was also hinted at on the poster designed by Toronto graphics artist David Buchan to advertise the symposium (see plate 1, following p 51). Instead of representing AIDS with sensationalistic media images of lesion-ravaged victims or grenade-like models of the virus, Buchan chose to allegorize it academically by reproducing the eerily quiet image of a neoclassical funeral urn from an eighteenth-century book of engravings entitled 'The Architecture of Death.' Surrounding the urn, as if to protect it from vulgar scrutiny, are the leafy branches of an old shadowy forest – a brooding ground for pensive questers.

This unexpected pastoral scene, at first glance so inappropriate to the crisis-world of the postmodern epidemic, serves to distance the viewer in time and space from the urban capitals of the plague. It suggests a contemplative retreat from the hysterics of 'media-ted' AIDS commentary, a turning inward to the shady glades of nostalgia and stoic apathy within the philosophic mind. Buchan, like Fabo, both applauds and criticizes this retreat. The latent metaphoric implications of the image turned out to be quite appropriate to the critical theme and academic setting of the symposium. As an aesthetic representation of death, a haunting memento mori in the groves of academe, the urn effectively represents the cultural products and hence the cultural process of representing AIDS.

Representation is simultaneously a re-creation and a disposal of the represented, Buchan implies, and he no doubt chose an urn to represent the common disposal of PWAs by cremation rather than coffin burial (which, according to many funeral directors in 1988, including several in London, Ontario, was like putting toxic waste in the ground!). In order to deal with the horror of death by AIDS, society must aestheticize death itself; yet the ironic loveliness of the 'architecture of death' can distract the contemplative viewer from the urgent needs of people still living with AIDS, and living longer than ever.

If the academic urn was more or less intact at the beginning of the symposium, it was surely shattered by the end: no one who took part in the London debates over aestheticism versus activism in AIDS representation came away from the conference without feeling that the limits of academic discourse had been touched, pushed, broken through. What had damaged the urn – so constructively – was our communal effort to reimagine 'the body under duress' (as Fabo would put it) in opposition to repressive social formulations of its value, function, and destiny. In retrospect, the morbidly chaste, unchanging, durable body of Buchan's funerary icon seemed to symbolize all that was conventionally wrong about our culture's erotophobic constructions of the body, and all that was unconventionally challenged by Fabo's silence-breaking apology for the erotic life in the Age of AIDS.

Though this volume in many ways proceeded from the 'Representing AIDS' symposium, it should not be narrowly construed as the proceedings of it. Its range of voices, for one, has been duly expanded to meet certain objections about the exclusivity of the original meeting.[4] Several people who attended it but did not speak from the platform – notably Jan Zita Grover, Jeff O'Malley, David White, Brian Patton, David Kinahan, and Jamelie Hassan – have added their internationalizing and decentralizing perspectives to the volume. Its contents, moreover, now include many more visual representations of AIDS than were originally shown or discussed at the conference. As even a quick glance over its pages will show, the anthology is too iconoclastic in its heterogeneous contents and design to pass for a 'purely' academic book.

If you are looking for a well-wrought urn preserving the lifeblood of a master-spirit, or a scholastic monument embodying the tasteful classical ideals of perfect proportion and doctrinal harmony dear to the hearts of most university anthologists, you will not find it here. To have fashioned such a book out of the fragments of the London symposium would have been to falsify its explosive spirit – and the radicalizing spirit of the times.

That does not mean that on entering the open-ended debates of this volume you will hear only the voices of a 'politically correct' minority chanting out their slogans like ACT UP zappers before the unhearing walls of the politically incorrigible Establishment. Far from it. What you will find here is a very mixed crowd of radicals and liberals conferring with each other across the old and now entirely outmoded divide between the Establishment and the Counterculture. The rhetorical result is an unpredictable and therefore lively heteroglossia (not an ideal harmony) of discourses opposed to the deadening monologism of the 'AIDS-Staat.' No rigid symmetry has been imposed on the verbal or visual contents of the book. No single aesthetic agenda trims its edges. No single ideology hardens its lines. Its asymmetrical parts fit together fluidly – like the perversely idiosyncratic speeches in Plato's *Symposium*, which vary in length, tone, and idiom to reflect the strongly (because freely) divergent viewpoints of the assembled speakers.

Hence the title of the volume: *Fluid Exchanges*. A 'symposium' in the ancient Greek sense literally meant a sharing of drinks, an exchange of fluids, which Socrates conceived and experienced in a fully

Dionysian way. Though there was no bantering, wine-logged Socrates at the AIDS symposium in University Hospital, his critical role seemed to be filled at times by the absent presence of Foucault.

Dionysian exchanges of fluids (in an erotic sense at least) are hard to enjoy or even to contemplate now in a free spirit without anxious recollection of the 'new facts of life' proclaimed for the Age of AIDS by Foucault's panoptical moralists, the public health boards.[5] Their sobering version of AIDS awareness has ushered in a profoundly anti-symposiastic age. As more than one public-health poster put it in the reeling eighties, the party's over, and as the nineties dawn, it's time to call it a day. A new day of sobriety, self-control, and silent meditation on the virtues of a sex-free lifestyle: that's what many conservative 'prevention' campaigns are unapologetically hailing in the sex-charged idiom of modern commercial advertising. 'Three good reasons not to go out with the boys,' declares an ad in the massive America Responds to AIDS campaign: the reasons (revealed in a family album photo) turn out to be a charming wife and two innocent kiddies. Another ad from the same series, showing a single woman resolutely crossing her legs, proclaims that the Centers for Disease Control have discovered 'a simple way to prevent AIDS.' That's right: 'Don't have sex.'

Read as a kind of erotic invitation, the title of this volume calls into question the repressively puritanical message of such signs and the anti-symposiastic spirit behind them. Besides suggesting the etymological meaning of 'symposium,' *Fluid Exchanges* is of course also a take on the official AIDSpeak phrase 'exchange of bodily fluids' – which has deviously translated sex into a kind of high-risk commerce, a commodity transaction. By echoing the public-health discourse that all the authors in the anthology challenge, the title effectively proclaims our critical concern with the political reinventions of the erotic life in the wake of the epidemic. Far from trivializing the 'AIDS tragedy,' the very serious puns in the title counter the fatalistic reading of the epidemic promoted by the erotophobic Right.

That artists and critics have much to exchange – theories, images, terminologies, experiences, strategies – in their common engagement with the issues raised by AIDS and AIDS-discrimination is also implied by the title of this volume. Such exchanges are evident all through these pages: for instance, Fabo using Foucault to attack the public-health notion of the 'AIDS victim,' or Somerville alluding to Fabo in her critique of AIDS legislation. As the subtitle urges, the flow of ideas and images between 'Artists and Critics in the AIDS Crisis' must remain unhampered by rigid dogmas and inflexible pieties if it is to be sustained during the coming decades.

Though bodily fluids pose the greatest moral threat to anyone who has swallowed even a small draught of such official information, fear of infection has tainted many other sociable liquids that used to be thought quite harmless. Drinking-fountain water, salad oil, and even communion wine can seem as dangerous now as the contents of a shared syringe. Back in classical Athens, a city with no centre for disease control to calm its plague anxieties, Socrates himself had something to say about the exchange of fluids. He was not one to stop the flow. 'It would be nice,' he remarked at the prototypical symposium for academics and artists, 'if wisdom were a sort of fluid, and flowed by contact out of a person who has more of it into one who has less, just as water can be made to pass through wool from a full cup to an empty one. If that's what wisdom is like, then I count it an honour to take my place next to you' (*Symposium* 175D). He said this with a sly nudge to his host Agathon, a literary bon vivant who thought himself wise in the mysteries of love and death because his latest tragedy had just won a prize at a drama festival. Everyone at the party had seen how Socrates made a point of reclining next to him, and this no doubt pleased Agathon enormously. But the tragedian was not taken in by the old philosophical satyr's satiric suggestion that mere adjacency at a symposium, with the thin thread of social chit-chat and love talk connecting them, was enough to fill the guests to the brim with their host's highbrow wisdom. Socrates, not Agathon, was surely the full cup from which all the symposiasts would take their fill of inebriating thoughts.

So Socrates cannot have been entirely joking when he suggested that people from different backgrounds, with different points of view, cannot begin to gain wisdom about any aspect of life and love until they are willing to sit down together and drink in each other's reasonings. For what was Socratic dialectic, after all, but the fluid exchange of definitions, terminologies, beliefs, theories, and visions between minds in intimate contact? If Socrates had been an AIDS activist, he would surely have promoted dialectic as an advanced kind of safer sex.

NOTES

1 See Simon Watney's introduction (written in 1986) to *Policing Desire: Pornography, AIDS, and the Media* (Minneapolis: University of

Minnesota Press 1987) 3–4. See also Douglas Crimp 'AIDS: Cultural Analysis / Cultural Activism' in *October* 43 (winter 1987) 3–16. To avoid confusion between the latter essay and the anthology it introduces – they bear the same title – I shall indicate the essay with quotations marks and the anthology with italics. In reprinting the journal issue as an academic book, MIT Press retained the original title *AIDS: Cultural Analysis / Cultural Activism* (Cambridge, MA: MIT Press 1988).

2 For the 'Founding Statement of People with AIDS/ARC (The Denver Principles),' see *AIDS: Cultural Analysis / Cultural Activism* ed Crimp, 148–9. For the 'Manifeste de Montréal,' see pp 211–13 of this volume.

3 With Adam Rolston, Douglas Crimp offers a militantly Foucauldian defence of his activist aesthetic bias in favour of graphic art in *AIDS demo graphics* (Seattle: Bay Press 1990) 13–24. This visually compelling monograph – 'a do-it-yourself manual, showing how to make propaganda work in the fight against AIDS' (p 13) – clearly illustrates why in the specific context of New York City, with its constant blitz of advertising images and media replays, bold visual signs of AIDS resistance are an effective way to get messages across from small affinity groups to a broad socially mixed audience. Words must be turned into pictures, as in the 'Silence = Death' logo, in order to compete with the barrage of propaganda produced by big government and the pharmaceuticals. But what about smaller cultural settings far from the crowded streets of New York? Would the shock-tactic graphics of ACT UP work as well in London, Ontario, say, or Chapel Hill, North Carolina? Perhaps AIDS literature (in the non-propagandistic sense) is more likely to 'invade' these quieter spaces – local bookstores, university seminar rooms, church basements, suburban living rooms – than Gran Fury's sophisticated parodies of Big City advertising.

4 See Tom Folland's review of the conference, 'Representing Acquired Immune Deficiency Syndrome' *Vanguard* 18.1 (February/March 1989) 22–7. In his reconstruction of the conference, Folland divides the speakers into two opposing camps: the radical Foucauldian theorists (whom he commends) and everyone else (whom he dismisses). By pitting gay radical speakers like Andy Fabo and Douglas Crimp against liberal speakers like Michael Ruse and Margaret Somerville, Folland unfairly implies that there was little or no communication between them during the conference. But 'Representing AIDS' was more than a series of papers read from strongly defined ideological standpoints: after each session the speakers and delegates had a chance to question, challenge, modify, and defend their viewpoints in a discussion period that tended to open up communication between gays and straights, radicals and liberals, academics and artists, critics

and activists. Folland simply ignores the bridging work done in the discussion periods, and fails to mention speakers like Ruth Wilson and John Gordon who contributed to the aestheticism-vs-activism debates without fitting neatly into either of his opposing camps.

5 For its 1987–8 AIDS awareness campaign, the Canadian Public Health Association produced a militaristic poster with the caption 'The New Facts of Life,' beneath which was the injunction 'Join the Attack on AIDS' in red lettering. The latter slogan appeared to be spray-painted in blood by inner-city delinquents eager to join the right-wing attack on gays, prostitutes, immigrants, addicts, and anyone else branded as a 'high risk' to the health of the general public.

Visible Lesions: Images of the PWA in America

JAN ZITA GROVER

> The camera invariably seeks out the 'victims' of the most spectacular battles. Its instinct for the sensational leads it to prefer the bald and wasted AIDS patient with the feverish, haggard look, lying in his hospital bed (preferably with a few tubes up his nose), to his companion who is still able to take care of himself and speak articulately about his condition ... Everyone knows it's best not to give us a chance at the microphone and that pictures deceive even better than words.
>
> Emmanuel Dreuilhe *Mortal Embrace: Living with AIDS*[1]

What do 'the picture of health' and 'the picture of sickness' look like? A stupid question, to be sure, unless we refine it: *whose* picture of health/sickness? and *for whom*? and in the service of *what*? So let's refine the question, narrow it down some: What does 'the picture of health/sickness' look like in relation to AIDS within three separate discursive fields – those of medicine (directed toward physicians), newspaper and periodical photojournalism (mainstream and gay), and art photography (directed toward curators and patrons of museums and commercial galleries)?

For the sake of this argument, we will use AIDS – acquired immunodeficiency syndrome – as the measure of 'sickness' by which health is defined, just as masculinity can only be understood in relation to femininity, heterosexuality in relation to its supposed opposite, homosexuality. It is through these oppositions that we can name a term, a condition.[2]

It has been almost eight years since Marcus Conant, MD, stood outside the annual meeting of the American Academy of Dermatologists handing out a pamphlet he had produced with a $500 grant from Neutrogena, illustrated by photographs of patients with Kaposi's sarcoma (KS). This was one of the first representations of AIDS, a condition that both then and now has been partially identified with *appearances*. Photographs 'of AIDS' first appeared in medical (*New England Journal of Medicine*, *Lancet*, *Journal of the American Medical Association* [*JAMA*]) and basic research (*Science*, *Nature*) journals. These photographs were not concerned with humanizing AIDS; they were largely close-ups of affected organs or microphotographs of cells, tissue, virus. They were made to identify AIDS's signs and symptoms for purposes of surveillance, diagnosis, and treatment.[3]

But as popular media became preoccupied by AIDS – most markedly, after Rock Hudson admitted his diagnosis in July 1985 and then died that October – other images of AIDS appeared, this time amidst the scenes of catastrophe, celebrity, horror, and novelty that constitute mass media's photographic archives. Like many of the photographs that appear in tabloids, these 'images of AIDS' were mostly unremarkable pictures in any sense: their subjects were obviously ill, usually shown seated on couches or lying in beds. It was the words surrounding these photographs that gave them their particular resonance: the words told us that these were people *doomed to die*, much as others sharing their pages told us that this unremarkable-looking boy had wed and divorced five women twice his age or that this woman had borne sextuplets or owned a three-headed cocker spaniel.

Broadcast/newspaper journalists and gallery ('art') photographers do not make their images only in response to the inherited traditions or conventions of their medium; they also incorporate their own understanding of events, authorities, and institutions related to the objects they depict. The ways that scientists and physicians understand AIDS have as great an impact on the ways that, for example, newspaper photographers depict PWAs (persons with AIDS) as do existing photojournalistic conventions for depicting the chronically ill. It is only through seeing the complex relations between medical/scientific 'facts' and modes of visual representation that we can assess the significance of the *choices made* by people who make images. For example:

1. What does it mean in 1989, when the average life expectancy of a person diagnosed with AIDS is over 20 months, for a photographer to

consistently depict PWAs as debilitated, disfigured, *in extremis*? Does it mean the same thing(s) as it did in 1983, when the average life expectancy of a person diagnosed with AIDS was only eight months?

2. What does it mean in 1989, when there are well-organized cadres of PWAs nationwide who protest government inaction on drug trials, understaffing in clinics and hospital wards, discrimination in employment and housing, to depict PWAs *as victims*? Does it mean the same thing(s) it did in 1983?

3. What did it mean in 1986–7, when the most dramatic increases in diagnosed cases of AIDS were among black and Latino men and women, that the plight of heterosexuals with AIDS was epitomized largely in terms of white suburbanites?

4. What does it mean throughout the period 1985–9 that children with AIDS (1 per cent of total U.S. AIDS cases) received more media attention than the 61 per cent of diagnosed cases among gay men?

My aim here is to periodize medical-scientific-epidemiological events and political-cultural-media representations of AIDS in such a way that these questions can be answered. This essay is intended to propose some grounds from which they can be asked. Most criticism of photographs treats images as if they were made and can be assessed within a continuous historical moment. As short as the history of AIDS in the United States is, there have been sufficient permutations in scientific, medical, epidemiological, political, media, and artistic responses to make historical differentiations crucial even within this brief eight-year period. What AIDS *is*, what it has been made to *mean*, and how those two interpretations have been *represented* at any given time is rather like the parable of the blind men and the elephant: everyone has an opinion of the elephant's shape, but it depends on where they are positioned in relation to it.[4]

Two premises underlie the discussion of representation that follows. The first is that media representations spiral outward from the most specialized and 'authorized' (in this case, those of science) toward the most dependent and 'opinionated' (that is, those depending most heavily on the authority of representations already made at higher orders of influence). Meyrig Horton and Peter Aggleton, in their study 'The Cultural Production of an AIDS Research Paradigm,'[5] make a persuasive case for this model, employing Ludwik Fleck's paradigm for the trajectory of scientific discourse (developed in Fleck's *Genesis and Development of a Scientific Fact*).[6] In Horton and Aggleton's application of Fleck (see plate 2, following p 51), the data published in science journals (for example, *Science* and *Nature*) possess the greatest authority and prestige to readers who subscribe to the authority and prestige of research science. This includes not only other research scientists, but also physicians, surgeons, nurses, and other health-care workers, *although these may never even read the journals in question.* This group may also include newspaper and periodical science reporters and other reporters assigned to 'cover' AIDS and those activists and patients for whom scientific activity is the preeminent authority on AIDS. By contrast, for researchers, physicians, et al who reject the findings of research science (for example, those who reject the hypothesis that HIV is the causative agent of AIDS, whether they believe it stems from other causes, such as a different virus or 'lifestyle' factors, or regard the issue as moot and instead focus on other concerns, such as attitudinal healing), the work of journal science is not at the core of authority and prestige. Rather, the 'cone of influence' is inverted: that-which-is-not-debated in the research-science model (for example, etiologic agents other than HIV) moves to the centre of debate, while what was previously the core (for instance, HIV as primary etiologic agent) moves to the periphery as that-which-is-no-longer-debated.

This paradigm is equally useful in looking at other worlds of discourse (general-circulation periodicals, television news, and so forth), where similar levels of dependence and influence are in operation. For example, within the world of general-circulation weeklies, *Time* and *Newsweek* possess greater 'authority' than *National Enquirer* and *The Star*; so the latter are more likely to refer to the former as 'proof' of their claims than vice versa. Similarly, the *New York Times* has greater influence as an authority publication than *USA Today*, so the latter is more likely to quote the former than the other way around.[7]

The second premise underlying this discussion is that AIDS in the United States must be differentiated year by year and locality by locality in order for us to understand it (this is of course true for AIDS anywhere else as well). Before 1989, AIDS in the United States was very unevenly distributed. Instead, it was concentrated – a distinctly coastal phenomenon, whether considered from an epidemiological or media-coverage viewpoint. In 1986, for example, 40 per cent of all reported cases of AIDS in the United States were in metropolitan New York and San Francisco.[8] These cities were closely followed by Los Angeles, Houston, and Miami. Together, these five American metropolises reported most of the country's AIDS cases. For the majority of Americans living outside these communities, AIDS appeared to be someone else's problem – something freakish and citified, related not only to an exotic homosexuality but to the corruptions of downtown city life. Despite warnings from both gay activists and the right, before 1985 AIDS seemed unlikely to invade the (attempted) suburban refuges where most middle-class Americans lived.

Significantly, the federal Centers for Disease Control (CDC) recently announced that the greatest number of cases reported in 1989 are in communities outside the cities previously reporting the greatest case loads. The coastal cities of the American empire have now been surpassed in sheer numbers of reported cases by other metropolitan areas – Washington, DC, Chicago, Indianapolis, Denver, Boston. By 1991, the CDC predicts that New York and San Francisco will account for only 20 per cent of all reported AIDS cases.[9]

Our periodization begins by looking at the epidemic on two different fronts: events in medicine-science-epidemiology and representations in media-politics-culture.

Medicine, Epidemiology, Scientific Research	**Media, Politics, Culture**
1981	1981
– Syndrome largely reported in gay men; perceived as gay disease by epidemiologists and clinicians; given various names – GRID, CAID, AID, gay plague, WOG[10]	– reports largely in medical journals
1982	1982
– CDC announces surveillance definition and name: AIDS – Diagnosis of AIDS commonly precedes death by < 9 months	– meagre coverage in gay press – first voluntary AIDS service organizations are formed: Gay Men's Health Crisis (New York City) and Kaposi's Foundation (San Francisco)

1983	1983
– French researchers isolate LAV – first pediatric cases, transfusion cases, and hemophiliac cases (involving fraction VIII/IX)	– popular media discover AIDS – *JAMA* publishes report on 'casual' transmission of AIDS – medical press covers AIDS – gay press increases coverage – voluntary AIDS service organizations formed in large U.S. cities – Advisory Committee of People with AIDS formed – first gay safer-sex publications

1984	1984
– HTLV-III argued as causative agent for AIDS – reports of transfusion and hemophiliac cases increase	– medical and gay press coverage increases

1985	1985
– HIV antibody test put on market for blood-banking; begins being applied by insurance companies – first international AIDS conference held in Atlanta	– Rock Hudson dies – heterosexual panic ensues in popular media – gay press begins covering AIDS extensively – PWA Coalition formed in NYC

1986	1986
– cases involving heterosexuals, children, IV drug users, and transfusion patients widely publicized – drug trials in coastal cities	– heterosexual panic continues – LaRouche Initiative proposed for quarantining PWAs in California

1987	1987
– AZT licensed for use – Presidential Commission on HIV epidemic appointed – Project Inform (San Francisco) urges people to get HIV antibody tests – aerosolized pentamidine prophylaxis for pneumocystis pneumonia begun in NYC	– Helms Amendment – second LaRouche initiative in California – NAMES Project Quilt unveiled in Washington, DC – publication of trade and pocketbook heterosexual safer sex guidebooks[11]

1988	1988
– disputes over estimates of HIV infected – presidential commission returns report – extent of HIV/AIDS in black and Hispanic communities becomes evident	– Masters and Johnson furore – third LaRouche initiative in California – ACT UP and other activist groups mount media actions – mainstream media highlight AIDS and the arts, but otherwise back off widespread AIDS coverage

Anyone involved in the struggle against AIDS will have many amendments to make to this rough chronology. But I would argue that it is useful for beginning discussion of many strands in the evolving history of *how AIDS has been depicted*. It points out some of the push-and-pull between dominant and counterdiscourses about AIDS over time. (In saying this, I am not suggesting that the many constructions placed on AIDS can be understood solely in historical terms; there is far too much of the transhistorically irrational about the shaping of AIDS to propose that.)[12] Paula Treichler's chronology of dominant media discourses is also useful and briefer for these purposes:[13]

1 evolving biomedical understandings of AIDS (1981–5)
2 Rock Hudson's illness and death as a turning point in national consciousness (July 1985–December 1986)

3 AIDS perceived as a pandemic disease to which sexually active heterosexuals are vulnerable (fall 1986–spring 1987)
4 diversification of discourse about women and AIDS (spring 1987–present).[14]

1981–1985

In 1981, the yet-unnamed syndrome was also unimaged. Although many gay men (and, we now know, heterosexual intravenous drug abusers) in New York and San Francisco were already suffering from inexplicable illnesses, there was no discernible pattern except for a marked increase in persistent generalized lymphadenopathy (swelling of the lymph glands, particularly in the neck and groin) that had been noted by physicians with large gay practices since 1979. In winter 1981, several of these physicians reported anomalous cases of Pneumocystis carinii pneumonia (PCP) and KS among their patients to the CDC in Atlanta. PCP and KS are rare conditions among young middle-class men, yet cases were showing up on both coasts. What struck CDC epidemiologists most forcibly about these cases was that all of the first patients reported were gay.[15] From this fact U.S. epidemiologists and medical researchers concluded that the condition these men suffered from was either sexually transmitted or somehow related to what came to be called 'homosexual lifestyle.' As Jacques Leibowitch, a French researcher immune to the peculiarly American obsession with gay-plague theory, put it: 'The "homosexual mystery" will dominate the beginning of the story: a notion that will shackle the minds of those too closely concerned with it ... [the] first (false) lead: the lavender peril.'[16] For the next four years, American medical, political, and social responses to AIDS were dominated by the hypothetical equation of AIDS and homosexuality, an association that also had long-term effects on how the syndrome was depicted visually.

In 1981–2, while AIDS as a clinical and epidemiological entity was still very much in flux, it was 'visible' only in the pages of research and medical journals, where it joined other pathologic conditions as radically abstracted from the human beings suffering it: microscopic views of biopsy specimens, X-rays, and close-ups of KS lesions. As Horton, using Fleck, has argued, the pivotal influence of scientific research journals had a determining role in setting the terms of the central discourse on AIDS at the time, in the scientific press and elsewhere.

This influence, moreover, was of a distinctly Anglo-American kind:

although in 1983 Luc Montagnier's group at the Pasteur Institute announced that they had isolated and named a retrovirus, LAV (for lymphadenopathy-associated virus), present in cells from persons with AIDS, their discovery received little play in the pivotal American scientific journals until Robert Gallo of the National Cancer Institute announced *his* discovery of HTLV-III (human T-cell lymphotropic virus type III) the following year. (This discovery was immediately followed by enterprising Reaganite Health and Human Services Director Margaret Heckler's announcement that a cure for AIDS was just around the corner.)[17] These discoveries were quickly applied to the commercial production of assay kits for detecting the many-named virus[18] in blood-banking, the cultural outcome of which was a profound disturbance in popular beliefs about who might be *at risk* and what they might look like (see below). Hysteria now extended not only to the visibly ill but to the invisibly ill/infected – the sick homosexual *redux*.

Early articles on AIDS in the gay press, which was the only other medium interested in AIDS in 1982, duplicated the visual icons of the medical, with the result that AIDS was represented almost wholly in medicalized terms. The same microscopic views of KS lesions and PCP-infested lung tissue dominated visual coverage in gay journals, making it possible for us to gauge the influence that medical/scientific discourse initially had for gay communities.[19] After the American 'discovery' of HTLV-III in 1984, the virus became a familiar image in both scientific/medical and popular media (see plates 3, 4).

What is most striking about the non-scientific media's visual coverage of AIDS in 1981–3 is the virtual absence of the *subjects of AIDS*. Several political factors played a role here. In the years before and immediately after the virus was isolated and designated as the primary etiologic agent for the syndrome, widespread ignorance about how 'AIDS'[20] was contracted mobilized all the old fears about toilet seats, doorknobs, infected waiters and cooks, contaminated silverware, handshaking, and coughing strangers. As the late Nathan Fain, an AIDS activist, wrote in 1983: 'The result [of mainstream media coverage] plant[s] ... the idea in the general population that AIDS risk groups are like walking Three Mile Islands.'[21] Identifiably ill PWAs (and in the early years of the epidemic, about one-third of PWAs were diagnosed with the often-visible lesions of KS) suffered employment, housing, and benefits discrimination, but there were no government statutes or ordinances as possible sources of redress until 1984. Thus PWAs' reluctance to make themselves visible to camera crews and inquiring photographers was understandable. To their credit, a number of PWAs in New York and San Francisco none the less chose to appear publicly on local television programs and in newspapers, although in several instances their participation was halted by nervous camera crews.[22] Their aim, perhaps naïve and certainly optimistic, was to speak *for themselves* (victims are *spoken for*)[23] and to 'humanize' themselves for a public that viewed them as a threat to 'the general population.'

Two visual broadcast/photojournalistic conventions undercut PWAs' attempts to represent themselves and instead worked to entrench their status as threatening outsiders. Broadcast television has developed conventions for depicting persons whose identity needs to be guarded – heavy backlighting, isolation of the subject in deep shadow. These have most commonly been used with felons or potential felons – such as rapists, child abusers, and drug abusers. These same conventions were often used to protect PWAs against backlash, with unintended secondary consequences: they made PWAs look *as if they had something to hide, as if they were criminals.*[24] If the PWA became in some sense more visible in such encounters, he did not become *more-like-'us'*: his status as pariah was if anything reinforced. Even when the coverage is intentionally 'sympathetic,' the visual tropes of isolation used in journalistic coverage emphasize the PWA's status as radically different, as cut off from life (see plate 5).

In addition, television and photo journalists frequently sought out the most debilitated PWAs they could find. ABC's May 1983 '20/20' coverage of AIDS is typical of such sensationalizing coverage. The segment's producer, Joe Lovett, contacted Gay Men's Health Crisis (GMHC) in New York 'and promptly found several eloquent and very ill men. They didn't *look* very sick, though. In fact, some of them looked downright handsome. Lovett kept searching until he found Kenneth Ramsauer, who at 28 was dying of Kaposi's sarcoma with an unusual – and ghastly – disfiguration of his once-winsome face.'[25]

Kenny Ramsauer was subsequently featured in double-page photo spreads in *Paris Match*, *Photo* (Paris), and the British tabloid *Sunday People* (see plate 6). The uses Kenny Ramsauer was put to are the most grotesque examples of the mainstream media's penchant for seeking out the most visibly ill,[26] but similar sensationalizing coverage characterized most of the media's belated 'discovery' of AIDS in 1983.[27]

While there were clearly many factors involved in the new attention paid to AIDS during 1983 in the mainstream media, probably the most influential was the 6 May issue of the conservative, general-medicine

Journal of the American Medical Association, which provided the 'hook' on which non-medical newspapers and networks hung their subsequent stories. *JAMA* suggested, in several articles and an editorial, that the syndrome might be transmitted through *casual* (that is, household) contacts. If this were so, then 'the general population' (that is, heterosexuals) might also be 'at risk' for AIDS.

All hell broke loose in the popular media: AIDS briefly became a topic of wide concern. In the quarter following *JAMA*'s speculations, for example, the *New York Times* published 20 articles in May, 28 in June, and 21 in July. In the four months *preceding JAMA*'s 6 May issue, they had published a total of only 12 articles on AIDS.[28] Geraldo Rivera, with his customary restraint, upped the ante on 26 May when he proclaimed on '20/20' that 'every single one of us' was at risk for AIDS from contaminated blood. 'You have heard right,' he brayed. 'There is now a steadily growing fear that the nation's entire blood supply may be threatened by AIDS.'[29] From this time until Rock Hudson's death in October 1985, the mainstream media found an image for the illness: the moribund *AIDS victim*, who was also (magically) a demon of sexuality, actively transmitting his condition to the 'general population' even as he lay dying off-stage.

During 1981–5, several kinds of images countered this mainstream one. Some were private: the loving snapshots and formal portraits, home movies, and videos made by families, lovers, friends as someone sickened, was diagnosed, lived on, died. Such images can be found in the archives of gay and lesbian history societies, hospital AIDS-unit albums, AIDS service organizations, and family/personal albums. Unlike the mainstream media images that began to appear in this period and swelled throughout the following years, these photographs emphasized *the continuities* in a PWA's life as he moved toward and through diagnosis. They deserve our careful attention but unfortunately they are difficult to locate and reproduce (see list of resources at end of this article).

The major source of public counter-images between 1983 and 1985 was the gay and lesbian press and AIDS service organizations (the San Francisco Kaposi Foundation, now the San Francisco AIDS Foundation, and Gay Men's Health Crisis, New York, were both founded in late 1982). Representations of AIDS were addressed by these groups almost exclusively in terms of *text* in the early years (their chief publications in 1983–4 were text-heavy safer-sex pamphlets) in the gay press. For them, AIDS was part of the evolution of their communities. They did not seek out subjects to picture simply because they had been diagnosed with AIDS. They were photographed because they were active, whether in gay communities at large or in emerging AIDS communities. Thus, when PWAs appeared in the gay press and AIDS service-organization newsletters and fund-raising appeals, they commonly appeared as whole people, not simply as *AIDS victims*: they were shown with lovers, families, caregivers. Pleasurable activities that marked their lives before and after diagnosis (gardening, weight-lifting, pets, music, leather culture) regularly figured in interviews and photographs. In the gay media, PWAs' identities were not wholly collapsed into their illness as they usually were in the mainstream media coverage.

This suggests some fundamental differences between the mainstream media's hit-and-run approach, which records only the *current* appearance of it objects (see plate 7) and which can draw attention to their *past* only through the device of before-and-after photographs, and a community's coverage of its own. Kenny Ramsauer was quite literally *the victim* of '20/20,' which did not encourage viewer identification *with* him, but in fact discouraged it by reducing him to his present physical grotesqueness (plate 6) and contrasting that with a photograph of him *before* his illness. Community coverage by AIDS service organizations and gay newspapers, in contrast, encouraged readers' identification with the PWA because of shared history and concerns.

Such identification would of course have been possible in the mainstream media's coverage; in fact, in 1985–7 it was regularly produced in covering white heterosexual PWAs and their families – AIDS's 'innocent victims.' It is ritually invoked every year in the ghastly 'human interest,' down-and-out stories that appear in city newspapers and on night-time news between Thanksgiving and Christmas. For a single month, members of America's underclass are briefly rehabilitated as 'the worthy poor,' their problems treated for once as understandable and lamentable, before being returned to their usual status as invisible and incomprehensible.[30] For a host of reasons, it does not serve the mainstream media's interests to regularly promote identification with the poor, gay, dying, or otherwise disenfranchised. When individual reporters do follow 'victims' long enough to develop strong sympathies with them, this deviation from standard journalistic practice creates ethical problems that the more customary 'hit-and-run' approach does not.[31]

1985–1988

Remarkable shifts in both the quantity and nature of depictions of AIDS took place in 1985. Publicity surrounding blood banks' use of anti-HIV antibody tests because of the growing number of transfusion-related cases focused public attention on AIDS, epitomized in *Life*'s July 1985 cover story, which proclaimed 'Now No One Is Safe from AIDS.' Rock Hudson's public admission that month that he was suffering from AIDS made the syndrome seem immediate and threatening to much of the American public, for whom Hudson was a familiar figure, the quintessential manly American. If *he* could contract AIDS, couldn't anyone?[32] The fact that Hudson had continued to act – more, to *kiss* Linda Evans while taping the next season's episodes of 'Dynasty' without the cast's suspecting that he was mortally ill – produced a massive outpouring of outrage and anxiety on television news and in the popular and tabloid press (plate 8).[33]

I would argue that this anxiety was a factor in producing the increasing emphasis upon rigid categorizations of 'risk groups' (low, high) and 'the general population' (that is, the population presumed *not* to be at risk). The advent of a method for detecting HTLV-III infection meant, among other things, that the threat of AIDS was no longer embodied only in people with visible lesions: it might also be your neighbour (who looked a little effeminate), your boss or secretary ... The invisibility of infection threw into question the comfortable categories that had kept anxieties manageable for many 'low-risk' people and reinforced the need to shore them up. The anti-HTLV-III antibody assays were introduced at a time coinciding with increased reports of transfusion and hemophiliac cases of AIDS, marking the nation's invisible 'carriers' of HTLV-III as internal security risks. A conservative, anti-Communist federal administration invoked containment methods recycled from ferreting out ideological impurities in the 1940s and 1950s for purposes of epidemiologic containment: *test, test, test.*

Photographically, the (illusory) boundary between who was at risk and who was not was stressed in various ways. The media repetitiously threw up images of street prostitutes (plate 9) and stereotypically gay men as paradigmatic 'risk group' members. 'Innocent victims' – adult heterosexuals and children with AIDS tended to be photographed surrounded by family members and animals (living or stuffed) (plate 10), as if gay men lacked both. 1985 was also the year of the first made-for-television movie about AIDS; *An Early Frost* (NBC) enforced existing prejudices by returning its PWA protagonist to the bosom of his family. Evidently he lacked long-term, close-knit friends back in Manhattan; it was only after being shorn of his sexuality and his identity as a gay man that he could be returned, neutered, to his mother and father, enfolded once again within the nuclear family, and die in peace.[34] *Newsweek* also mined this rich vein of sentiment (the gay man returned to his boyhood place in the nuclear family; see plate 11), as did countless 'heart-warming' local newscasts.[35]

The increasing divisiveness of mainstream-media coverage in 1985–6 was countered in gay communities by massive campaigns affirming the values of gay liberation: *re*-sexualizing gay men by *re*-defining sexual pleasure and sexual acts. Safer sex, as theorized by AIDS activists, could not only prevent transmission of HTLV-III (as it was still known) but also act as a cohesive force in communities increasingly under fire from the Right (now under the guise of AIDS prevention).[36] Gay safer-sex advice, begun in 1982, changed over time to accommodate new knowledge about transmission.[37] Safer-sex publications before 1985 had been exclusively textual. In 1985–6, GMHC, the San Francisco AIDS Foundation, and other AIDS service organizations began producing lively, graphically illustrated safer-sex materials. Glenn Mansfield, a Chicago gay photographer, produced a 'safe sex' nude male calendar (plate 12). GMHC produced *Chance of a Lifetime*, a 42-minute 'erotic' videotape picturing a smorgasbord of safe sex (vanilla, leather, solo/masturbatory) between men of different classes, races, and what mainstream medicine/media would now term 'antibody status.' Recruitment materials for 'The Study' (GMHC's prospective study of gay men's sexual practices) and public-service announcements depicted the male body as a focus of erotic pleasure (plates 13, 15). GMHC's Safer Sex Comix, which came to public attention when Jesse Helms used them to win support for a 1987 amendment to the Senate appropriations bill to prohibit any public monies being spent on AIDS preventive education for gay men,[38] were commissioned and produced pro bono by gay artists, then distributed in New York bars (plate 14).

All these materials reaffirmed the pleasurability of gay sexuality and gay identity in the face of medicine, epidemiology, and (in their wake) the popular media's massive assault on gay sexuality. At the pinnacle of medical-scientific influence, CDC epidemiologists at the first International AIDS Conference in Atlanta told gay men that they should all take the anti-HTLV-III antibody test and stop having sex with anyone whose 'antibody status' differed – 'as if,' Cindy Patton has observed, 'gay male culture is little more than a giant dating service.'[39]

Health and life insurance companies began calling for wholesale screening of applicants in 'high-risk areas' and 'high-risk occupations' (such as hairdressers, florists, interior designers). The military began planning their own massive screening programs of recruits and people overseas. The federal prison system began mandatory testing programs.

'Mandatory testing,' the rubric under which such government programs were enacted, was in keeping with the Reagan administration's penchant for technological fixes – like the Strategic Defense Initiative ('Star Wars') and mandatory drug-testing of federal employees. I do not intend to suggest a simple cause-and-effect linkage between the increased emphasis upon the erotic as *a medium of information* for gay men and the distinctly chilly atmosphere created by Big Brother antibody surveillance programs in federal, state, and corporate systems: the relationship between the two is much more complex. Epidemiologists, clinicians, and media 'experts' advised sexually active straights and gays to find 'safe' (that is, proven antibody-negative) partners and then enter into 'mutually monogamous' relationships with them. Such a model made *any* multiple-partnered sex (at this point everyone not monogamous became *promiscuous*), no matter how unrisky in terms of its practices, appear intrinsically unsafe. Heterosexual panic coloured movies about marital infidelity (*Fatal Attraction*) and threatened to reduce sexual pleasure and sexual choice between men and women to the dimensions of a mortally serious job interview.[40] Yet at this time, gay institutions chose to visibly reassert the plurality and plenitude of their sexual pleasure and sexual practices *if carried out safely*. Thus the eroticized videotapes, films, and photographs that circulated increasingly after 1985 in AIDS education must be seen as a counterdiscourse to the dominant messages of science, medicine, and the mainstream media.

A second counterdiscourse also became visible. People with AIDS became increasingly active in AIDS political actions and organizations, demanding that they have a voice in policy rather than being treated merely as 'clients.' Local PWA groups, meeting at the annual AIDS Forum at the Lesbian and Gay Health Foundation conferences, founded the National Association of PWAs. As the need for organized opposition to draconian measures like the California LaRouche initiatives[41] became clear, PWAs led media-savvy 'zaps' and other direct actions. In 1987–8, new drugs/treatments that appeared to delay the onset and severity of AIDS-related infection, such as AZT and aerosolized pentamidine, were released slowly by the federal government and were too expensive for most PWAs to purchase. ACT UP, the AIDS Coalition To Unleash Power, was founded in 1987 in reaction to federal foot-dragging at the National Institutes of Health and the Food and Drug Administration. It conducts AIDS direct actions in many U.S. cities. In short, the 'AIDS victim' stereotype has never been less accurate (though probably in consequence of that all the more necessary: these people are *so unruly!*) than in the period extending from 1987 to the present.

As counters to the mainstream media's one-note depiction of PWAs as *victims*, individual photographers working on self-assignment as well as for leftist photojournals and AIDS service organizations produced portraits of PWAs that were recognizably 'positive images' reflecting the historical moment. The work of two women photographers suggests the sorts of uses such photographs have been put to. Gypsy Ray (Santa Cruz, CA) and Jane Rosett (Brooklyn, NY) began making photographs of PWAs in the mid-1980s. Both Ray's and Rosett's photographs were intended primarily to serve instrumental purposes: Ray's illustrated fundraising and other appeals for the San Francisco AIDS Foundation and Hospice of San Francisco (plate 16) and Rosett's appeared, for example, in left press coverage of AIDS activism and the PWA Coalition (NYC)'s valuable guide to living with AIDS, *Surviving and Thriving with AIDS* (plates 17, 18).[42]

Significantly, neither of these photographers' work was originally produced for viewing outside contexts sympathetic and committed to the struggle around AIDS. Nor were they designed to be viewed as images independent of text: Ray's were framed by the institutional message accompanying them, while Rosett's were captioned in photojournalistic style. Unlike mainstream press and TV images of PWAs in 1985–8, Ray's subjects were usually photographed in domestic settings (rather than backlit against windows or silhouetted against studio backdrops), which emphasized their participation in life rather than their isolation from it.[43] Unlike mainstream media-makers, Ray directed attention to PWAs as people living with a medical condition rather than dying from it. She also directed attention to their caregivers – the people who assisted them in living independently: health-care workers, volunteers from Shanti and Hospice, lovers and friends.

I don't mean to suggest that Ray's work lacked problems or that it presents a model to be emulated;[44] only that whatever problems it had derived from the tradition of formal photographic portrait that Ray used and not from an unfamiliarity with her subject or a naïveté about her photographs' possible uses.

Rosett's photographs also filled in many gaps in the mainstream's usual representations of PWAs. They documented PWAs' political and social activity: testifying before New York State legislative committees, picketing and protesting, partying, goofing off. As a counter to the widespread (I'm tempted to say definitive) media image of the PWA-at-the-window-watching-life-go-by-without-him, Rosett's photographs constituted a significant body of evidence for AIDS not as an identity, but as a condition that people live with.

> ... The marks on the face of a leper, a syphilitic, someone with AIDS are the signs of a progressive mutation, dissolution; something organic.
>
> Susan Sontag *AIDS and Its Metaphors*[45]

It was also in 1985–6 that photographers working primarily within the artisanal system of galleries, museums, and art schools/colleges began circulating their photographs of AIDS. In the world of art, often viewed by its participants as 'above' or 'away from' the fray of politics, photographs expressed different things about AIDS. The photographic strategies employed by, for example, Duane Michals, Rosalind Solomon, and Nicholas Nixon, were all different, as were their politics and their experience with AIDS and the mostly gay men who appeared in their AIDS photographs. But all three spoke the central discourse of modernist art photography – that the subject of art is the artist's feelings.

There are undeniable attractions to such a stance at this time. One of the things that living on any sort of familiar terms with AIDS does is dull one's feelings, make numbness seem intermittently desirable. In theory, I have come to like the idea of photographs that court feelings, that speak to communal and personal loss. I think Duane Michals' AIDS images are a step in this direction (plate 19) – acts of mourning, affirmations of the persistence of desire in the face of death.

This brings me to the portraits of PWAs by Nicholas Nixon and Rosalind Solomon (plate 20).[46] Critics, particularly gay ones,[47] have had a difficult time pinpointing the unease these photographs produce. During Nixon's 1988 MOMA show, members of New York's AIDS activist group, ACT UP, staged a protest in the gallery where Nixon's AIDS portraits were hung. They handed out a flyer:

> NO MORE PICTURES WITHOUT CONTEXT
>
> We believe that the representation of people with AIDS (PWAs) affects not only how viewers will perceive PWAs outside the museum, but, ultimately, crucial issues of AIDS funding, legislation, and education.

> The artist's choice to produce representational work always affects more than a single artist's career, going beyond issues of curatorship, beyond the walls on which an artist's work is displayed.
>
> Ultimately, representations affect those portrayed.
>
> In portraying PWAs as people to be pitied or feared, as people alone and lonely, we believe that this show perpetuates general misconceptions about AIDS without addressing the realities of those of us living every day with this crisis as PWAs and people who love PWAs.
>
> FACT: Many PWAs now live longer after diagnosis due to experimental drug treatments, better information about nutrition and holistic health care, and due to the efforts of PWAs engaged in a continuing battle to define and save their lives.
>
> FACT: The majority of AIDS cases in New York City are among people of color, especially women. Typically, women do not live long after diagnosis because of lack of access to affordable health care, a primary care physician, or even basic information about what to do if you have AIDS.
>
> The PWA is a human being whose health has deteriorated not simply due to a virus, but due to government inaction, the inaccessibility of affordable health care, and institutionalized neglect in the forms of heterosexism, racism, and sexism.
>
> We demand the visibility of PWAs who are vibrant, angry, loving, sexy, beautiful, acting up and fighting back.
>
> STOP LOOKING AT US; START LISTENING TO US.

ACT UP is undoubtedly right to challenge Nixon's motives in choosing his particular subjects, since his choice amounts to a statement that AIDS is identical to a death sentence.[48] Such a proposition is medically and historically inaccurate. It depends for its 'power' on a highly selective process of choosing subjects and on people's credulity before 'documentary' images. I also question the ethical value of building up a body of such single-mindedly bleak work *as a project*: '[It] may stop in a year or so ... when I figure I have enough for a book.'[49] But the challenge to Nixon's work should be aimed even deeper – at the ways that Nixon (and Solomon) use these photographs to foreground *their own experience* in photographing PWAs: they make it sound as if they were stalking rare animals at great emotional cost to themselves. The photographs then become the evidence of their bravery.

Solomon began photographing PWAs after completing projects on nursing homes and the homeless.[50] She recalls conversations with PWAs 'about art exhibits, rafting trips, and Fellini films ... There was little talk of death; the tone, the words were life.' How strange ... Nixon found the same thing: that several of his subjects were witty, educated, enjoyable men. This discovery, of course, made the project more difficult *for him*: we are in the land here of photographs-as-mirrors-of-the-artist's-soul.

It is this, finally, that makes Solomon's and Nixon's work so inadequate, so irrelevant: it tells us nothing about the historic battles surrounding AIDS and its representation; it challenges none of the existing conventions that have led to PWAs being shunned, snubbed, hurt; it leaves us with very little to grasp but the photographer's sensibility.

But that tiny gift is precisely what art photography encourages. 'Nixon has reached out to his subjects with his honesty and concern,' one critic wrote; and another, 'Nixon literally and figuratively moves in so close we're convinced that his subjects hold nothing back. The viewer marvels at the trust between photographer and subject.' Thomas Sokolowski tells us that Solomon '*enabled the sitter* not only to participate ... but also to shed *the expected role of victim* [expected by *whom*? – my emphasis].' Solomon, he writes, '*lets* [each PWA] ... shout out, "I'm still here!" [my emphasis]'[51] *Photographer-as-lion-hearted-explorer-of-emotional-jungles, our-surrogate-witness-to-pain, enabler-of-victims ...*

The photographer may be an intrepid explorer of the unknown, but even while critics supportive of Nixon and Solomon praise them for taking us to *terra not very cognita*, they are quick to deny that there's anything distinctly different about the condition of the photographers' subjects: it's the *human condition*, isn't it? Owen Edwards approvingly quotes a friend looking at Nixon's work in San Francisco: '"This show isn't about AIDS, it's about mortality."' Edward himself writes: 'These six people, who know they are dying, are not really much different from each of us, who are dying, too, but (if we're lucky) don't have to think about it just yet.'[52] Rosalind Solomon tells us, 'Because all life leads inevitably to death, these pictures are about all of us,'[53] and Thomas Sokolowski, curator of her exhibition, tells us that Solomon's portraits are 'portraits *of the human condition* [my emphasis].' The title to his essay on her work is 'Looking in a Mirror.' Precisely: this is what art photography encourages its practitioners and viewers to value – the artefact as mirror to its maker's soul.

If we accept these confused propositions at face value, we're to believe on the one hand that these photographs have merit because it took extraordinary courage to obtain them, and on the other that what they represent is something we all know and live everyday. Formulations like 'each of us ... [is] dying, too' function not to console the dying (they don't) or to acknowledge their difference but rather to cancel it out, to deny it. Critics and curators who tell us that these photographs are about all of us do so at the expense of people who are currently ill and dying.

These photographs belong to no current discourse on the representation of the PWA, dominant or counter. They reflect no understanding of the complicated history of PWAs' attempts to *name themselves*, to assert their rights, or of the accumulated meanings surrounding the mainstream media images that PWAs struggle to oppose. Their crude emphasis upon physically debilitated or disfigured PWAs most closely resembles the choices made by popular media three and four years ago in emphasizing *their difference* from the rest of us. For all these reasons, these photographs are irrelevant to current attempts to define what AIDS means – whether by organized AIDS activists/PWAs, mainstream journalists, Bush administration policy-makers, the federal Immigration and Naturalization Service, the Social Security Administration, ad infinitum. Nixon's and Solomon's photographs appeal to audiences who believe that art *is* about 'timeless realities,' 'enduring values,' 'the human condition' – viewers who prefer wispy abstractions to the historical and specific. The specific historical formations – such as those of class, gender, politics, medicine, culture – that make the position of PWAs different from mine are precisely the differences that art photography is said to transcend. These are precisely the differences that it does not.

This essay originally began here. Now it is a more fitting ending.

One of the most commonly voiced convictions among photojournalists and art photographers making portraits of PWAs is that such images can teach lessons: help other people avoid a similar fate, teach us our common fate, 'humanize the disease, to make it a little bit less something that people see at arms length [sic].'[54]

This is a goal that has never been reached. Even in a city as saturated by media images of PWAs as San Francisco, researchers at the City and County Department of Public Health have concluded that media messages (posters, television and radio spots, billboards, newspaper advertisements) do not account for the decline of new HIV infections after 1985. What did it was watching one's friends and lovers grow sick and die.[55] Other cities that began their AIDS prevention media campaigns earlier in the course of their epidemics have found the same thing: media messages have no significant impact on the rising incidence of AIDS in their communities. The experience of watching friends and lovers grow sick and die does.

There is no reason to think that other didactic purposes are better served by photographs. A telling example of the importance of personal experience appeared last week in *Advertising Age*, this time in relation to AIDS in the workplace. Crane Publications, *Ad Age*'s publisher, surveyed the opinions of senior executives from advertising agencies, media, and marketing companies. Ad executives' responses were divided into those from agencies who had had employees dying from AIDS and those who had not:

	Agencies who had employees who had died from AIDS	Agencies who had *not* had employees who died from AIDS
Would your agency hire an 'openly homosexual' job candidate today?	78% yes	50% yes
Would you allow an HIV-infected employee with no symptoms to remain on the job?	91% yes	63% yes
If an employee exhibited AIDS symptoms, would you retain him/her?	74% yes	47% yes
Do you agree with current medical opinion that AIDS is transmitted in three ways: through sexual contact, exposure to infected blood/blood components, or prenatally from mother to unborn child?	83% yes	54% yes
Do you believe the presence of an employee with AIDS might cause co-workers to leave the agency?	13% yes	48% yes[56]

This survey, like the San Francisco studies, shows that *personal experience,* not media messages (and who would have more of an investment in crediting the power of media messages than advertising executives?), makes the critical difference in changing people's beliefs and behaviour.

This is not a heartening message for public-policy officials or photographers who justify making portraits of PWAs in the belief that 'everyone who sees the photographs will be changed ... and our collective understanding be advanced.'[57] But it does justify our reply to all such assertions: *Then you're naïve: what you want to accomplish has no basis in our experience.*

APPENDIX

AIDS ARCHIVES AND RESOURCES FOR VISUAL RESEARCHERS

The following list of resources for visual research on AIDS is a result of my own research, so I cannot claim that it is comprehensive. It is biased towards the West Coast because that is where I live and do most of my work.

Archives and Collections in AIDS Service Organizations and Lesbian/Gay Archives

Unfortunately, most of these are not officially open to the public; staff and space are too overtaxed to permit much public use. These resources are identified with an asterisk (*).

D.A.I.R. (Documentation on AIDS Information and Research). Small archives on AIDS-related issues; volunteer-run. 2336 Market Street, San Francisco, CA 94114 (415) 928-0292.

**Gay Men's Health Crisis* (New York). Well-organized archives of media, medical, political materials on the epidemic as well as on gay men. Organized by subject category. P.O. Box 274, 132 West 24th Street, New York, NY 10011 (212) 807-7517.

Lesbian Herstory Archives. A magnificent archives in Manhattan. Publishes newsletter on an irregular basis. Photo collections housed separately from other materials. Efficient, friendly staff. P.O. Box 1258, New York, NY 10116 (212) 874-7232.

**National Association of People with AIDS.* Maintains Washington, DC, office that distributes publications. I've never been to the office, so I do not know what other resources it may house. 1012 14th Street, N.W., Washington, DC 20005 (202) 347-1317.

NAMES Project. Houses materials on the development of the NAMES Project Quilt, including a massive archives of photographs and letters accompanying contributions to the Quilt. Always busy; write or telephone. 2362 Market Street, San Francisco, CA 94114 (415) 863-5511.

**San Francisco AIDS Foundation.* Extensive archives of photographs, print materials, but not organized or accessible. Closed to the public. Education Dept.: 333 Valencia Street, San Francisco, CA 94103 (415) 864-4376.

Finally, many cities have informal lesbian/gay archives but lack the money to house them permanently. Ask around; several old archives (New York, Los Angeles) recently lost their homes, but they still own materials critical to researchers.

AIDS Films/Videos for Visual Researchers

These are databanks for videotapes on AIDS, both broadcast and independent video. They are far more accessible resources; most publish lists of their holdings and rent/sell copies of them.

AIDS Films. Distribute the same as well as do production work. 50 W. 34th Street, Suite 6B6, New York, NY 10001 (212) 629-6288.

AIDS Film Project. A film/video distribution company associated with Frameline, producers of the San Francisco International Lesbian and Gay Film Festival held each June. Catalogue; rents and sells. (415) 861-1404.

AFI Video Festival. Bill Horrigan is a mine of information on current as well as in-production AIDS videotapes. 2021 N. Western Avenue, Los Angeles, CA 90027 (213) 856-7600.

Los Angeles International Gay & Lesbian Film/Video Festival. Catalogues of recent festivals, which have included many AIDS tapes, some of which previewed there. Catalogues: GLMC, 4391 Sunset Boulevard #522, Los Angeles, CA 90029 (213) 665-4464.

Media Network. Distribution company with an extensive listing of AIDS films and tapes that may be annotated by the time this book is published. Catalogue. 121 Fulton Street, 5th Floor, New York, NY 10038 (212) 619-3455.

I would appreciate hearing from people knowing of other resources so that I can compile as complete a listing as possible.

NOTES

This essay was first printed in *Afterimage* 17, no. 1 (summer 1989).

1 Drueilhe *Mortal Embrace: Living with AIDS* (New York: Hill and Wang 1988) 122

2 Unfortunately, the term by which sick-gay-man-(with AIDS) is opposed – ie, healthy homosexual – has yet to be conceded in most of the fields we will look at, including the gay press. The opposite of gay PWA remains sick homosexual; the idea of healthy homosexual remains apparently inexpressible. This is no less true in gay communities (*pace*, Susan Sontag), where psychologizing the 'sick' nature of the PWA has produced *internalized homophobia, repressed anger, Type-A personality*, etc, as symptoms of the underlying (ie, gay) illness.

3 See my 'AIDS: Keywords' *October* 43 (1988) 17–30, repr in *AIDS: Cultural Analysis / Cultural Activism* ed Douglas Crimp (Cambridge: MIT Press 1988), for notes on the distinction between disease as sign and symptom of AIDS *versus* sign/symptom as a disease itself.

4 Several thoughtful attempts to make sense out of the bewildering volume of data on the AIDS epidemic can be recommended: Dennis Altman's *AIDS in the Mind of America* (Garden City: Doubleday 1985); Cindy Patton *Sex and Germs: The Politics of AIDS* (Boston: South End Press 1985); Randy Shilts *And the Band Played On: Politics, People, and the AIDS Epidemic* (New York: St Martin's Press 1987), though this should be read critically in light of Shilts's method and biases; Paula Treichler's 'AIDS, Homophobia, and Biomedical Discourse: An Epidemic of Signification,' in Crimp *AIDS: Cultural Analysis* 31–70, and 'AIDS, Gender, and Biomedical Discourse' in *AIDS: The Burdens of History* ed Elizabeth Fee and Daniel M. Fox (Berkeley: University of California Press 1988) 190–266 are gold-mines of references as well as provocative interpretations.

5 Horton and Aggleton 'Perverts, Inverts, and Experts: The Cultural Production of an AIDS Research Paradigm' in *AIDS: Social Representations and Social Practices* ed Peter Aggleton, Graham Hart, and Peter Davies (Barcombe, East Sussex: Falmer Press 1989) 74–100

6 Fleck *Genesis and Development of a Scientific Fact* (Chicago: University of Chicago Press 1935, repr 1979)

7 See also Noam Chomsky and Edward Herman *Manufacturing Consent: The Political Economy of the Mass Media* (New York: Pantheon 1989), which comes at the same problem from a different perspective. Chomsky and Herman locate what Fleck/Horton-Aggleton see as the prestige of related discourses as the prestige of particular experts/authorities. This begs the question of how x becomes designated as an expert and y does not, a question that Fleck et al's analysis of institutional discourses answers more effectively.

8 Institute of Medicine, National Academy of Sciences *Confronting AIDS: Update 1988* (Washington, DC: National Academy Press 1988) 4–5

9 Ibid

10 GRID = gay-related immune deficiency; CAID = community acquired

immune deficiency; AID = acquired immune deficiency; WOG (a gay black-humour term) = wrath-of-god

11 See J.Z. Grover 'Safer Sex Guidelines' *Jump Cut* 33 (1987) 118–22 and 'Reading AIDS' in Aggleton, Hart, and Davies *AIDS: Social Representations* 252–63

12 Simon Watney's work on AIDS employs a psychoanalytic framework and provides some very persuasive readings of the seemingly *homophobic* reactions to AIDS as arising instead from defence of the (seemingly a-)historical heterosexual family unit. See Watney *Policing Desire: Pornography, AIDS, and the Media* (Minneapolis: University of Minnesota Press 1987) and Jeffrey Weeks *Sexuality and Its Discontents: Meanings, Myths and Modern Sexualities* (London: Routledge & Kegan Paul 1985).

13 Treichler 'AIDS, Gender, and Biomedical Discourse'

14 Ibid 196

15 The whole question of what is and isn't significant in epidemiological surveillance is a fascinating subject and one explored with great subtlety by Jacques Leibowitch in *A Strange Virus of Unknown Origin* [1984] (New York: Ballantine Books 1985). Leibowitch was one of the immunologists responsible for the isolation of LAV (the Pasteur Institute virus known in the United States as HTLV-III and now known internationally as HIV-1).

16 Leibowitch *A Strange Virus* xvi

17 A second example of the distinctly Anglo-American (and homotropic) bias in defining AIDS in the United States was the medical-scientific establishment's dismissal of evidence from Africa and former African colonial powers (such as Belgium and France) that AIDS was evenly distributed between the sexes in Central Africa.

18 *Naming* in science is a means of establishing ownership, hence the multitude of names under which this retrovirus has been known: LAV (Montagnier, Pasteur Institute), HTLV-III (Gallo, NCI), ARV (AIDS-related virus) (Jay Levy, University of California–San Francisco), IDAV (immune deficiency-associated virus), HTLV-III/LAV (an American compromise acknowledging the equivalence of the French virus to the American) and LAV/HTLV-III (a French compromise acknowledging the equivalence of the American virus to the French), culminating in that internationalist, HIV (human immunodeficiency virus), christened in 1986 as a replacement for HTLV-III/LAV and LAV/HTLV-III. Most clinicians and just about everyone else has cut right through all that to the dreaded heart of the matter: they call it 'the AIDS virus.' Problems with this are discussed in Grover 'AIDS: Keywords' 21.

19 I'm not suggesting here that what publishers choose to print is necessarily what readers want or embrace. The *New York Native* is an interesting case in point. Its AIDS coverage through 1986 was far more

comprehensive than that of any other gay paper and was followed closely in cities such as San Francisco and London, despite the fact that it is basically a Manhattan 'city' paper.

When its publisher's personal conviction that HIV has nothing to do with the etiology of AIDS resulted in the paper altering the emphasis of its AIDS coverage to searches for new 'causes' for AIDS, including swine flu, mosquito-borne viruses, malaria, and syphilis, those readers who believed that HIV was the principal causative agent of AIDS ceased reading the paper. The *New York Native* still publishes and is still read, but the *audience* for its AIDS coverage has changed markedly. Its pre-eminent AIDS reporter, Ann Guiducci Fettner, who had no use for Ortleb's theories, also left. Thus any account of the gay press's response to AIDS would have to factor in a complex interaction between what is published and how it is received.

20 I call attention to this term because 'AIDS' is *not* itself transmissible, despite the mainstream media's reckless use of such phrases as *catching AIDS*, *taking the AIDS test*, and *the AIDS virus* suggest. For more on this distinction, see my 'AIDS: Keywords' in Crimp, *AIDS: Cultural Analysis* and revised in *The State of the Language* ed Leonard Michaels and Christopher Ricks (Berkeley: University of California Press 1989), forthcoming.

21 Fain 'How Infectious Is AIDS?' *The Advocate*, 23 June 1983. Fain's article was occasioned by the 6 May 1983 *JAMA* issue I discuss below.

22 Eg, Randy Shilts 'TV Studio Turmoil over AIDS' *San Francisco Chronicle*, 15 June 1983, 8; Michael Hechtman and Jack Peritz 'TV Crew Nixes Show with an AIDS Victim' *New York Post* 31 July 1985; Jay Sharbutt 'TV Crew Facing the AIDS Issue' *Los Angeles Times* 10 Sept 1985, VI:1, 8. Stuart Marshall comments sarcastically on these episodes in his important AIDS videotape *Bright Eyes* (1984).

23 See 'The Denver Principles' (1983) of the group that became the National Association of People with AIDS: 'We condemn attempts to label us as "victims," which implies defeat, and we are only occasionally "patients," which implies passivity, helplessness and dependence upon others. We are "people with AIDS."' National Association of People with AIDS pamphlet (Washington, DC: NAPWA n.d.).

24 Stuart Marshall uses/inverts this device in *Bright Eyes*. See also Martha Gever's discussion of the tape, 'Pictures of Sickness: Stuart Marshall's *Bright Eyes*' in Crimp, 122–3.

25 Nathan Fain 'AIDS and the Media: Rating the Crisis Coverage' *The Advocate* 29 Sept 1983. Stuart Marshall decisively deconstructed the media's use of Kenny Ramsauer in *Bright Eyes*. See also Simon Watney's discussion in *Policing Desire*.

26 Eg, Jean Carlomusto, audiovisual director of GMHC, reports that she decided to become actively involved in producing counter-images to

the mainstream media's after she saw a *New York Times* reporter reject the host of GMHC's New York cable show as the subject of a PWA report 'because he looked too healthy.' Similarly, Michael Callen, diagnosed with AIDS in 1983, has spoken frequently of being rejected as a subject for media reportage because he 'doesn't look like a PWA' (ie moribund).

27 See Dorothy Nelkin *Science in the Streets: Report of the Twentieth Century Fund Task Force on the Communication of Scientific Risk* (New York: Priority Press 1984) 87–95.

28 Nelkin, 87

29 Rodger Streitmatter 'The Bad-News Bearers: Lowlights of AIDS Summer '83' *The Quill* 72, no. 5 (May 1984) 25

30 The classic text discussing this in relation to photographs is Martha Rosler's 'In, around, and afterthoughts (on documentary photography)' *Martha Rosler, 3 Works* (Halifax: The Press of Nova Scotia College of Art and Design 1981) 59–89. For local examples of traditional documentary in action, see J.Z. Grover 'The Inadequacy of Systems' *Artweek* (24 Jan 1987) 11; 'Representing the "Victim"' *Artweek* (6 Sept 1986) 14; 'Documenting Documents and Processing Reality: The photographs of Jim Goldberg' *In These Times* (29 Jan–4 Feb 1986).

31 Laurie Garrett 'When Death Is the End of the Story: Reporters describe the troubling problems they face in covering the mortally ill' *Columbia Journalism Review* 27, no. 5 (1989) 41–2

32 Treichler 'AIDS, Gender, and Biomedical Discourse' quotes a man 'interviewed by *USA Today*,' who said: 'I thought AIDS was a gay disease, but if Rock Hudson can get it, I guess anyone can' (p 205).

33 Eg, 'Fear & AIDS in Hollywood' *People Weekly* (23 Sept 1985) 23:13; 'AIDS Panic: Fury in Hollywood over Suspect Stars on Top Television Shows' *Star* (10 Sept 1985); 'Has Linda Anything to Fear?' *Globe* (13 Aug 1985) 20; 'Linda Evans & *Dynasty* Cast Terrified – He Kissed Her on Show' *National Enquirer* (13 Aug 1985); 'AIDS Panic on *Dynasty* over Rock's Last Love Scenes' *Star* (13 Aug 1985); 'He Vows: Doctors Cleared Me for *Dynasty* Love Scenes' *Star* (24 Sept 1985) (where no page numbers are given, these are cover quotations). Letters poured in to the popular newsweeklies; readers clearly felt betrayed by Hudson's suddenly changed 'identity.' How much of their anger was displaced from this source onto the 'Dynasty' kisses (or vice versa) isn't clear.

34 For a broad survey of broadcast television and independent video work on AIDS through 1987, see Timothy Landers 'Bodies and Anti-Bodies: A Crisis in Representation' *The Independent* 11, no. 1 (January–February 1988) 18–24.

35 Eg, 'A Family Gives Refuge to a Son Who Has AIDS' *Newsweek* (12 Aug 1985) 24

36 See Patton *Sex and Germs* and 'Resistance and the Erotic: Reclaiming

History, Setting Strategy as We Face AIDS' *Radical America* 20, no. 6 (September 1987) 68–78; Douglas Crimp 'How to Have Promiscuity in an Epidemic' in Crimp *AIDS: Cultural Analysis* 237–70.

37 Richard Berkowitz, Michael Callen, and Richard Dworkin's *How to Have Sex in an Epidemic* (New York: News from the Front 1983); Lawrence Mass, MD's several editions of *Medical Answers about AIDS* (New York: Gay Men's Health Crisis 1983–); and GMHC's *AIDS Newsletter* (1983, 1984) provide documentary evidence of the sophistication of gay men in evolving safer sexual practices without benefit of the federal government's testing programs.

38 See Grover 'Safer Sex Guidelines.'

39 Patton 'Resistance and the Erotic' 69

40 A striking feature of the pop 'safer-sex' manuals written for heterosexuals after 1986 is their emphasis upon the necessity of 'interviewing' sexual prospects. Dr Art Ulene ('*The Today Show*'s Physician') actually provides 'the questions you should ask to help determine just how risky your partner is for the AIDS virus' (pp 34–5), 'hypothetical cases to test your savvy at risk assessment' (39–53), and a table for 'Estimating a Sex Partner's Risk for AIDS' (64–5) in *Safe Sex in a Dangerous World* (New York: Vintage 1987). Helen Singer Kaplan jumps through similar hoops in *The Real Truth about Women and AIDS: How to Eliminate the Risks without Giving up Love and Sex* (New York: Fireside Books/Simon & Schuster 1987).

41 These were proposed measures for mandatory testing/reporting and optional quarantine of PWAs that appeared on the general-election ballots in California in 1986 (Proposition 69), 1987 (Proposition 64), and 1988 (Propositions 96 and 102). All but Proposition 96 were voted down by California voters by resounding majorities.

42 Michael Callen, ed, *Surviving and Thriving with AIDS* vol 2 (New York: PWA Coalition 1988); vol 1 was published in 1987 and is out of print.

43 I spent six months working with Tom Waddell, founder of the Gay Games, after his diagnosis with AIDS. Because of Waddell's prominence in San Francisco's gay community, he was frequently interviewed, taped, and photographed. His house was a huge turn-of-the-century *Turnverein* in the Mission District – a distinctive and novel home, with the old gymnasium serving as a living room used for many fund-raising and political events.

When the *San Francisco Examiner* sent a reporter and photographer to interview Waddell about four months before he died, the photographer chose to seat Tom in front of a backlit, venetian-blinded window, posed at a right angle to the window. Although I could see the classic *AIDS victim* shot that the photographer was setting up, I had no right to intervene in the shoot. I can't describe the peculiar pain it gave me to know what was happening and yet to say nothing. The resulting photograph showed a gaunt man in high, Rembrandt sidelighting with the bars of the blinds cutting dramatically across his face and upper body.

44 See my review of her work in Grover 'Representing the "Victim."'

45 Sontag *AIDS and Its Metaphors* (New York: Farrar, Straus and Giroux 1989) 41

46 Nixon's photographs of PWAs appeared in his retrospective exhibition at the MOMA last fall as well as at his dealers' galleries. One series of these appears in *Nicholas Nixon: Pictures of People* (Boston: Little, Brown / New York Graphic Society 1988). Rosalind Solomon's photographs of PWAs appeared in a May–July 1988 exhibition at the Gray Art Gallery, New York University. A selection of these appears in the catalogue, *Portraits in the Time of AIDS*, with text by Thomas W. Sokolowski (New York: Gray Art Gallery & Study Center, NYU, 1988).

47 Here I am speaking of Douglas Crimp, Robert Atkins, Deborah Bright, and myself.

48 In an informal talk at MOMA last October, Nicholas Nixon said that he had turned down some of the PWAs who had contacted him about participating in his project because he didn't find them interesting-looking. If his exhibition is any indication, *interesting* PWAs are ones who bear visible signs of their mortality.

49 Nixon, audiotape made at MOMA, 11 Oct 1988

50 Solomon 'Artist's Statement' *Portraits in the Time of AIDS*

51 Sokolowski 'Looking in a Mirror' *Portraits in the Time of AIDS*

52 Edwards 'Mortal Vision: Nicholas Nixon Shows Us the Condition We're in' *American Photographer* (December 1988) 19

53 Solomon 'Artist's Statement'

54 Nicholas Nixon, artist's statement, *People with AIDS: Donald Perham* (1987), in *AIDS: The Artists' Response* ed Jan Zita Grover [exhibition catalogue] (Columbus, OH: University Gallery of Fine Arts, Ohio State University, 1988) 45

55 Patricia E. Evans, G.W. Rutherford, J.W. Amory, and N.A. Hessol 'Does Health Education Work? Publicly Funded AIDS Education in San Francisco,' presented at IV International AIDS Conference (Stockholm: 1988) 1; 364 (abstract 6044). See also Stephen F. Morin 'Behavior Change and Prevention of Sexual Transmission of HIV,' presented at IV International AIDS Conference (Stockholm: 1988) 1, 368 (abstract 6058), which found 'perceived threat' the most critical early factor in gay men's changes in sexual behaviour.

56 Questions paraphrased to save space. Thomas J. Tyrer 'AIDS: *AA* Survey Shows Workplace Concern' *Advertising Age* 60, no. 15 (3 April 1989): 1, 22, 27

57 Sokolowski, n.p.

1

REPRESENTING
AIDS:
CRISIS & CRITICISM

An interdisciplinary conference on the impact of the AIDS crisis on contemporary art, culture and thought.

FRIDAY EVENING, SATURDAY, SUNDAY MORNING
NOVEMBER 11-13, 198

AUDITORIUM A, UNIVERSITY HOSPITAL
UNIVERSITY OF WESTERN ONTARIO
LONDON, ONTARIO

REGISTRATION FEE $50 (Canadian)

For further information, contact the Office of Continuing Medical Information, Faculty of Medicine, University of Western Ontario, London, Ontario N6A 5C1. Tel. (519) 661-2074

The conference committee is pleased to announce the generous support of the Embassy Cultural House, Burroughs Wellcome Inc., the [illegible] Council, the Social Sciences and Humanities Research Council of Canada, the Faculties of Arts and Medicine, the Departments of English and Visual Arts, and the Centre for the Study of Theory and Criticism at the University of Western Ontario.

POSTER DESIGN BY DAVID BUCHAN
COMMISSIONED BY THE EMBASSY CULTURAL HOUSE

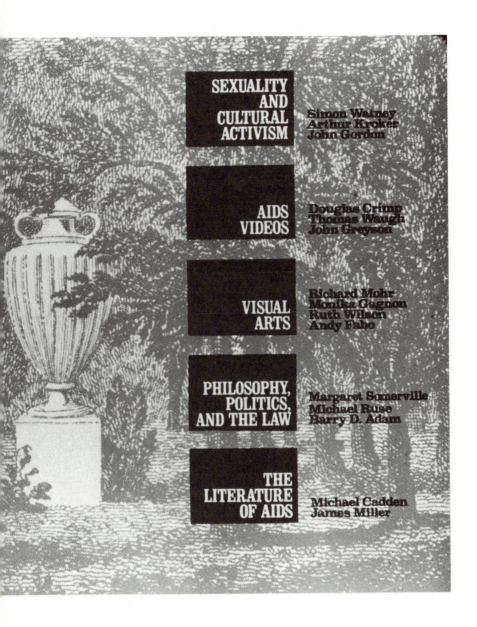

1 David Buchan, poster commissioned by Embassy Cultural House for *Representing AIDS* symposium (University of Western Ontario, Nov. 1988)

2

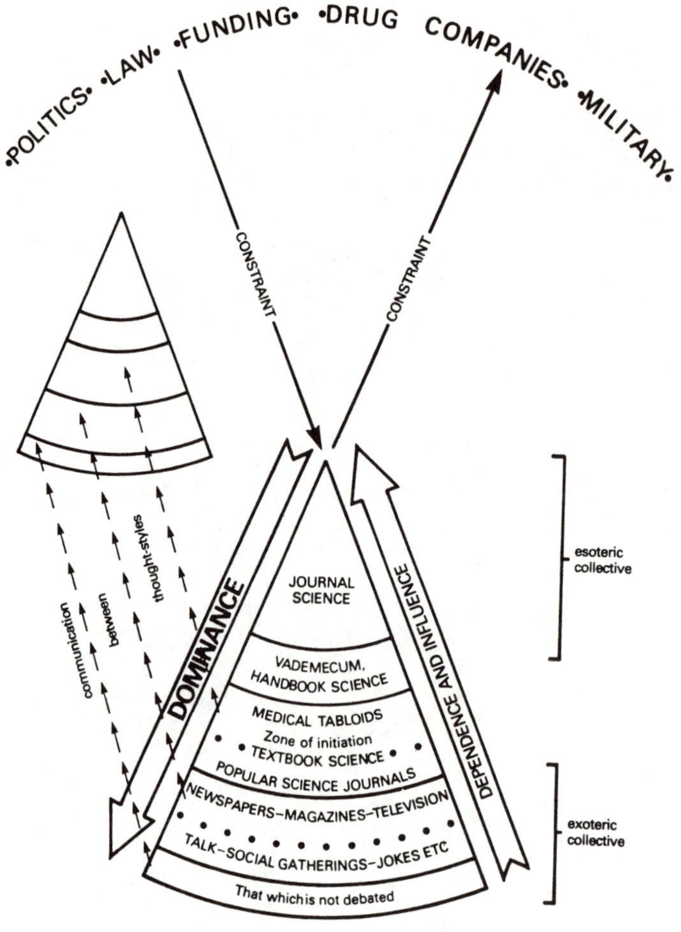

2 Meyrick Horton and Peter Aggleton 'Preliminary model of the thought-collective of the AIDS world' from *AIDS: Social Representations, Social Practices* ed Aggleton et al, 93

3 Lennart Nilsson, 30,000× magnification of human helper T cell 'under attack by the AIDS virus,' *National Geographic* 169:6 (June 1986) 707. Gendered wars at the subcellular level.

4 'The AIDS Virus,' cover of *Scientific American* (Jan. 1987). Paula Treichler calls this schematic image 'virus as grenade.'

3

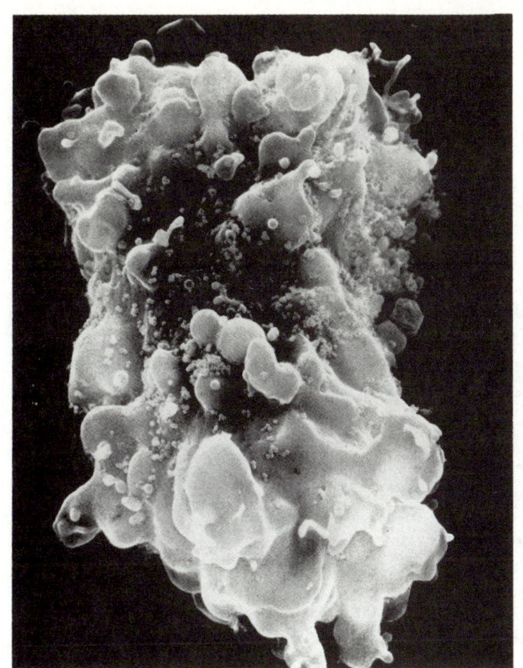

4

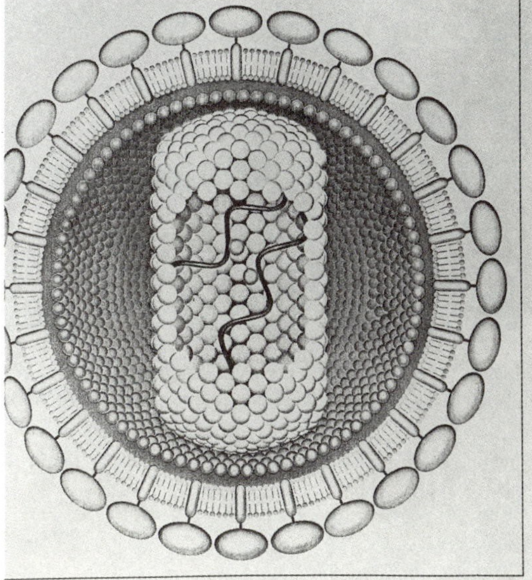
SCIENTIFIC AMERICAN

THE AIDS VIRUS $2.50

January 1987

5

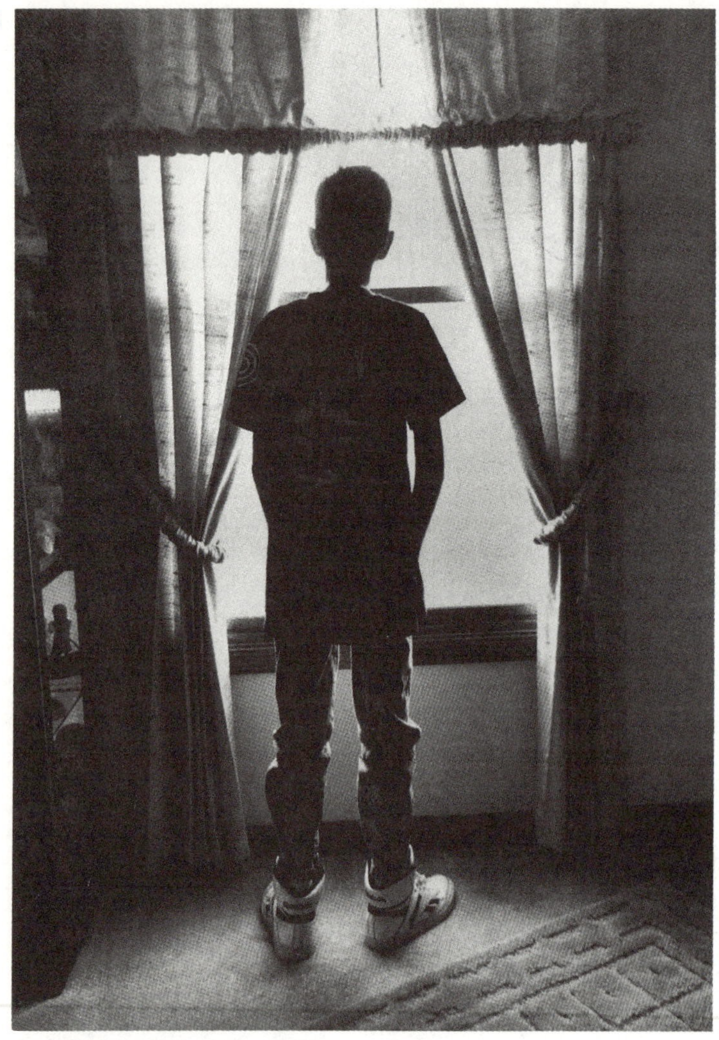

5 Taro Yamasaki, photograph of Ryan White, *People Weekly* 29:21 (30 May 1988) 96

6 Photograph of Kenny Ramsauer, from Simon Watney and Sunil Gupta 'The Rhetoric of AIDS' *Screen* 27:1 (Jan.–Feb. 1986) 81

7 Peter Sterling, photograph of David Chickadel, *People Weekly* 28:5 (3 Aug. 1987) 73

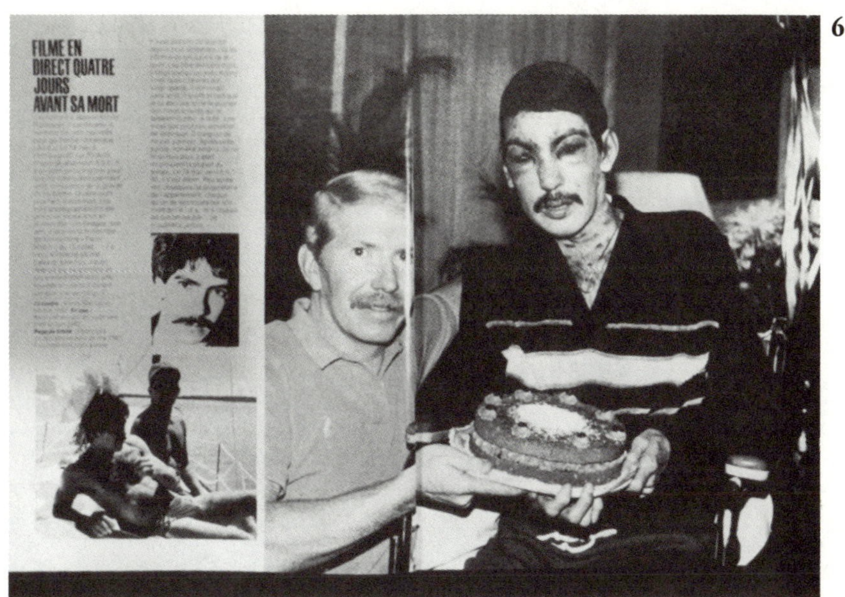

6

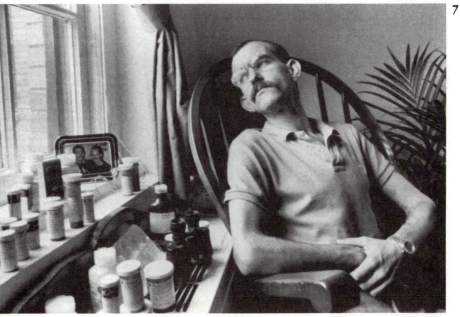

7

8 Photograph of Rock Hudson and Linda Evans, *Globe* (13 Aug. 1985) 20

9 Prostitutes as guilty 'carriers,' photograph by Ethan Hoffman, *Newsweek* (12 Aug. 1985) 28

10 'The most blameless victims': Ryan White (*left*), photograph by Max Winter; Matthew Kozup and mother (*right*), photograph by Tim Dillon, in *Newsweek* (12 Aug. 1985) 29

8

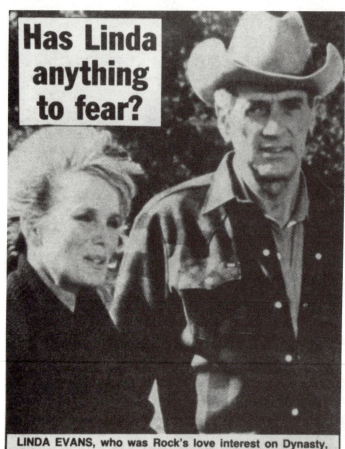

Has Linda anything to fear?

LINDA EVANS, who was Rock's love interest on Dynasty, doesn't have to worry about catching his fearful disease through kissing, a medical expert says. Dr. Alan Cantwell, of Los Angeles, points out that AIDS is transmitted through a transfer of bodily fluids during intimate sexual activity, blood transfusions and the use of contaminated hypodermic needles, but not during kissing. An insider on the Dynasty set confirms that there is no panic among the actors — just great sadness that Rock is so frightfully ill.

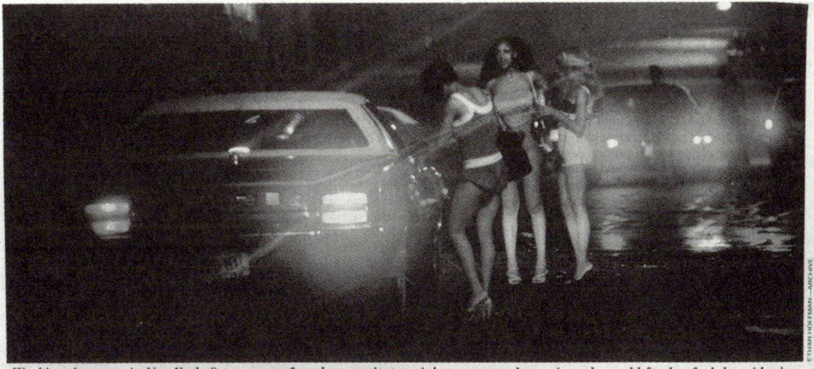 9

ETHAN HOFFMAN—ARCHIVE

Working the streets in New York: Some experts fear that prostitutes might turn out to be carriers who could further fuel the epidemic

The Social Fallout From an Epidemic

A 'safe sex' movement—and an aura of fear.

In West Hollywood, Calif., a city heavily

blameless of its victims. "The stigma is tre-

There are also sharp disparities in awareness of the disease around the country. While 96 percent of the poll respondents said they did not personally know anyone who had AIDS, in cities like Los Angeles and New York, which have large homosexual populations, many people not only know AIDS victims but have been to their funerals. In Hollywood, where the news of Rock Hudson's AIDS illness has kindled rumors of more such disclosures to come, a virtual siege mentality has taken over. "It's here, folks, it's all around us and we should stop pretending otherwise," says comedienne Joan Rivers, who has lost three friends to AIDS and has been active in fund-raising benefits for research on the disease.

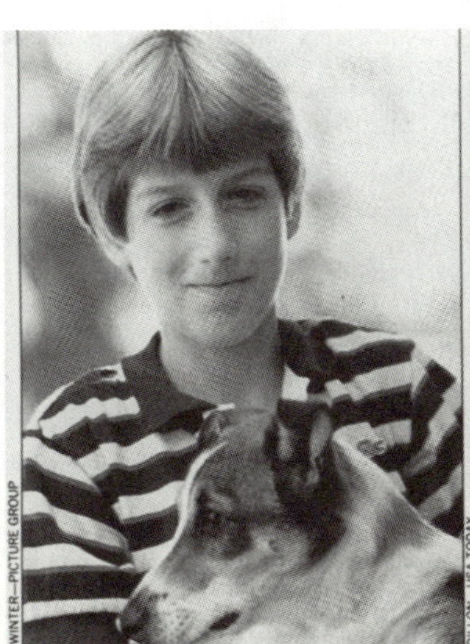

MAX WINTER—PICTURE GROUP

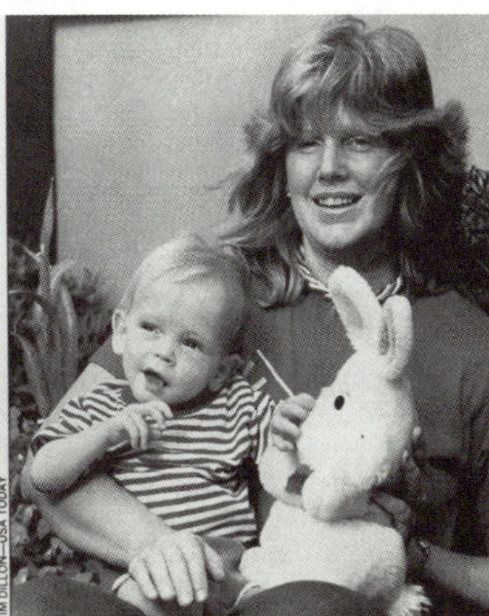 10

TIM DILLON—USA TODAY

Ryan White (left), Matthew Kozup and his mother: The most blameless victims

11

A Family Gives Refuge To a Son Who Has AIDS

Despite initial shock, there is understanding.

Although Helenclare Cox had known for years that her son Andrew was gay, she was still shocked when she found out he had AIDS. But there was never any question in her mind that if Andrew, now 34, was sick, he belonged at home in Altadena, Calif. In that respect, Andrew Hiatt (his mother has remarried) is lucky: horror stories abound of families who, unable to cast aside their own fears or prejudices about AIDS, leave their sons to lonely deaths in strange hospitals or force them to seek support solely from friends, lovers and even concerned strangers.

By the summer of 1983 Andrew had ended a six-year homosexual relationship and moved to San Francisco. He was working as a flight attendant for Continental Airlines when he first noticed the little bluish spot on his right ankle; initially, he figured he must have bruised himself while pushing a food cart. He knew about Kaposi's sarcoma, the skin cancer that strikes AIDS victims, but he couldn't believe the bruise was a telltale lesion. When he moved in with his sister Linda and experienced the intense fatigue and night sweats that are hallmarks of AIDS, she was also reluctant to acknowledge what was going on. "AIDS happened to other people, to decadent gays," she says. "It didn't happen to your little brother."

By Christmas Andrew had lost 15 pounds and was in excruciating pain from Burkitt's lymphoma—a rare but fast-growing cancer. At the family holiday celebration, he could barely get out of bed. After discussing it with her husband, Bill, Helenclare persuaded Andrew to come home with them to Altadena (a suburb of Los Angeles).

But the doctor his mother consulted wanted Andrew to be hospitalized immediately. As he lay close to death at Cedars-Sinai Medical Center in Los Angeles, Helenclare remained by his bedside all day, every day, the one constant in what he remembers as a nightmarish blur of chemotherapy injections and visitors who had to wear gowns, gloves and masks, so that all he could really see was "the shock in their eyes." One day in a half-sleep, Andrew heard the word "AIDS," and he thought to himself, "So it's really true. This is it." When he got well enough to look out of the window, he discovered a bizarre sight: his room overlooked a gay bathhouse. "I'd watch guys going in," he recalls, "and I'd automatically equate sex with illness—and then with death."

Dramatic Recovery: When it was time to return to his family's home, still weak and helpless, still taking chemotherapy, Andrew had mixed emotions. "I'd always stayed close to my family," he explains, "but I didn't always need them. Then, all of a sudden, I needed them for everything." His mother and stepfather put Andrew in their master bedroom overlooking the garden and the hills next to the pool, and they moved into the guest bedroom. Helenclare fed him, bathed him and tried to comfort him. Andrew's 88-year-old grandmother, who lived with the family, was another, surprising, source of solace. She died last spring, avoiding her fear that she might survive her only grandson, whom she adored, but she lived long enough to see him make his dramatic recovery.

There were some rocky times. An extended visit by his young niece and nephew had to be cut short because their father feared that they might be threatened by Andrew's condition. The sterilized dishes and separate towels Andrew had to use sometimes made him feel "like a piece of crawling crud that no one could touch." But today he feels quite healthy and is optimistic. He has moved into his own apartment in the Hollywood Hills, a departure that has been difficult for Helenclare. "I was never the kind of mother who minded when my kids left home," she explains, "but we're talking about a kid with a life-threatening illness." Still, Andrew himself believes that he has put the disease behind him. His only symptoms now are three lingering Kaposi's sarcoma lesions, and his body has fought off a series of infections, including pneumonia. "It's a new life," he declares, "and however long it lasts, it's going to be a really good one."

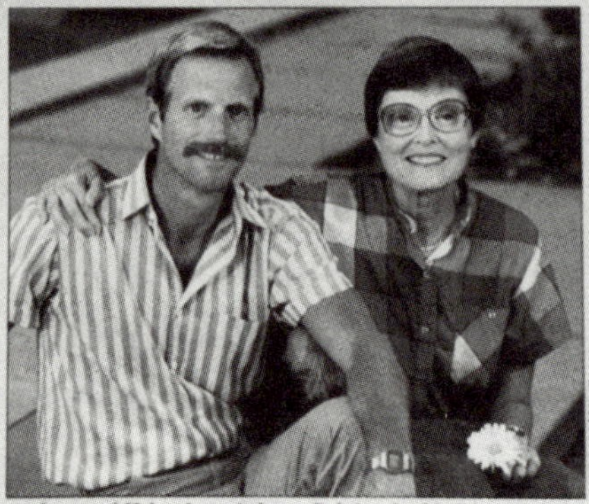

Andrew and Helenclare: At home fighting for his life

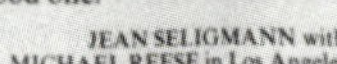

JEAN SELIGMANN with MICHAEL REESE in Los Angeles

24 NEWSWEEK/AUGUST 12, 1985

11 James D. Wilson, photograph of Andrew and Helenclare Cox, *Newsweek* (12 Aug. 1985) 24

12 Glenn Mansfield, *Safe Sex Calendar 1986* (Chicago: Gay Chicago Magazine 1985)

13 'Join me in THE STUDY' (New York: Gay Men's Health Crisis 1985)

14 *Safer Sex Comix #2* (New York: Gay Men's Health Crisis 1986)

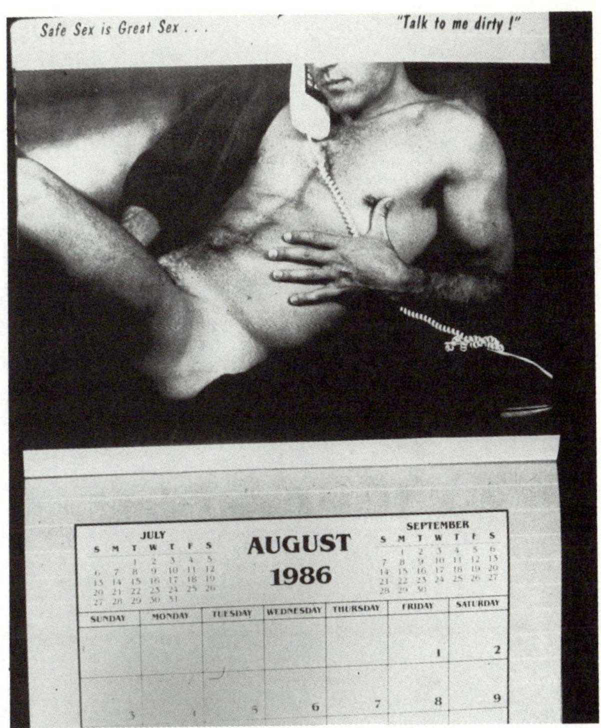

Safe Sex is Great Sex . . .
"Talk to me dirty!"
JULY
AUGUST
1986
SEPTEMBER
SUNDAY MONDAY TUESDAY WEDNESDAY THURSDAY FRIDAY SATURDAY

12

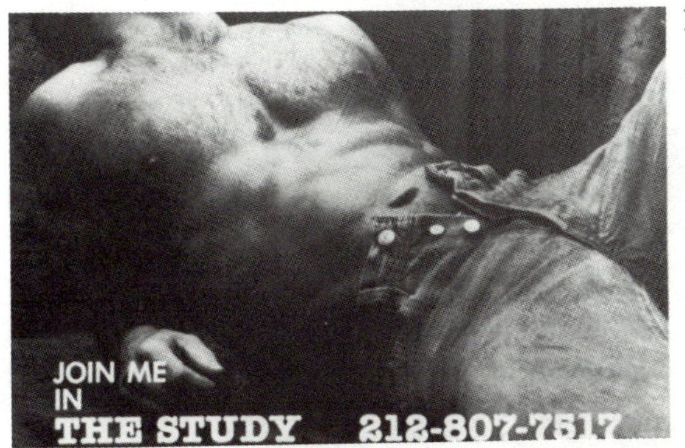

JOIN ME
IN
THE STUDY 212-807-7517

13

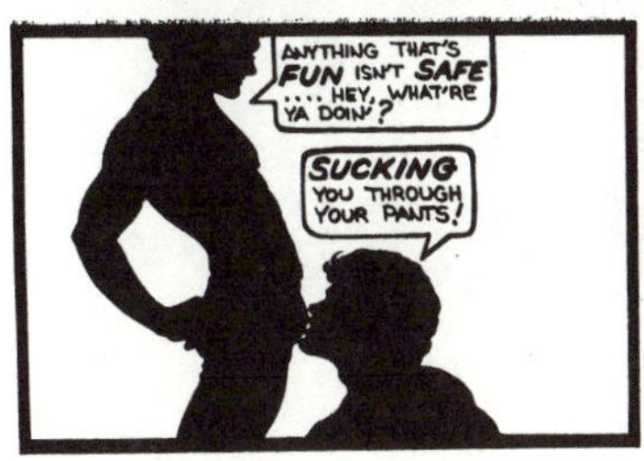

ANYTHING THAT'S FUN ISN'T SAFE .... HEY, WHAT'RE YA DOIN'?
SUCKING YOU THROUGH YOUR PANTS!

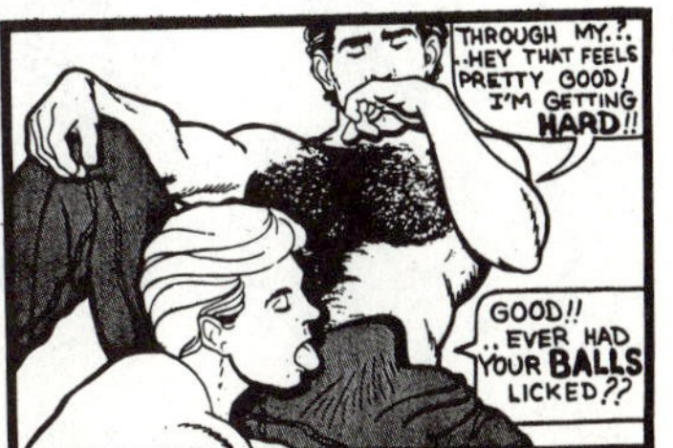

THROUGH MY..?.. HEY THAT FEELS PRETTY GOOD! I'M GETTING HARD!!
GOOD!! .. EVER HAD YOUR BALLS LICKED??

14

15

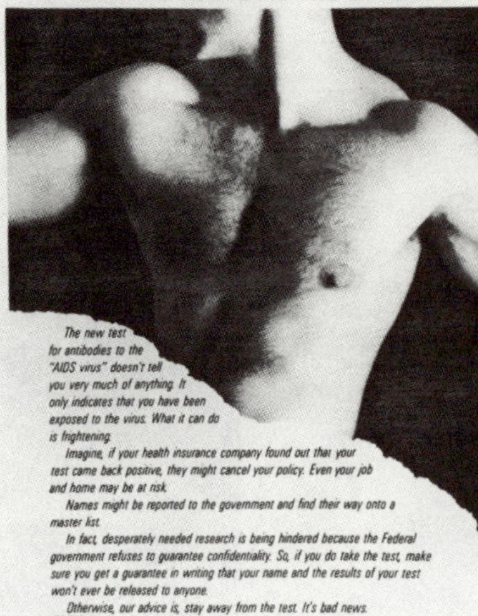
THE TEST CAN BE ALMOST
AS DEVASTATING AS THE DISEASE
The new test for antibodies to the "AIDS virus" doesn't tell you very much of anything. It only indicates that you have been exposed to the virus. What it can do is frightening.
Imagine, if your health insurance company found out that your test came back positive, they might cancel your policy. Even your job and home may be at risk.
Names might be reported to the government and find their way onto a master list.
In fact, desperately needed research is being hindered because the Federal government refuses to guarantee confidentiality. So, if you do take the test, make sure you get a guarantee in writing that your name and the results of your test won't ever be released to anyone.
Otherwise, our advice is, stay away from the test. It's bad news.
GMHC Hotline 212-807-6655

16

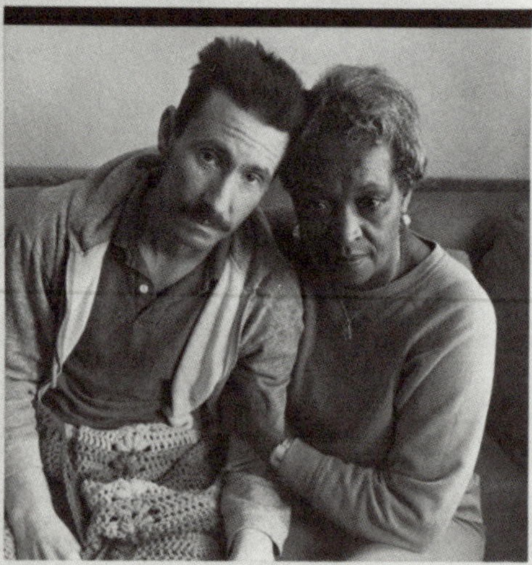
AIDS HOME CARE AND HOSPICE MANUAL
Developed by the AIDS HOME CARE AND HOSPICE PROGRAM
VNA of San Francisco
Sponsored in part by grants from
The Robert Wood Johnson Foundation and Caremark/Home Health Care of America

15 'The Test Can Be Almost as Devastating as the Disease' (New York: Gay Men's Health Crisis 1985)

16 Gypsy Ray, photograph from 'AIDS Home Care and Hospice Manual' (VNA of San Francisco: no date)

17 Jane Rosett, photograph of PWA David Summers (*left*) and his lover Sal Licata (with berets, *centre*) protesting *New York Post*'s inflammatory AIDS coverage, from *Surviving and Thriving with AIDS* 1:88

18 Jane Rosett, photograph of David Summers wearing mask and pearls outside his hospital room at NYU Co-op Care, *Surviving and Thriving with AIDS* 1:98. 'Rumors of my death have been greatly exaggerated,' he informed the press when a mix-up over names resulted in a false report that he had died.

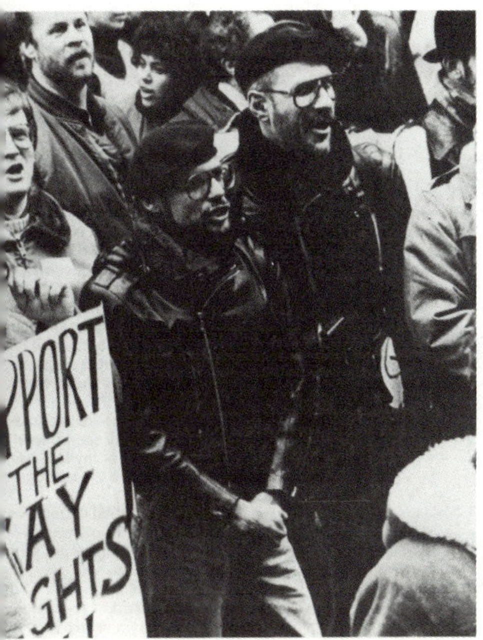

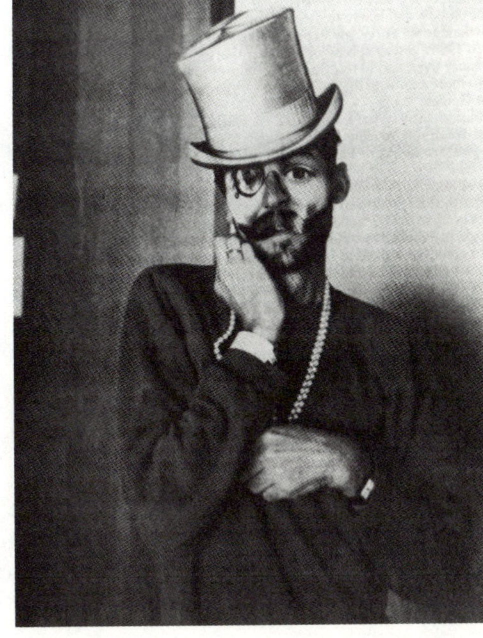

17 **18**

19

ALL THINGS MELLOW IN THE MIND,
A SLEIGHT OF HAND, A TRICK OF TIME.
AND EVEN OUR GREAT LOVE WILL FADE.
SOON WE'LL BE STRANGERS IN THE GRAVE.
THAT'S WHY THIS MOMENT IS SO DEAR.
I KISS YOUR LIPS, AND WE ARE HERE
SO LET'S HOLD TIGHT, AND TOUCH AND FEEL
FOR THIS QUICK INSTANT WE ARE REAL.

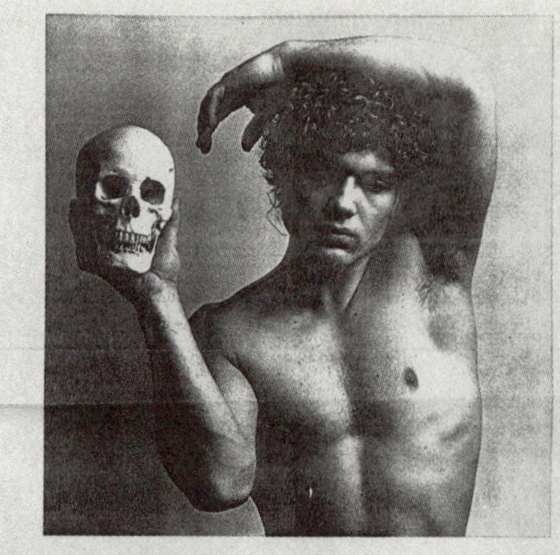

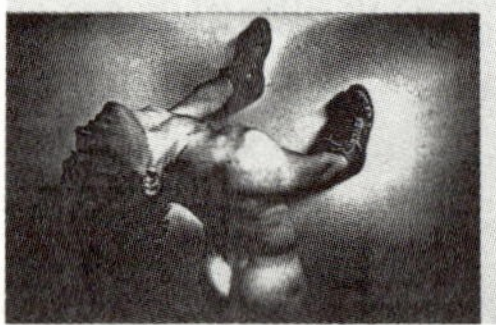

The unfortunate man could not touch the one he loved. It had been declared illegal
by the government. Slowly his fingers became toes and his hands gradually
became feet. He began to wear shoes on his hands to hide his shame.
It never occurred to him, to break the law.

19 Duane Michals, 'All things mellow in the mind ...' and 'The unfortunate man ...' [photographs untitled]

20 Nicholas Nixon, photograph of Donald Perham, *People with AIDS*

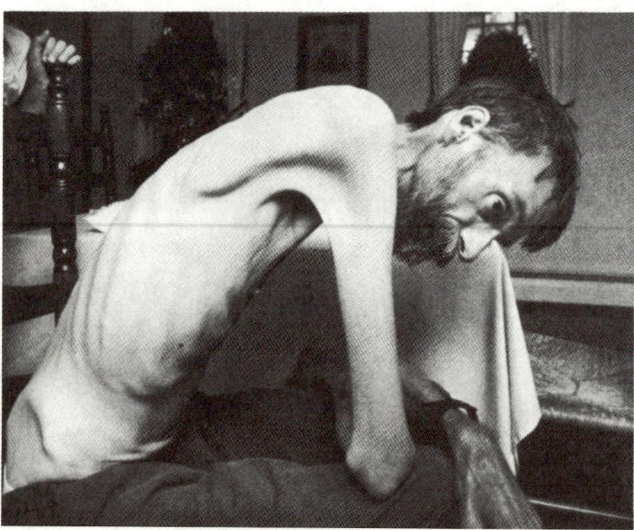

20

21

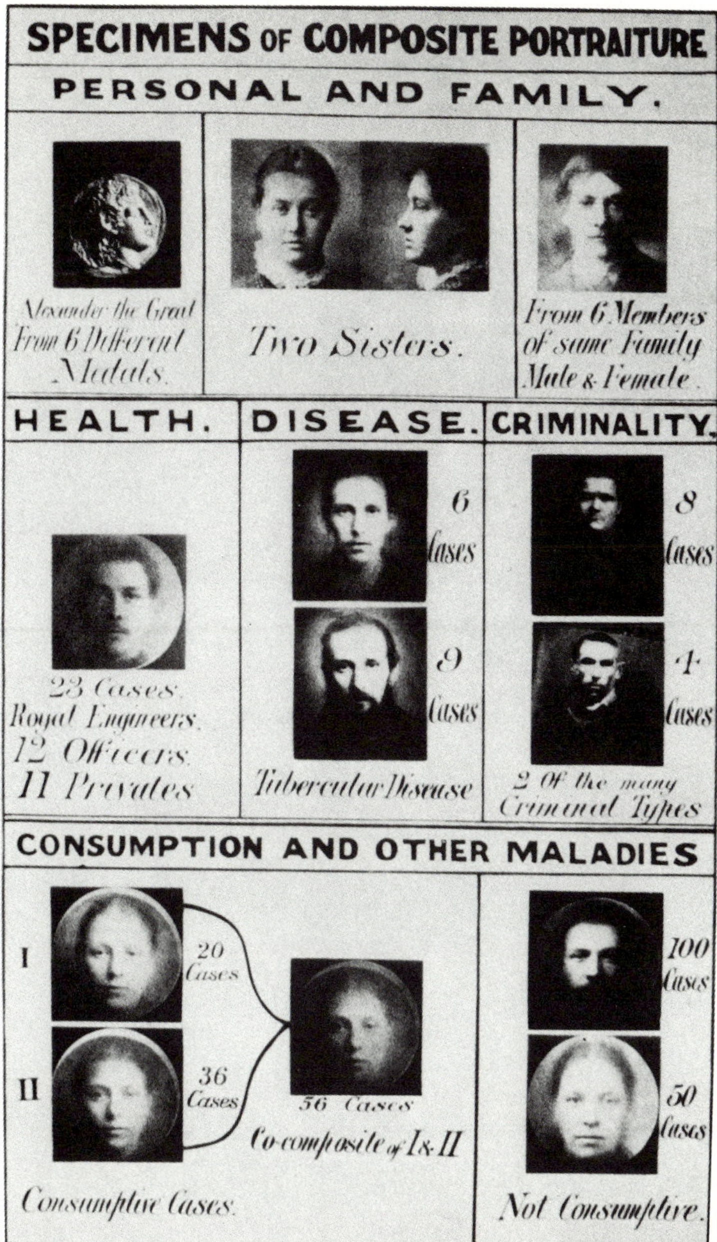

21 F. Galton, 'Inquiries into human faculties and its [sic] development' (1883)

22

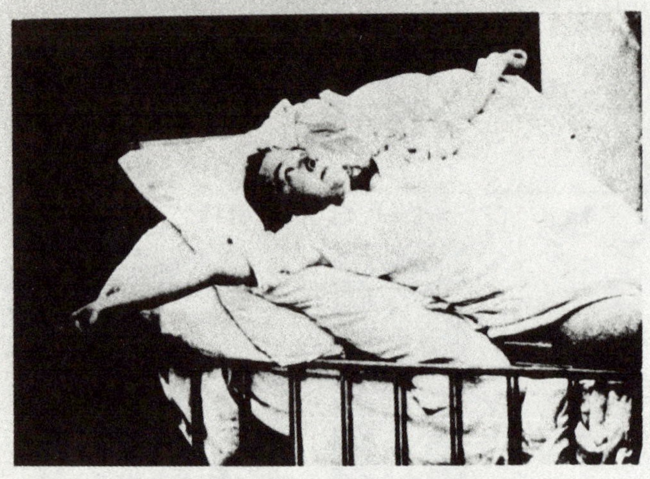

Planche XXV.

ATTITUDES PASSIONNELLES

CRUCIFIEMENT

Fig. 107. Régnard. Photographie d'Augustine
Iconographie... Tome II.

22 Paul Régnard, photograph of Augustine, *Inconographie photographique de la Salpêtrière* tome II (1878)

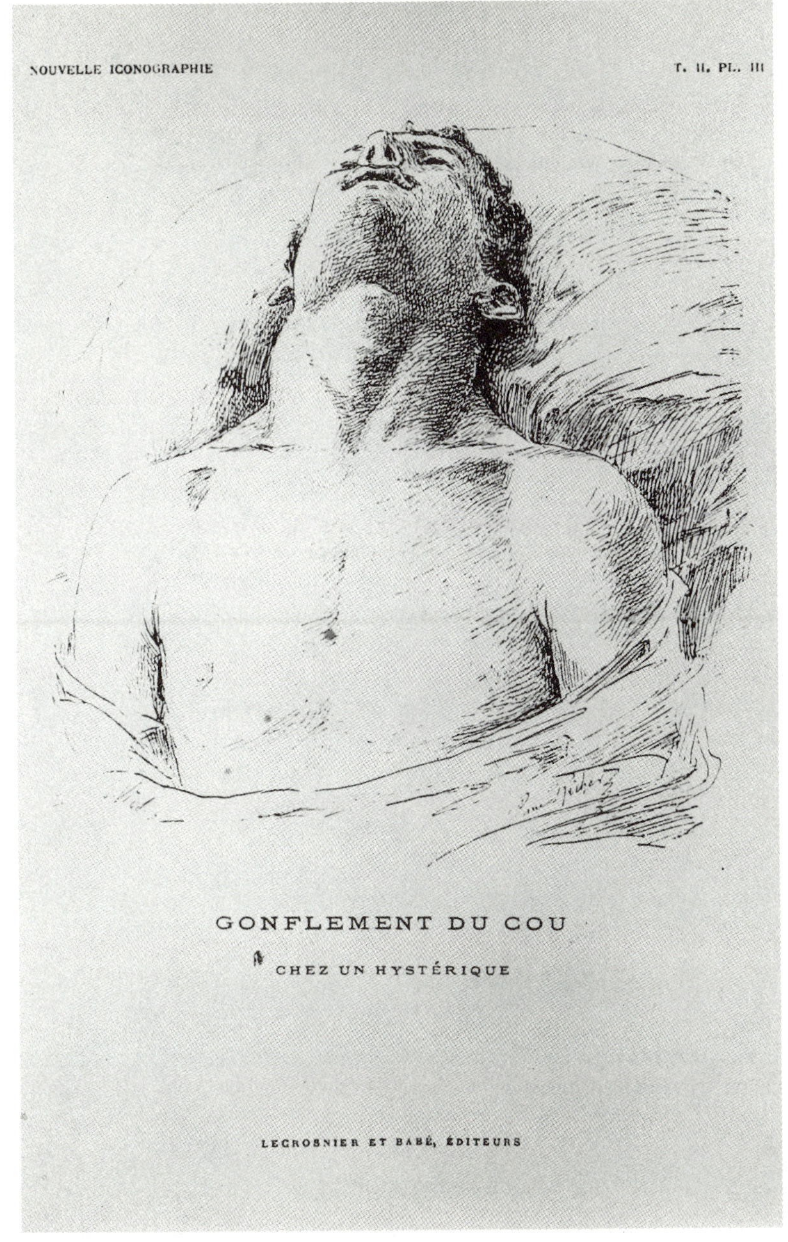

23

23 'Swelling of the Neck in a Hysteria Patient,' *Nouvelle Iconographie de la Salpêtrière* (1889)

24

si nettement de la précédente que la 2ᵉ de la 1ʳᵉ, l'expression du visage varie avec les hallucinations qui obsèdent le malade; chez notre sujet, ce qui prédomine ce sont les images de la vie militaire, envisagée surtout sous ses côtés sombres. Il se bat avec un ennemi invisible, le

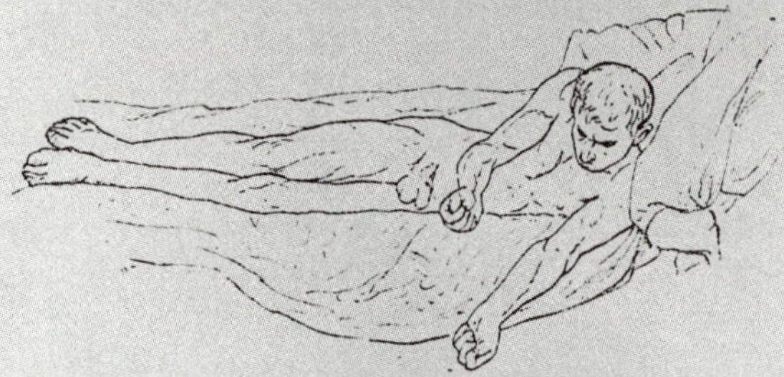

FIG. 92. — Periode der Hallucinationen.

terrasse; il exécute admirablement tous les mouvements du combat à la bayonnette, il met en joue, etc. Tout cela finit généralement par l'attitude du crucifiement.

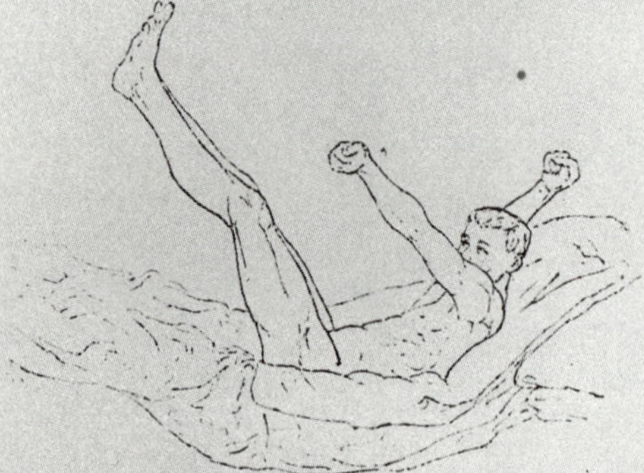

FIG. 93. — Periode der Hallucinationen.

Dans cette 3ᵉ période, les yeux sont également ouverts d'ordinaire et la pupille réagit bien. Toutes les attaques, spontanées ou provoquées, présentent cet aspect typique; l'attaque entière se subdivise en une série d'attaques (3-6) séparées par un intervalle de une demie à plusieurs

24 'Hysteria in the German Army,' *Nouvelle Iconographie de la Salpêtrière* (1889)

A Convergence of Stakes: Photography, Feminism, and AIDS

MONIKA GAGNON

I

'The Body & Society' was the series title for three group exhibitions organized by the London artists' group Embassy Cultural House during the fall of 1988. Conceived in tandem with a series of seminars, 'AIDS and the Arts,' held at the University of Western Ontario, these exhibitions were anticipated to coincide with the 'Representing AIDS: Crisis and Criticism' conference. The twelve Canadian and American artists in these shows were not selected because their work could be related strictly to AIDS; rather, they were included because of the consistently progressive engagement of their work with issues generally concerning the placement of the body in the social world (see pp 215–21 in this volume). Quoting from Bryan Turner's book *The Body and Society*, the exhibition predicated an expanded social scope, and it is thus to bodies in representation that my own comments are addressed. What body is being invoked? Whose body?

As Paula Treichler has observed, 'Perhaps it would be helpful, in rewriting the AIDS text, to take "[Bryan] Turner's Postulates" into account: (1) disease is a language; (2) the body is a representation; (3) medicine is a political practice.'[1] My observations on nineteenth-century medical discourses on female and male hysteria attempt to take these 'postulates' into account and consider how static gender roles in the social realm had determined the separate trajectories – practical and theoretical – that their respective treatments had taken.

The nineteenth-century medical determination of 'homosexuality' as an organically based 'disorder' prompted conceptualizations more aligned with female hysteria than with the concurrent socially based analyses of male hysteria. In all instances, rigid models of masculinity and femininity within a strictly heterosexual paradigm appear to underpin the framework and limits of medical research and theory itself.

Like the imaging of the body in 'The Body & Society' exhibitions, the term 'body' itself escapes descriptive reduction: from Nancy Spero's repetitive lino-print scrolls of tortured figures in *Tow IV*, to Andy Fabo's poignant exploration of the public and private effects of AIDS in his personal and political *The Body Under Duress: A Manual For Those Who Suffer the Syndrome*, to Mary Scott's 'exotic' performer in *Untitled (quoting Irigaray, Paley, image V. Burgin)*, these works all attest that the body is not merely a self-evident or universalized possibility. Rather, the body is always, in some sense, 'spoken' through language, in representation. Upon its entry into the world, the body is necessarily framed (by gender and sexuality, by family, by the state), constructed, fantasized, constrained, disciplined, punished, socialized, educated, enjoyed, destroyed, and imaged in different ways and toward different ends. There is no bodily essence, then, that we might have recourse to behind the word, behind the image, no essence that might be conceived as existing outside of representation.

Feminism has insisted that the body is invested with relations of power. Dealing fundamentally with women's corporeal placement within the social world, feminism has insisted that the body is a site of political inscription and of struggle.[2] I reiterate here what is probably redundant, and as a feminist critic speaking with usually specialized concerns, I am perhaps also eliding the many differences, contradictions, and conflicts of feminists' positions. I simply want to underline how the varied and significant contributions by feminism to what we understand as a politics of the body may often be underestimated once located outside a strictly feminist context.

The marginalization of feminism itself is frequently paralleled by a literal marginalization of women; that in one sense was evident at the conference 'Representing AIDS: Crisis and Criticism,' as three women contributed formally as speakers to a weekend of discussions that included *fifteen* speakers. The precarious future of feminism becomes only too apparent when the important contributions made by feminists to cultural analysis, critique, and activism seem not only marginalized, but made virtually invisible and therefore irrelevant. It is not simply because HIV infection, ARC, and AIDS are democratic conditions that this point is crucial, nor is this to subvert the very devastating effects that AIDS has had on gay men very specifically. But if the critical analyses of AIDS as a socio-medical and cultural crisis is to significantly broach and expand analyses of heterosexism, homophobia, and racism, as well as contribute to ongoing critiques of dominant institutional apparatuses (government, medicine, mass media), unusual affiliations between otherwise disparate groups and their specific practical concerns and goals must be seen as both productive and necessary. Lynne Segal notes in 'Lessons from the Past': 'AIDS has fuelled the already growing new Right backlash against gay liberation and sexual permissiveness, against women's equality and abortion rights, and against the feminist rejection of all forms of male domination. There is nothing at all surprising about homophobia and the reassertion of male power. Both are a defense of the dominant form of heterosexual masculinity enshrined in marriage, a "masculinity" which oppresses women and gay men alike.'[3] If AIDS is not to be detrimentally assigned and perceived as being a male 'homosexual' issue, as it has been consistently reinforced by the mainstream popular media, it is imperative that a sexual politics rigorously insist that the 'problem' of HIV – its social, political, and medical production – not remain a male issue either.

It is a convergence of stakes that I wish to consider.

II

> Somewhere every culture has an imaginary zone for what it excludes, and it is that zone we must try to remember *today*.
>
> Catherine Clément, 1975[4]

> The 'homosexual body' would thus evidence a fictive collectivity of perverse sexual performances, denied any psychic reality and pushed out beyond the furthest margins of the social.
>
> Simon Watney, 1988[5]

As the 1980s wore on, it became painfully clear that the production of knowledge and representations, as well as critical analyses, with regards to the AIDS crisis could not be left unattended and unchallenged, left merely to be dealt with practically by government, medical bodies, and the popular media. The development of counterdiscourses to mainstream 'AIDS commentary' affirmed what feminist, lesbian, and gay activists, working across the fields of medicine and law as cultural producers and critics within academic institutions, have consistently foregrounded and insisted upon: that representation is not neutral but thoroughly invested with relations of power. This is a convergence of stakes that enables us to understand the way in which power and knowledge are written across the body in complex and often invisible ways.

Perhaps it would be useful to consider how the current abjection of the gay body – an abjection produced across a variety of institutions – finds a precedent in the general subjection and abjection of the woman's body. This analogy perhaps runs the risk of oversimplifying and reducing a gay specificity, but none the less provides important evidence of the way in which fear and fascination are simultaneously evoked in confrontation with one another, by bodies that are (to be) marked by difference. While the specific constructions of these bodies involve different social and psychical motivations, different operations, different effects, these are bodies bound and confined by the language of Western patriarchy, and hence relegated to fields outside of a sanctified white, heterosexual terrain. Outside, perhaps, but in their otherness or 'alterity,' they are strictly managed, and thereby known and dominated.

For many contemporary feminist writers and artists, the site of the hysteric's body has been emblematic of the way in which the containment of what is perceived as threatening to so-called 'natural' femininity and the social role of woman – as mother and wife – is achieved. In the works of French feminist Catherine Clément, American feminist Elaine Showalter, artists Mary Kelly and Nicole Jolicoeur, amongst many others, the historical exploration of the female hysteric has productively allowed for complex analyses of how the subjection of women is achieved, not only through medical/scientific discourses, but with its attendant reaffirming effects in the social and political spheres. As Kelly remarked in relation to the research and production of her 1985 work *Corpus*: 'I was intrigued by the idea that hysteria is no longer represented clinically, but somehow remains very present in a popular sense ... In *Corpus* I'm also attempting to establish a unity in the way that the body is constructed, how it is hystericized and made *visible in its symptomic consequences* [my emphasis].'[6]

French neurologist Jean-Martin Charcot's treatment of female hysterics from 1872 until his death in 1893 exhibits the 'containment' and explanation of women's 'disorder' within a framework posited on the truth of vision – disorder characterized by an extremely expansive range of symptoms from coughing, loss of speech, fainting, chronic sleeping, to the theatrics of the *grande hystérie*, fully documented in dozens of photographs produced at the Salpêtrière hospital in Paris (see plates 21–4, following p 51). The treatment of hysteria as an organically based disorder, the search for lesions and other signs of physical disturbance particularly during autopsies, the systematic organization of phases of the hysterical attack, the literal mapping of the body, and finally the use of hypnosis and photography to document these signs – all confirmed the necessity for science to assign to disease *a visible truth*. It is important to recall that this so-called disease would later be seen by Freud (once himself a student of Charcot) as rooted in psychic trauma, opening the way for his radical theory of the unconscious.

In attempting to locate the manifestations of the hysteric's behaviour within the realm of sight, Charcot articulated the profound power of vision: to see was to know and understand. The birth of the hospital and modern medical discourse is roughly coterminous with the development of the modern prison and of photography, and as Michel Foucault has underlined, these 'inventions' evidence a profound shift in the surveillance of the individual by the state. That Charcot employs photography in the service of his investigations and inventions signals how within the sanctified field of science, knowledge – in this case knowledge of the woman – was produced through the prism of a highly specialized terminology that ultimately reduced the disorder of the hysteric to the spectre of her own body: to anchor is quite clearly in this instance to construct, define, and contain behavioural deviations and disorders within the realm of the visible, and therefore within a powerful circuit of surveillance. His well-documented prescription of chloroform and amyl nitrate, his use of cauterizing instruments and ovarian compressors, as well as suggestive hypnosis, all remained well out of frame of the photographic documentation, and paled in the presence of his patients' spectacular, well-attended performances in the amphitheatre on the hospital grounds – case histories and the *Leçons* themselves reading like theatrical plays.

Returning to Catherine Clément's encapsulating description of the hysteric's symbolic function, we should note that she underlines a crisis of sexual identification:

> ... the hysteric embodies somewhere an incompatible synthesis – bisexuality. And like all subgroups that are unsituated in the complex of symbolic systems, women are threatened by the

> reverse of mobility, by symbolic repressions that are ready to limit the effects of symbolic disorder ... In *Tristes Tropiques*, Lévi-Strauss distinguishes two forms of repression (or two forms of integration one could say). The anthropoemic mode, ours, consists in vomiting the abnormal ones into protected spaces – hospitals, asylums, prisons.[7]

The crisis in gender identification produced a range of complex and provocative problems when an analogous symptomology was exhibited by the male subject, what Charcot had termed the 'virile' hysteric. As Michele Ouerd comments in her introduction to a re-publication of Charcot's case histories on male hysteria *Leçons sur l'hystérie virile*, originally written between 1885 and 1891, '[les leçons] qui sont consacrées à l'hystérie virile sont curieusement restés dans l'ombre ([the case histories] consecrated to male hysteria remained curiously in the shadows).'[8]

Ouerd underlines how the etymology of hysteria posed a primary problem: the symptomology of hysteria had since the time of Hippocrates been associated quite literally with a disorder of the woman's reproductive system, a problem attributed to her womb (*hystera*) and her fragile feminine constitution. This etymology clearly posed problems of applicability to the male subject, and Ouerd further suggests that while hysterical behaviour could produce impotence or lack of sexual desire, the male subject's sexuality generally would not come under question or examination to the extent that it had with hysterical female subjects.

The concept of male hysteria was not new to Charcot, but had been posited by Charles Lepois as early as the seventeenth century. It was left to Charcot, whose specialty had become the treatment of female hysteria for over ten years, to first shift emphasis away from the womb as a specific site of hysterical problems to the brain, thus enabling the transportation of his model of hysteria from one sex to the other, and thereby also insisting on the possibility of a male hysteria proper. In 1881, Charcot began his first treatment of masculine hysteria, which he presented in research in 1885. It was, however, received with a certain reluctance, a reluctance that a Dr Briquet had expressed some twenty years earlier:

> Supposons un homme doué de la faculté d'être affecté à la manière de la femme, il deviendrait hystérique et conséquemment impropre à remplir le rôle auquel il est destiné, celui de la

> protection et de la force. *Un homme hystérique, c'est le renversement des lois constitutives de la société* (italics mine).[9]
>
> Supposing a man were endowed with the option to be affected in the manner of a woman, he would become hysterical and consequently unable to fulfil the role to which he is destined, that of protection and of force/power. A hysterical man is a reversal of the constitutive laws of socicty.

In her essay 'Male Hysteria and Early Cinema,' Lynne Kirby argues that what 'male hysteria shows is not so much the coding of men as women, as the uncoding of men as men.'[10] The implicit emasculation of the male hysteric within hysteria's discursive history produced telling ideological correctives that attempted to redefine what was, in effect, a rupture in strict conceptions of masculinity. Charcot's *Leçons* cover instances of male patients' suffering from traumas inflicted by railway travel – what was termed 'railway spine and brain' and already extensively under research by medical communities in England. Charcot, however, proposed and maintained that 'railway spine and brain' could be assimilated to hysterical symptomology. Gilles La Tourette, working under Charcot in 1889, published a paper describing a case of male hysteria in the German army, citing hallucinations and re-enactments of combat scenes under the same organizational schemata of *grande hystérie* assigned to female sufferers at the Salpêtrière.[11] Charcot's premises were contested by Oppenheim and Thompsen in Germany, who preferred the term 'traumatic neurosis,' insisting 'that railway trauma gave rise to a nerve condition, with electricity coursing through the nerves as the causative agent,' despite symptoms analogous to classical hysteria.[12]

Clearly, the shift away from organic explanations – explanations rooted in the body and based on degenerative or hereditary theories – toward socially motivated attributions for hysterical behaviour appears to be triggered by the incidence and appearance of male hysteria. Elaine Showalter goes so far as to suggest that the diagnoses of 'shell shock' made twenty-five years later during the First World War, and the masculinity crisis effected at a moment when masculine heroism was essential for the ideology of war, precipitated the era of psychiatric modernism: 'The efficacy of the term "shell shock" lay in its power to provide a masculine-sounding substitute for the effeminate associations of hysteria and to disguise the troubling parallels between male war neurosis and the female nervous disorder epidemic before the war.'[13]

The absence of photographs of male hysterics amongst the vast documentations of female hysterics produced at the Salpêtrière photo studio by Paul Régnard and Albert Londe (published in the *Iconographie photographique de la Salpêtrière* in 4 volumes dating from 1876–80) can be explained by the fact that Charcot's work on masculine hysteria did not begin until 1881. Besides the images of female hysteria in these volumes there are photo documentations of spinal lesions and of epileptics' muscle and limb contortions, and the strange presence of a detail from a Rubens painting depicting the contorted face of a woman possessed by a demon. Charcot's fascination with demonic possession and physical deformities, his authoring of *Les Démoniaques dans l'art* with Paul Richer (laboratory head of the clinic for nervous disorders and also an extensive illustrator for many of the *Iconographie* volumes), lends a cryptic slant to his penchant for the systematic and influential ordering and mapping of hysteria. Charcot's one essay on the subject of 'homosexuality' and its attempted cure with hypnosis was co-authored with Victor Magnan in 1889, and was entitled 'Inversion du sens genital et autres perversions sexuelles.'

The absence of photographic representations of male hysterical subjects become more curious in the *Nouvelle Iconographie* published in 1889, a volume in which La Tourette's essay on hysteria in the German army appears. While a handful of somewhat nondescript line drawings of a hysterical subject with a swollen neck and diagrams documenting the bodily contortions and poses of a hysterical attack illustrate the accompanying presentation papers, no photographic images of male hysterics appear to exist; indeed, none has been reproduced within the *Iconographies*, despite the extensive photo documentation of female hysterics throughout the volumes of the 1870s, and despite photographs of male epileptics and patients with spinal deformities.

Until Freud, the examination and definition of female hysteria remained mapped to the woman's body, a mapping that failed to acknowledge the ideological role of femininity and the woman's placement and function within the patriarchal family; the spectacular images documenting her attacks, which are over-produced and in excess, present and re-present her fascinating 'disorder.' Studies on male hysteria, alternatively, could not tolerate the crisis of masculinity that was implicitly suggested, necessitating the positing of specific social events to account for what were none the less behaviours analogous to those exhibited by female hysterics. That photographic evidence of such behaviours is generally absent is simply confirmation of both the precariousness and danger of the dependancy of hysteria on the visible: like the structure of fetishism that Freud describes, what reveals and subverts – the *image* of woman as embodiment of disorder – threatens also to remind the viewer that *he* too may be implicated in the psychic drama.

III

In his essay 'The Spectacle of AIDS' Simon Watney points out how the popular media have represented AIDS either with medical images magnifying HIV (hundreds of thousands of times in an abstraction otherwise invisible to the naked eye) or with visual documentation of the ravages on the body that are the signs of complications only in the very advanced stages of infection. 'AIDS,' Watney concludes, 'is thus embodied as an exemplary and admonitory drama relayed between the image of the miraculous authority of clinical medicine and the faces and bodies of individuals who clearly disclose the stigmata of their guilt.'[14] The imperative to visualize, confirm, and fix AIDS on the body solves the 'problem' of how to know the disease – how to understand what is in fact an invisible cellular disorder within the body – yet again, situating the confirmation of knowledge in the visual field, a visuality that is itself a discursive production. Knowledge, then, can be produced visually, and knowledge of HIV infection and AIDS is produced, in many ways invented, by the photograph. In dominant representations of HIV infection, we find its conflation not only with the fatal, final stages of AIDS itself, but dominantly embodied by photography across the figure of the 'homosexual.'

Nineteenth-century society, through the cipher of the medical gaze, turned the woman's body into spectacle; by making hysteria a visible symptom it was able not only to contain a threatening 'otherness' but also to turn that threat into a source of fascination and voyeurism. The entire concept of male hysteria is not merely a lexical problem, but more generally, as Showalter suggests, a crisis in masculinity, in which the rigid gender roles appear to be in collapse. Similarly, the insistence on the location of AIDS as a visible symptom on the 'homosexual' body provides the opportunity for macabre fantasies about homosexuality in an ideological continuum that not only allows the spectator to pity the subject – a classic and redundant response typical of 'concerned' photography – but, importantly, provides re-affirmation of a fantasy that marks the underlying homophobia of our culture, in conformity with nineteenth-century characterizations of 'homosexuality' as 'criminal deviation.' The far-ranging complexities of AIDS are reduced to the spectre of the PLWA's body, which in turn is frighteningly identified with the generic gay man's body and further reduced to the one-dimensional characteristics of his sexuality.

Contemporary theory in art and cinema, with significant contributions by feminist cultural producers and critics, has produced a politics of representation that understands how the image is determined in part by power relations in the social world within which images are produced, exchanged, and consumed. If, as Douglas Crimp has insisted, we are to think of the production and possibilities of art beyond their capacities as saleable commodities generating money toward AIDS research, beyond an aesthetic idealism that would dismiss art's capacity for cultural intervention,[15] we must equally recognize that such practices are neither programmatic nor formulaic, but rather are in a constant state of invention and reinvention.

We might, for instance, consider what such a practice *would not be*.

In the work of two American photographers, Nicholas Nixon and Rosalind Solomon, we find the tradition of 'concerned' social photography unfortunately alive and well after more than twenty years of critical work on the photograph. Two series of Nixon's 'Pictures of People,' one on people living in old-age homes, the other on PLWAs, were shown in 1988 at New York's Museum of Modern Art in a travelling exhibition accompanied by paperback and hardback catalogues.

Nixon's and Solomon's images, in the classic tradition of documentary photography, take as their subject the so-called downtrodden victim; we can identify the collusion of language and its spectacularization within the realm of sight in the relations of power operating between the masterful command of the photographer and the placement of her or his subject. That People Living with Aids have strongly rejected their subjection as AIDS *victims* has immediate political significance for visual representations as well. Like Nixon's photographs, Solomon's images clearly demonstrate the sheer objectification of the PLWA within a sanctified 'aesthetic' discourse – that is, documentary – revealing the veneer of objective documentation as a fictional discursive construction. That Solomon's subjects are either in severe states of weight loss, or afflicted with Kaposi's sarcoma, underlines the fear and fascination that dominant institutions, represented here by MOMA, may have in the 'homosexual' body. It is precisely the victimizing voyeurism of this type of social documentary, for instance, that prompted Martha Rosler to eliminate the body and foreground the discursive properties of photography and language in her photo-text work *The Bowery: Two Inadequate Sign Systems* (1974).

The historical overdetermination of the woman's image across a range of visual representations – in art, medicine, popular media – has prompted many feminist artists to problematize, and in many instances, completely eliminate the site of the woman's body, precisely in order to draw attention to the conventions of its ubiquitous spectacularization, and critically to address how such images have become so normalized. Bodies infected by HIV or afflicted by AIDS have also become 'normalized' images within popular culture, and like women's bodies are subject to the disintegrating gaze of the patriarchal spectator. Here a mottled arm or leg is shown – there a shrunken cheek or swollen neck – as if these dissected parts of the diseased body somehow 'proved' the dominance of the medical viewpoint by their apparent abjection and virtual dismemberment. Their significance as parts depends, of course, on the determining totality of patriarchy as a cultural system privileging white heterosexual males. If we are to rupture this dual process of normalization and victimization, we need to problematize the discursive construction of AIDS in the popular media (including photography) by recognizing the powerful history of oppressions to which such subjection and abjection belong.

NOTES

1 Paula Treichler 'AIDS, Homophobia, and Biomedical Discourse: An Epidemic of Signification' *October* 43 (Winter 1987) 65

2 The recent court cases of Barbara Dodd and Chantal Daigle, for instance, have focused feminist concern in Canada primarily on the struggle for reproduction rights. Other issues provoking feminist criticism of the definition and control of women's bodies by the state include access to safe birth control, sexual violence, and physical abuse.

3 Lynne Segal 'Lessons from the Past: Feminism, Sexual Politics and the Challenge of AIDS' in *Taking Liberties: AIDS and Cultural Politics*, ed Erica Carter and Simon Watney (London: Serpent's Tail 1989) 133

4 Catherine Clément 'The Guilty One' in *The Newly Born Woman* trans Betsy Wing (Minneapolis: University of Minnesota Press 1986) 6

5 Simon Watney 'The Spectacle of AIDS' *October* 43 (Winter 1987) 79

6 Mary Kelly, quoted in my article 'Texta Scientiae: Mary Kelly's *Corpus*' *C* 10 (Summer 1986) 30
7 Clement 'The Guilty One' 8
8 Jean-Martin Charcot *Leçons sur l'hystérie virile* intro Michele Ouerd (Paris: Le Sycamore 1984)
9 Michele Ouerd 'Introduction' to Charcot *Leçons* 19
10 Lynne Kirby 'Male Hysteria and Early Cinema' in *Camera Obscura* 17 (May 1988) 126
11 Gilles La Tourette 'L'hystérie dans l'armée allemande' in *Nouvelle Iconographie de la Salpêtrière* (Paris: Lecrosnier et Babe, Libraires-Editeurs 1889) 318–26
12 Kirby 'Male Hysteria' 123
13 Elaine Showalter *The Female Malady: Women, Madness and English Culture, 1830–1980* (New York: Penguin Books 1985) 164
14 Watney 'The Spectacle of AIDS' 78
15 Douglas Crimp 'AIDS: Cultural Analysis / Cultural Activism' *October* 43 (Winter 1987) 6–7

'The Soul is the Prison of the Body': Fabo on Foucault

DAVID WHITE

> We believe, in any event, that the body obeys the exclusive laws of physiology and that it escapes the influence of history, but this too is false. The body is molded by a great many distinct regimes; it is broken down by the rhythms of work, rest, and holidays; it is poisoned by food or values, through eating habits or moral laws; it constructs resistances ... Nothing in man – not even his body – is sufficiently stable to serve as the basis for self-recognition or for understanding other men.[1]

Andy Fabo was born in Calgary, Alberta, in 1953. He studied at the University of Calgary (1970–1) and at the Alberta College of Art, Calgary (1973–5). He began exhibiting in Toronto at the A Space gallery in the group exhibition *Works By ...* (1978) and in a solo exhibition, *Male à la Mode* (1979). In 1978 he was an employee at The Barracks, a Toronto bathhouse that was raided by the police in one of their periodic purges of the 'gay underworld.' Fabo, along with one other employee and the three owners of The Barracks, was charged as 'a keeper of a common bawdy house.' (On 12 June 1981, a provincial court judge found the employees guilty of the charges against them, while acquitting the owners.)[2] Fabo's 1980 solo exhibition *Self-Portraits of An Alleged Keeper of A Common Bawdy House* (The Funnel, Toronto) addressed the problem of gay self-representation in a society that systematically denies gay people the possibility of establishing recognized social and cultural institutions.

During the early 1980s, Fabo was a member of the ChromoZone Gallery. In addition to exhibiting works in their Toronto gallery, the ChromoZone group exhibited in galleries across Canada and also in West Berlin (Das Institut Unzeit, 1982). ChromoZone 'was the first gallery to take a serious interest in the new figurative art that has come to typify the decade,'[3] and the artists connected with the gallery were exploring the figure in a country where figure painting had been, for the most part, of secondary importance to the major Canadian art movements. In the mid-1980s, Fabo had a residency in the Canadian Studio at Public Studio One, New York (1984–5). Since 1986 Fabo's solo exhibitions have included *Western Flesh and Blood* (Garnet Press, Toronto, 1986), *Landscape of Loss* (Garnet Press, Toronto, and Forest City Gallery, London, Ontario, 1987), and *Technologies of the Self* (Garnet Press, Toronto, 1989); and he has participated in the group exhibitions 'The Body & Society' (Embassy Cultural House, London, Ontario, 1988) and *Homogenius* (Mercer Union, Toronto, 1989).

In December 1986, Andy Fabo's lover, artist Tim Jocelyn, died of illnesses contracted as a result of AIDS. Fabo, who is seropositive, went through a period, as he explains in a letter to James Miller, in which he produced elegiac art: 'In my work I have tried to confront the personal issues straight on, to give a notion of the complexities of gay love and the reaction to the loss of the loved one(s). I went through a period of elegiac art, which I consider to be very important during this plague-remembering.'[4] Elegy is also present in the second phase of Fabo's artistic response to AIDS, the representation of activism, just as, in part, it informs his work as an activist. To a certain extent, Fabo's development as an artist in the Age of AIDS confirms Jan Zita Grover's observation that 'none of us can simply transcend this level of reaction to the loss of friends, lovers, family members. Only later is it possible to make the social connections, touch the anger and harness it to social purposes. That occurs in second-generation AIDS artwork – the activist, largely collectivist work that has appeared in the past two years in the U.S. coastal cities first hit by AIDS.'[5] In his book-works, Fabo explores the relationship between elegiac and activist art and suggests that elegiac art is the site of rupture from which the activist challenge to conventional representation emerges in the Age of AIDS.

An early painting by Andy Fabo indicates his awareness of the problems of representation involved in the depiction of gay identity. *The Wall* (1980) is, in part, a self-portrait that expresses the impossibility of conventional portraiture for those who are recognized as members of a marginalized group primarily through stereotypes. If the aim of conventional portraiture is to express some aspect of the inner life of the individual through the external signs of the body, the portrait presented in *The Wall* underlines not only the impossibility of such a practice when the external signs are limited to stereotypes, but also raises the issue of the way in which stereotyping can influence not only the perceptions of the mainstream but those of the marginalized as well.

In the painting, the actual 'portrait' occurs at the extreme right of the canvas. The head that is represented from the chin to not quite the crown is cut in half by the edge of the canvas. The eye is obscured by one half of a pair of sunglasses. While the moustache, close-cropped hair, and sunglasses are signs that are not limited to gay men, the background, a wall of graffiti, indicates the field of conflicting messages within which the stereotyping occurs. Occupying the centre of the canvas, in large letters, imitative of spray-painted slogans, are the words 'Fuck' and, beneath it, 'Off.' Inserted between the two and in smaller letters is the phrase 'Me Please' while at the bottom of the canvas is the phrase 'Kill All Fags!' In the upper left corner we find 'For a good blow phone Eric' and a telephone number, while in the opposite corner there is the name 'Tom' and another telephone number. The interplay of conflicting meanings that these words represent is further emphasized at the left edge of the canvas, where the initial phrase 'Gays Are Sick' (only a part of the 'S' is visible and the first letter of 'Gays' is absent in order to indicate the continuation of the wall and the sentiments expressed on it beyond the range of the painting itself) has been altered to 'Breeders Are Sick.'

As Richard Rhodes has observed, Fabo's 'self-portraits are never so much portraits of an inner self as they are portraits of a man who is aware that because he is gay, he is forced to live out a kind of public stereotype of himself.'[6] But as the wall of graffiti in the painting indicates, while stereotyping occurs as a result of one's marginalized position in a heterosexist society, it is not necessarily the exclusive act of the dominant members of society. The painting is an analysis of the power of iconography, here represented in its least complex form, to shape the perceptions not only of those who adopt the majority stance but also of those who are marginalized by such a stance. The bifurcated self-portrait in Fabo's painting indicates the artist's unwillingness to participate in the stereotyping process while it underlines his commitment to engage in an analysis of the portrait's iconographic significance.

The analysis of iconography and the problems it poses to the act of representation occupies a central position in Fabo's practice as an artist. This is perhaps most powerfully seen in those works that deal with the problematic nature of AIDS representations. The works that I shall discuss were presented at the third 'Body & Society' exhibition at the Embassy Cultural House (10 November to 8 December 1988; see pp 215–21 in this volume) in London, Ontario; the opening of the exhibition coincided with the conference 'Representing AIDS: Crisis and Criticism' at the University of Western Ontario. The works are in the form of books, and while I will cite their titles at this point I will also acknowledge that the visual nature of the 'text' in these works, even in such matters as the title, requires a certain unfortunate compromise in order to be included in a text such as this essay. I will begin with a discussion of some of the common features of the books, which bear the following provocative titles: *the dying slave/the desiring machine; Conduct Sheet, Mil. Bk. 43; The Body Under Duress: A Manual For Those Who Suffer The Syndrome*; and *a figure, a flame, a subject, a name: A Catalogue of Accusations & Counter-Actions.*

The choice of the form itself says a number of important things about the representation of AIDS. Perhaps the most important of these is the way in which the books stress the inability of representing the crisis by a single image. An individual painting (or even paintings in a series that can then be easily separated and distributed among various galleries) cannot confront the crisis as effectively as the indivisible multiplicity of images in each of these books. This stance seriously challenges the 'masterpiece' mentality; while this mentality has been the subject of attack in the visual arts for some time now, Fabo's work urges us to consider that the quest for a masterpiece is an untenable position given the current crisis. Since the desire for the masterpiece seems to inform the statements of St Martin's Press editor Michael Denneny, as cited by David Kaufman in 'AIDS: The Creative Response,'[7] and author Edmund White,[8] it would appear that the criticism inherent in Fabo's choice of form would apply equally well to other branches of the arts.

Besides calling into question the Romantic quest for the single transcendent all-expressive masterwork, the book form places the viewer in a different relationship to the work than that traditionally imposed by academic painting. If the conventional posture for viewing a painting is to stand back, almost reverentially, Fabo's work requires the viewer to approach, to touch, and to be involved in the process of representation by the act of turning the pages. Given the untouchable status of persons with AIDS (PWAs) in the phobic mind-set of the general public, Fabo's work physically denies the viewer the inexcusable posture of aesthetic detachment. In this regard, Fabo's position is not unlike that of Jamelie Hassan, one of the founders of the Embassy Cultural House. 'I want my work to be in accord with my own political beliefs,' Hassan has stated, 'but I don't identify with the didactic approach of a lot of political art because it doesn't really allow the viewer to come to his or her own understanding of the issues. For me, knowledge occurs when one unravels things for oneself and arrives at an understanding independently. In other words, there may be a starting point in some event or encounter which is then integrated into one's own sense of the world so that it becomes a felt experience.'[9] I am certain that, for both Hassan and Fabo, coming to that understanding and achieving that felt experience are prerequisites to the adoption of an activist position but not substitutes for it. By requiring the viewer to participate in the process of representation, Fabo initiates a process of understanding that, as the images unfold before the viewer, can only find its logical conclusion in an activist position.

Before turning specifically to the books, I would like to point out one other characteristic of the works that highlights some of the issues I have mentioned thus far. If the works are reminiscent of anything, it is of an artist's sketch-book, and throughout the books actual sketches torn out of sketch pads are pasted onto the pages in juxtaposition to more elaborate representations. In some cases, Fabo has been careful to preserve the ripped perforated edges that would normally be lost in the coil when the sheet is torn free from the pad. His care in these instances to preserve that which would in the normal course of events be lost without much concern speaks eloquently of the true nature of loss experienced by those of us who are, so far, survivors in the midst of the epidemic. We have been able to save scraps of paper but not loved ones.

Some of the sketches seem to have originated in a different context than the field of AIDS representation and draw our attention to the way in which AIDS has altered our perceptions of many previous contexts, at least for those of us who are gay, whether we assent or object to these imposed retrospective re-contextualizations of our own immediate histories. In addition to the use of sketches on a medium other than the actual pages of the books, those on the page (even the most elaborate representations) retain an element of the sketch. This undoubtedly contributes to the impression of the urgency of these representations as well as emphasizing the inadequacy of the 'masterpiece' impulse. A further reason for the choice of a form that is reminiscent of the artist's sketch-book might be that, just as a sketch-book is a place in which the artist works towards solving certain problems before executing the most finished work, these books are working through certain problems of iconographic representation in order to facilitate the artist's work. In the case of these books, however, the work that is being prepared for is activism itself, both for the artist and, I am certain he would hope, for his viewers as well.

Although I indicate the title of the first work that I wish to discuss in a linear fashion as *the dying slave / the desiring machine*, the words are superimposed on the endpaper of the front cover; 'the dying slave' printed in silver forms a background or undersurface for the words 'the desiring machine,' which are printed in black. The effect is that of a palimpsest, and as such it prepares us for the nature of this book, which the facing title page confirms. The book was (is still?) originally a textbook entitled *General Shop Work*. A pastel drawing based on Michelangelo's *Dying Slave*, the restraining bond now a blue T-shirt, is Fabo's addition to the original title page. This book, more than the others, relies upon a single iconographic image. By the time the viewer has finished moving through the book, the artist has been able to present an inventive series of iconoclastic distortions of the original image. The apparently obsessive repetition of the single image suggests that Fabo is searching over a long period of art history that stems from the original of the image in Michelangelo's statue up to a number of branches of modernism, searching for past examples that might be adequate to the current crisis of representation. In the last few pages of the book, after encountering the image as everything from a Rubenesque self-portrait (see plate 25, following p 88) to cubist distortion to a collage where the head of the figure is a cut-out of a magazine advertisement for a 'Ray-O-Vac Leak Proof Flashlight Battery' (an ironic allusion, no doubt, to the current fear of bodily fluids) to St Sebastian pierced by, in one drawing, drill-bits (plate 26) and, in another, tongs (plate 27) to mechanical figures composed of gears (plate 28), one feels, in spite of the undeniable power of the images, the failure of Western civilization's various conventions of representation to deal adequately with the present crisis. Those conventions finally appear to reveal their inadequacy in the last few pages, where the book moves towards portraiture.

I want to stress here that the failure of portraiture is not Fabo's but rather that of an iconographic tradition. But before I explore some of the problems with portraiture that Fabo exposes, I need to raise a few questions concerning the iconographic traditions that Fabo invokes. I will begin by citing from a familiar academic source: H.W. Janson's *History of Art*. The passages are from Janson's discussion of Michelangelo:

> As he conceived his statues to be bodies released from their marble prison, so the body was the earthly prison of the soul – noble, surely, but a prison nevertheless. This dualism of body and spirit endows his figures with their extraordinary *pathos*; outwardly calm, they seem stirred by an overwhelming psychic energy that has no release in physical action ...
>
> The 'slaves' are difficult to interpret: they seem to have first belonged to a series representing the arts, shackled by the death of their greatest patron; later, apparently, they came to signify the territories conquered by Julian II. Be that as it may, Michelangelo has conceived the two figures as a contrasting pair, the so-called *Dying Slave* yielding to his bonds, the *Rebellious Slave* struggling to free himself. Perhaps their allegorical meaning mattered less to him than their expressive content, so evocative of the neo-Platonic image of the body as the earthly prison of the soul.[10]

I cannot resist mentioning that what Janson refers to as 'expressive content' is also an allegory. While Janson draws our attention to the way in which the images have an existence independent of their function as potential memorials, his view, the 'party line' of so many general-survey courses in art history, is limited by his failure to consider that the allegorization of the body itself is a prison that effectively prevents the 'psychic energy' from expressing itself in 'physical action,' thus consigning the body to the realm of 'pathos.'

Although the figure of Michelangelo looms large in the gay pantheon, Fabo's invocation of the sculptor's work is not part of a naïve litany in the style of a Ned Weeks.[11] At one point in a series of transformations, the dying slave appears to metamorphose into the central figure of Picasso's *Demoiselles d'Avignon*; while in *Conduct Sheet*, another figure from the same painting appears as a self-portrait holding a sign that says 'ACT UP' (plate 29). Also in *Conduct Sheet*, Fabo engages in an often-amusing 'dialogue' with reproductions of drawings by Raphael. In *A Catalogue of Accusations & Counter-Actions*, the central figure from Gauguin's *D'où venons nous? Que sommes nous? Où allons nous?* recurs at intervals throughout the book, and at one point the St Sebastian pose is mocked by the substitution of suction-cupped toy arrows for the original weapons of his martyrdom (plate 30).[12] Since Gauguin and Picasso are 'notorious' heterosexuals, Fabo's intentions cannot be interpreted exclusively as allusions to gay history.

The use of Renaissance images in AIDS representations as opposed to medieval images of plague may, in part, stem from the conceptualization of AIDS as a venereal disease. As Sander Gilman has pointed out in his article 'AIDS and Syphilis: The Iconography of Disease': 'Icons of disease appear to have an existence independent of the reality of any given disease. This "free floating" iconography of disease attaches itself to various illnesses (real or imagined) in different societies and at different moments in history. Disease is thus restricted to a specific set of images, thereby forming a visual boundary, a limit to the idea (or fear) of disease.'[13] Examining the iconography of syphilis, Gilman indicates the extent of the use of this iconography in the depiction of PWAs. Fabo, himself, has encountered the media's use of this iconography in the form of an article in the Toronto *Sun* of 22 October 1988. The article, entitled 'AIDS in the Arts,' presents Fabo's lover, artist Tim Jocelyn, as an example of the 'exemplary suffering' that Gilman identifies as one of the iconographic images associated with males in the representation of syphilis that has now attached itself to AIDS representations. The Toronto *Sun* article is careful to isolate Jocelyn not only from the context in which he is presented but from the other individuals cited:

> It was, by any standard, Toronto's hottest party.
>
> The Queen St West's trendiest bands played back to back – Handsome Ned, then Micha Barnes then Alta Moda. The vanguard of Toronto's exciting new art scene danced and drank all night.
>
> On a balcony, to the side of the stage at Theatre Passe Muraille, the guest of honour, an exuberant but weakened Tim Jocelyn looked on, as the 400 guests partied.[14]

I will resist the temptation to perform the Watneyesque dissection that this piece of writing, with its echoes of Edgar Allan Poe, deserves but will note that five newspaper-style paragraphs separate the article's last reference to Jocelyn from its next citing of an individual. Andy Fabo is also referred to in the article that focuses primarily but not exclusively on the fund-raising abilities of the arts. While Fabo's activist stance is briefly noted by the reporter, there is no mention of his relationship to Jocelyn. Given the way in which the piece separates Jocelyn from the other people it presents, the mentioning of such a relationship would seriously undermine the iconography it employs.

When Fabo employs the iconography that has been attached to AIDS representations, he draws the viewer's attention to the powerful nature of its imagery and at the same time undermines its wholesale application by the media. The way in which Fabo accomplishes this is by conflating a number of apparently different iconographies. He is, in a sense, using the media's own practice of conflating images as a strategy of defiance against the media. Among the most powerful images in the book are those in which Fabo has transformed the dying slave into St Sebastian, an icon employed in, among other places, Derek Jarman's film *Sebastiane* in our immediate pre-AIDS history as an image of certain aspects of gay sexuality. Fabo expects his viewers to recognize the ease with which the iconography of the patron saint of 'plague victims,' a model of 'exemplary suffering,' can be grafted onto Michelangelo's image of Neoplatonic passivity, of the inability of the 'soul' to act as a result of its imprisonment in the 'body.' As the viewer recognizes the disparate sources of the composite image, there is also a recognition of their disturbing affinity that calls into question conventional models of representation. In addition, Fabo stresses his unwillingness to employ these iconographic images in the depiction of an individual in the (I at least hope) unthinking manner of the media.

First of all, with the references to a wide range of pictorial styles, Fabo draws our attention to the image not as a depiction of the progress of illness in the body of a particular individual but as an act of representation that has an existence independent of those on whom the iconography is projected. This visual self-reflexivity is also accomplished through the use of colour; in one instance Fabo indicates the body through a predominant use of green, while in another he uses orange. In each instance, Fabo invites the viewer to analyse the nature of the image rather than an individual person. When Fabo does turn towards portraiture it is after this long process of analysis, and I sense that for Fabo the failure of Western traditions of representation has contributed in some way to the progress of illness represented.

In creating the St Sebastian image, Fabo's drawing interacts with the printed text of the *General Shop Work* textbook. The figure is placed on the page in such a way that the tools represented in the textbook are seen to pierce the body in the manner of the arrows of St Sebastian. On a page in a chapter entitled 'Woodworking,' the text provides instructions for 'Boring': 'To do horizontal boring hold the head of the brace cupped in the left hand with the back of the hand against the stomach. To bore through without splintering the back of the wood, stop when the point of the screw shows through and complete the boring from the opposite side.'

In the textbook illustration of a man demonstrating the correct procedure, an acceptable representative of male sexuality as a right-handed skilled tradesman, the bore appears to rise out of the groin like a deadly phallus to pierce the body of the dying slave. By drawing the viewer's attention to the text, Fabo indicates one of the conceptualizations of gay men employed by, among others, the people who once used this textbook in order to learn their trade: the phallus can only cause suffering as it bores through the 'homosexual' body. It is an image in which, as Leo Bersani has phrased it in an article that Fabo quotes in *The Body Under Duress*, 'the rectum is a grave in which the masculine ideal (an ideal shared – differently – by men *and* women) of proud subjectivity is buried.'[15] As in his earlier painting *The Wall*, Fabo here demands an analysis of the iconographic conceptualizations of the 'homosexual' body, a body that is feared because 'male homosexuality advertises the risk of the sexual itself as the risk of self-dismissal, of *losing sight* of the self, and in so doing it proposes and dangerously represents *jouissance* as a mode of ascesis.'[16] Elsewhere in these books, Fabo presents the celebration of this aspect of gay sexuality as a 'Counter-Action' to the 'murderous' representation of our heterosexist culture.

I now want to turn to a figure that, as I mentioned earlier, occurs in both *the dying slave/the desiring machine* and *Conduct Sheet*. The figure from Picasso's *Demoiselles d'Avignon*, which Fabo presents as male, draws the viewer's attention to another aspect of the iconography of AIDS that Gilman has examined in his essay; Fabo's use of the figure connects Gilman's insights with those of Bersani. Gilman shows us that, in AIDS representations, 'already feminized in the traditional view of his sexuality, the gay man can now also represent the conflation of the images of the male sufferer and the female source of suffering traditionally associated with syphilis,'[17] while he also draws our attention to the nineteenth century's perception of the African origin of syphilis (as with AIDS in North America).[18] Both Gilman and Bersani (in addition to Simon Watney, whom Bersani cities) have noted the similarities between 'the public discourse about homosexuals since the AIDS crisis began' and 'the representation of female prostitutes in the nineteenth century.'[19] The demoiselles of Picasso's 1906–7 painting, originally intended as a 'temptation scene in a brothel,'[20] are prostitutes; and one of the features of the work invariably cited by art historians is the influence of African tribal masks in the representation of two of the prostitutes' faces. Another feature of the painting, of course, is its importance in the development of cubism.

Fabo's iconoclastic leap from the Neoplatonic image of Michelangelo's *Dying Slave* to the Cézanne-influenced 'progenitor' of cubism is perhaps not as arbitrary as it might first appear when we consider the following assessment of Cézanne and of cubism in Gleizes and Metzinger's 'Du Cubisme':

> He has plumbed reality with a resolute eye, and if he himself has not attained those regions in which the profounder realism is insensibly transformed into a luminous spiritualism, at least he has left, for those who desire steadily to attain it, a simple and wonderful method ...
>
> ... He prophesies that the study of primordial volume will open unknown horizons to us. His work, a homogeneous mass, shifts under the glance, contracts, expands, fades or illuminates itself, irrefragably proving that painting is not – or is no longer – the art of imitating an object by means of lines and colours, but the art of giving our instincts a plastic consciousness.
>
> To understand Cézanne is to foresee Cubism. Henceforth are we justified in saying that between this school and the previous manifestations there is only a difference of intensity, and that in order to assure ourselves of the fact we need only attentively regard the methods of this realism, which, departing from the superficial reality of Courbet, plunges, with Cézanne, into the profoundest reality, growing luminous as it forces the unknowable to retreat.[21]

I do not wish to suggest a simplistic continuity between the Neoplatonic representations of the soul imprisoned in the body and this vision of the 'luminous spiritualism' of 'our instincts' (no doubt heterosexual and male) liberated from the prison of 'superficial reality' by the 'masculine ideal of proud subjectivity.' Readers of Foucault will undoubtedly discern aspects of the modern *episteme* that Foucault explores in *The Order of Things* and *The Archaeology of Knowledge* in Gleizes and Metzinger's account of 'the great detour, the great quest, beyond representation for the very being of representation.'[22] What these images from Michelangelo and Picasso share, in their original contexts at least, is an implied dualism of inner versus outer, 'soul' versus 'body,' a dualism that, as I have indicated in my discussion of *The Wall*, Fabo has consistently questioned.

Acknowledging that Picasso's debts to Cézanne and to African art in the *Demoiselles* and the painting's role as a progenitor of later cubism 'are all overstressed,'[23] we might perceive a connection between the modernist movement of cubism and modern medical practice in light of the prevailing nineteenth-century conceptualizations of the prostitute. In a paper entitled 'Jack the Ripper: Race and Gender in Victorian London,' Sander Gilman cites a police autopsy report of a prostitute who had drowned in the Seine. According to Gilman, the figure of the prostitute was essential to the Victorian notion of 'woman' in so far as this figure was perceived as hiding the secrets of contamination (syphilis) as well as the 'true' nature of 'womanhood' within her body. The only way to discover the secret hidden within the prostitute was by opening her body either with a knife (the coroner's scalpel or the Ripper's blade) or with a penis. In the latter case, the hidden corruption was 'raised' to the surface and revealed by the visual signs on the surface of the penis.[24]

Compare this revelation with Foucault's account of the shift that occurred in medical perception at the beginning of the nineteenth century:

> The medical gaze must therefore travel along a path that had not so far been opened to it: vertically from the symptomatic surface to the tissual surface; in depth, plunging from the manifest to the hidden; and in both directions, as it must continuously travel if one wishes to define, from one end to the other, the network of essential necessities. The medical gaze, which ... was directed upon a two-dimensional area of tissues and symptoms must, in order to reconcile them, itself move along a third dimension. In this way, the anatomo-clinical range will be defined.[25]

If Foucault's description of the medical gaze is not unlike Gleizes and Metzinger's description of cubism, which views painting as drawing the hidden depth of reality up to the surface of representation, Guillaume Apollinaire makes the comparison explicit: 'A man like Picasso studies an object as a surgeon dissects a cadaver.'[26] In *Demoiselles d'Avignon*, Picasso, the surgeon, dissects five prostitutes and, discovering the secret hidden in their depths, draws it up to the surface of the canvas in the form of African tribal masks, associating the prostitute with the supposed origin of the disease.

It is not surprising, then, that Andy Fabo, 'legally' defined by the provincial court of Ontario as a 'keeper of a common bawdy house' after the police raid on The Barracks,[27] chooses the image of Picasso's prostitute for a defiant act of self-representation. The stylized self-portrait (only the goatee and the length of hair distinguishes the face from the original demoiselle) in the form of the figure second from the left in Picasso's painting is drawn in black and gold on a reproduction of Raphael's 'Anatomical study for the Virgin supported by the holy women.' In Raphael's drawing there are three female heads and the figure of the virgin holding a skeleton pietà-style. The four females of the Raphael drawing, together with the Fabo 'self-portrait,' remind us of the number of prostitutes in the Picasso. Fabo has also altered the image by extending the raised arm of the figure into a clenched fist, possibly following the example of the raised but open hand of the figure to the left in the painting. The torso of Fabo's drawing exaggerates the triangular nature of the original, presenting it as male rather than female. The hand that in Picasso's painting holds drapery in Fabo's drawing holds a sign that reads 'ACT UP!' Pasted above the head of Fabo's drawing is a black-and-white photograph of a piece of electrical wiring, a sign for the empowerment of activism. The thick black lines of the drawing contribute to the forcefulness of this 'portrait' of an AIDS activist who defiantly assumes the marginalized image of the prostitute (who is also, ironically, a central icon of modernism) and simultaneously criticizes conventional male assumptions concerning both women and gay men by superimposing the figure over the image of the passive suffering of the Virgin with her dead son in her arms.

The activist demoiselle is reinforced by a sequence of images that it initiates in a section of *Conduct Sheet*. The sections that precede it have such titles as 'Whose conduct and Whose controll? [sic],' 'dominion over corpus,' and 'conduct: A duct to another constraint'; the section whose first image is the demoiselle is labelled 'acting up/getting out of line.' On the page immediately following the Picasso image there is a simple drawing in black and gold on construction paper of a spearhead. The triangular shape, the point directed towards the top of the page like the pink triangle in the 'Silence = Death' poster is the reverse image of the torso that precedes it. The base of the spearhead suggests vertebrae. This is followed by a return to the image of the demoiselle; there is a drawing of the back of a head with close-cropped hair, neck, and a suggestion of the shoulders and spine on the construction paper onto which Fabo has pasted another drawing on gravure of the earlier image of his activist self.

Another drawing on gravure is found on the following page. Fabo's text at the bottom of the page reads 'philia, the archaic medium of friendship, is the nature of our dissent ...' (plate 31). On the upper portion of the plate that forms the surface on which Fabo has painted are architectural drawings of bridges labelled 'Blackfriars' and 'Westminster.' The painting superimposed upon this portion of the plate is of two same-sex couples; the two women facing each other on the right are holding hands while the two men on the left, one of whom is black, are about to embrace. The 'ground' on which these two couples stand is a giant eye painted over the plate's view of tall ships in harbour seen through a space between buildings. In the centre of the iris there is the outline of a maple leaf, an image Fabo takes from the endpapers of the book, where the almost infinite repetition of the maple leaf indicates the book's former existence as a government publication. The superimposition of the Canadian national symbol indicates which particular government (among so many possible candidates) is engaged in an act of surveillance of the two couples represented. The bottom of the plate has been burnt so that the outline of scorch marks reaches up towards the pupil of the eye. The scorch marks draw the viewer's attention to the similarity between the shape of the red maple leaf on the Canadian flag and stylized representations of flames. This also clarifies an image that appears in *the dying slave / the desiring machine* where flames appear to be shooting out from the side of the figure. While the image of the dying slave might be seen as a representation of the fevers that accompany illness, the unavoidable similarity between the outline of fire and that of the Canadian national symbol draws our attention to the contribution that this particular government's inaction has made to the fuelling of the AIDS crisis.

The next page presents the viewer with Fabo's 'completion' of a drawing by Raphael which is, in turn, based on Michelangelo's unfinished *St Matthew* (plate 32). Fabo has given the bearded man on the Raphael reproduction an enviable companion whose young arm rests firmly on the old man's shoulders. Fabo's text on this page is 'philia' printed above the pair and 'homo' printed beneath them.

If this suggests the comic nature of some of Fabo's work in these books, the following page in *Conduct Sheet* illustrates what Fabo refers to in *A Catalogue of Accusations & Counter-Actions* as a 'wicked wit.' Once again the drawing is on a reproduction of a Raphael drawing. The way in which Fabo has highlighted with gold the lines of the study of drapery assumed to be a version of the Sibyl suggests the vagina beneath the folds of the cloth. This is especially ironic considering that Fabo has drawn a monumental phallus rising from the drapery that unveils (according to the text) 'the continuing phallocentricism of enlightened survivors.'

The next page in *Conduct Sheet* shifts the focus from art history to Fabo's own history as an artist. The viewer is presented with a page taken from *Mandate* magazine (May 1987) (plate 33); the photograph is a coloured version of a Fabo linocut that accompanied an article entitled 'Love, and Money.' To the page taken from *Mandate*, Fabo has added the text, 'even as we examine the culture of our dissentience [sic] ...' The image is that of an artist at his drafting board. Fabo presents a back view of the subject who is wearing only a jock strap and white athletic socks and whose face is in profile. The pouch of the jock strap, visible above the outline of the right thigh, indicates the level of arousal that the work has caused its creator; this is also indicated by the way in which the left arm disappears beyond the left thigh, the hand presumably resting (or perhaps not exactly 'resting') in the crotch. The cause of the artist's arousal can be seen on the drafting board, where a smaller male figure rises up beyond the confines of the board itself, up into the light that shines down on the table, in a possible invocation of the Pygmalion myth. The pencil in the artist's hand points in towards the crotch of the figure on the drafting board. The pencil, an image of the artist's penis, rises from the drawing he is engaged in like an erection of the proportions of those in Beardsley's engravings for the *Lysistrata*. The way it is held in the artist's hand suggests masturbation.

This picture, which Fabo presents in two different versions on two consecutive pages, denies the stance expressed in Apollinaire's account of Picasso. It dissolves the distance between 'the masculine ideal of proud subjectivity' and the object of representation. With the back of the figure on the drawing board turned towards the artist, the form their potential sexual coupling may take is obvious. It might initiate a process whereby the artist comes to the understanding that 'it is possible to think of the sexual as ... moving between a hyperbolic sense of self and a loss of all consciousness of the self.'[28] In any event, the image suggests that engagement, arousal, and activism can be celebrated aspects of the artist's practice.

The final image of this section of *Conduct Sheet* is one that I want to touch on briefly because of its relation to the sequence that follows, a sequence that has in many ways determined the direction I have chosen to follow in this paper. The image is that of a naked male behind bars. The buttocks are turned towards the viewer and the head is turned looking over the right shoulder with the right arm extended horizontally, the hand gripping the bars. This is followed by Fabo's text 'conduct/conduit,' which is itself followed by a page that cites Foucault's 'the soul is the prison of the body' printed over an abstract design. After a page presenting an ambiguous image of bars or serpents or IV tubes (depending on how one wishes to interpret them in relation to similar images throughout the books), Fabo returns to the figure behind bars. The transformation of the figure is startling; the head is absent while the torso has taken the shape of a lyre and the bars now merge into the figure's arms. The use of blue at the bottom of the drawing, which relies primarily on the use of black crayon against the manila background, contributes to the viewer's identification of the figure as Orpheus, the dismembered artist. Seventeen pages later, Fabo reformulates Foucault and presents us with the aphorism 'the soul is the noose of representation.'

Fabo presents the Foucault text in a way that distinguishes it from most of the other texts in the books. Most of the quotations are included with some sort of pictorial representation of the body that indicates an aspect of Fabo's 'dialogue' with the original text. Almost all the texts that appear isolated from any pictorial representation are Fabo's own formulations. (It is only in *Conduct Sheet* and *A Catalogue of Accusations & Counter-Actions* that texts appear without immediate pictorial references.) The geometric shapes that form the background of the Foucault text present the viewer with an analysis of the Raphael plate that Fabo has altered later on in the book and to which he has added his own paraphrase of Foucault ('the soul is the noose of representation'). The abstract design accompanying the Foucault text is similar to cosmological representations that suspend the earth between heaven and hell. The Raphael drawing that forms the background of Fabo's re-interpretation is the 'Compositional Study for the Coronation of St Nicholas of Tolentino.' Fabo has obscured the Virgin and St Augustine of the original and replaced them in *Conduct Sheet* (plate 34) with the coiled 'spiritualized' bodies that also occur in *The Body Under Duress* and *the dying slave*, where they emphasize the loss of physical presence resulting from death. (In *A Catalogue of Accusations & Counter-Actions*, Fabo explores the effects of physical loss on the artist's practice and suggests that in the face of such loss the artist must 'reconstruct the body by remembering the gesture.') Fabo has also removed the wings and tail of Satan on whom St Nicholas is standing, thus 'humanizing' the figure of the fallen angel; and God the Father no longer holds the crown of sainthood but instead holds the eye of surveillance.

One critical appraisal of the Raphael drawing should indicate the degree of care with which Fabo has chosen this plate to serve his own analytical purposes: 'The proliferation of compass work demonstrates the mathematical exactness that underlies the clarity of Raphael's arrangement. The intersection of mandorla and arch, for example, is a brilliant device for isolating God the Father within the overall harmony, since his figure is designed to make productive use of the architecture that he conceals ... The geometrical designs that Raphael has devised here are numberless.'[29] (I will mention only in passing that another 'visionary' artist, William Blake, was highly critical of excessive geometrical representation and singled out the compass as an instrument of oppression in his representation of the Ancient of Days and of Newton.) Students of Foucault may be excused for perceiving a variation of the argument of *Discipline and Punish* in this account of the isolation of the omniscient God the Father who conceals the architecture that contains him. By placing the eye of surveillance in the hands of God, Fabo draws a parallel between Raphael's God and the observer in Bentham's panopticon.

The text following the 'Coronation of St Nicholas' in Fabo's work draws our attention to the 'modern soul' while suggesting the effect this 'noose' will have on the act of representation: 'The law makers attempt to steer us away from the uncertainty of the body/Product:/ towards the ease of geometry.' Geometric representation, as in Raphael, posits a certainty of knowledge concerning the body; the ability of the artist to execute a representation of the body with such geometric assurance provides an analogy to the techniques of constraint that power is able to enforce on the body as a result of the supposed certainty of its knowledge. In the paragraph cited by Fabo, Foucault writes:

> Rather than seeing this soul as the reactivated remnants of an ideology, one would see it as the present correlative of certain technologies of power over the body. It would be wrong to say that the soul is an illusion, or ideological effect. On the contrary, it exists, it has a reality, it is produced permanently around, on and within the body by the functioning of power that is exercised on those punished – and, in a more general way, on those one supervises, trains, and corrects, over madmen, children at home and at school, the colonized, over those who are stuck at a machine and supervised for the rest of their lives ... This real, non-corporal soul is not a substance; it is the element in which

> are articulated the effects of a certain type of knowledge, and knowledge extends and reinforces the effects of this power.[30]

Conventional representation of the body is truly an act of execution. The 'transcendence' of art is supported by a certainty of knowledge that reinforces power; in its geometric precision, the 'masterpiece' inscribes the body with the constraints that arise out of the certainty of power/knowledge.

The 'spiritualized' bodies are at once aspects of the 'modern soul,' which either executes bodies in conventional representation or obliterates them with a 'profounder realism,' and are also the remembered bodies of those who have died. These latter bodies, usually perceived through the construct of the stereotyped 'homosexual body,' are essentially absent from representation. In *A Catalogue of Accusations & Counter-Actions*, the eye of surveillance is an overhead light shining down on two lovers in a bed. The scene evokes, among other things, a hospital operating room. The text on the following page emphasizes the determination to prevent the executing absence to continue: 'We described our memories, gave image to our loss. / We do not have amnesia. We will not be neutralized / by the seductions of our times.' The defiance of the lovers before the all-seeing, 'illuminating' eye of surveillance is linked to the defiant act of remembering. A few pages later, Fabo presents a list of 'Problems' that must be confronted if the artist is to continue his act of defiance against conventional representation:

> (1) to retell the tale of Sisyphus except the mind becomes the rock;
> (2) to describe the mind by describing the body;
> (3) to recall the body by describing the gesture;
> (4) to reinvent the body by remembering.

In contrast to the conventional interpretation of the myth of Sisyphus as an image of futility and despair, Fabo's invocation of the myth suggests the perpetual struggle of the artist against conventional and exclusionary forms of representation. The mind the artist attempts to represent in his 'descriptions' of the body will refuse to be locked in the geometric certainty of power/knowledge. Both the mind and the body are in motion, described by individual gestures and not by fixed and archetypal poses that codify the body in the manner of the dying slave. Also, in the act of reinventing the body by remembering, the artist delivers the body from the 'spiritualization' enforced upon it by the 'modern soul' and, erasing the mind/body dichotomy of Cartesian systems of (medical) thought, attempts to restore the body to its as yet uncelebrated 'unstable' corporality.

If the artist's practice can be compared to the act of Sisyphus eternally struggling with the rock, Fabo consistently invokes another image of the artist throughout the books. As I have already suggested, in the transformation of the imprisoned figure in *Conduct Sheet* to the headless figure whose torso has become a lyre, the figure of Orpheus is a recurrent motif in these books. The figure can be seen in the simple 'Small World' drawings that recur in a *Catalogue of Accusations & Counter-Actions*. The small ink drawings depict a globe with two figures embracing at one pole and a solitary figure grieving at the opposite pole. As the image recurs in *A Catalogue*, Fabo 'rotates' the globe so that the grieving lover and the embracing couple are never fixed. Love, grief, and the restoration of loss remain as perpetual possibilities.

The image of Orpheus is presented not only as an image of the artist but also of the artist's subject. This is undoubtedly due to the personal reasons that underlie the use of the motif. In his keynote address at the 'Representing AIDS' conference, Fabo mentioned the similarity that his lover Tim Jocelyn perceived between himself and the image of Odilon Redon's *Orpheus*. If the images of Orpheus as they occur in the books, particularly in *A Catalogue* (simultaneously the most personal and the most political of Fabo's books), are representations of Jocelyn as the dismembered artist whom Fabo remembers in these various acts of representation, they are also potentially images of Fabo himself. As the grieving artist, Fabo is engaged in a courageous attempt at the restoration of loss even as he is confronted with the possibility of his own death ('the final dislocation,' as he refers to it in *The Body Under Duress*). While this identification between artist and subject arises out of the personal relationship between two artists, the act of identification is precisely what has been missing, as Simon Watney has so eloquently pointed out, in the media's accounts of people with AIDS. But, unlike the 'remembering' of a lost lover, Fabo's self-remembering is an act of defiance. By insisting upon the need to imagine his own survival, he defies the prevalent definition of AIDS as an invariably fatal illness.

Fabo's Orpheus, dismembered by the Bacchic frenzy of the homophobic media, is an artist of the technological society (plate 35). In both *A Catalogue of Accusations & Counter-Actions* and *The Body*

Under Duress, the head of Orpheus lies in a satellite dish, the ubiquitous lyre of modern mass culture. While the Ciconian women dismembered the ancient Orpheus because he scorned them and 'preferred to centre his affections on boys of tender years,'[31] Fabo's modern Orpheus is dismembered by a media industry that has, since the beginning of its coverage of the AIDS crisis, added its scrutiny to the traditional scrutiny that gay sexuality has suffered from the privileged gaze of the medico-criminological establishment. The 'message' of Fabo's Orpheus, 'Information = Survival,' most clearly represented in *The Body Under Duress*, is at odds with the mass-media messages that invoke the fear of the 'heterosexual spread' of AIDS (ignoring the fact that heterosexuals have been dying as a result of AIDS since the beginning of the epidemic) and preach 'Don't Die of Ignorance' to the presumably straight 'general' public.

Fabo's use of the image of the satellite dish also attacks what Cindy Patton refers to as the predominant erotophobia of contemporary society,[32] since the 'Information' necessary for survival involves a re-envisioning of the erotic possibilities as yet only faintly glimpsed in safer-sex education (plate 36). It is an irony that also serves as an indictment of the media in Fabo's presentation of the satellite dish that the radical gay artist is effectively denied access to mass culture. Rather than allow such access, the media dismember the artist and, by extension, all gay people through their active misinformation, hysteria, and silence. As the haven of conventional representations, the media are an efficient executioner.

In *The Body Under Duress*, Fabo begins his 'Manual for Those Who Suffer the Syndrome' by confronting some of the most widely disseminated images of AIDS, images that are reported by the media but never shown, never accorded the privilege of sight. In 'Taking the bad days with the good ...' and 'Confronting the fears ... (imagining your so-called worst-case-scenario)' Fabo presents images that, owing to the dictates of 'good taste,' are excluded from visual representations of AIDS, even though they are among the most commonly invoked 'symptoms' in written accounts of the syndrome. These 'tabooed' images of a person vomiting and a person with diarrhea are preceded by another image also censored in the name of 'good taste,' a penis sheathed in a condom, entitled 'Eroticising latex.' The juxtaposition of a method of preventing HIV infection with images of illness that may result from that infection, following the first page of the book with its message of 'Information = Survival' and its image of the satellite dish, serves not only as instruction for those who suffer the syndrome but as a reminder of the schizophrenic nature of media censorship.

An image that is 'acceptable' for visual representation follows the 'tabooed' images. 'Or choosing drug protocols oneself' shows an emaciated figure lying on a bed with an intravenous drip attached to his arm. Fabo questions this iconography of the 'thin' PWA by making the arm that is receiving the solution the same size as the torso of the figure. The distorted proportions of the figure suggest the possibility of PWA empowerment through such acts as choosing one's own drug protocols as well as by wresting control of the selective images of the media. The voice and vision of the PWA, so skilfully edited out of most media and medical accounts of AIDS, is essential to our understanding of the epidemic if we are to escape the enforced dualities that separate the body of the patient from the illness that affects that body. Denying PWAs the authority to represent themselves will undoubtedly be as devastating to our society as the epidemic itself.

Towards the end of *the dying slave,* Fabo moves hesitantly towards portraiture. The facial features of most of the figures in the book are schematic in nature and only rarely, as in the case of the Rubenesque self-portrait, do they express individual characteristics. The final series of images in the book present us with an emaciated but distinctly individualized dying slave whose features resemble those of the Orpheus drawing in *A Catalogue of Accusations & Counter-Actions*; however, Fabo's consistent questioning of conventional representation is evident even in these 'portraits.' On a page torn from the textbook and pasted onto another page of the text, Fabo has edged the torn page with gold paper as if to indicate that conventional drawing techniques are incapable of expressing the worth of the person represented. The gold paper also suggests the gold leaf of a medieval illuminated manuscript, and yet the coloured paper indicates a haste and a transience that are the antithesis of medieval (and Renaissance) representations.

The original text of the page from the motor-mechanics section of the *General Shop Work* textbook begins with instructions for 'Assembling a Leaf Spring' and draws our attention to the recurring motif of leaves as symbols of regeneration or government oppression. At the beginning of the second column and visible through the raised arms of the dying slave is a series of definitions of 'Engine Terms': 'The stroke is the movement from one dead centre to the other. The length of the stroke is expressed in inches. The throw is the distance, measured in inches, from the centre of the crank pin to the centre of the crank shaft. The stroke of the engine must always be twice the throw.' The similarity between the technical language of motor mechanics and colloquial expressions of sexuality underlines an aspect of the image of the dying slave that is certainly present even in Michelangelo's original as well as in Fabo's various explorations of the image. In this drawing towards the end of the book, the loved one, even in the process of dying, retains his sexual attractiveness.

It does not surprise the viewer, therefore, when on the penultimate page of the book, Fabo breaks away from the sequence of the dying slave and presents an earlier drawing of the person represented in these final images (plate 37). In this drawing the figure, no longer thin, stands with both arms raised above his head in a classic pose of seduction. The pose is also that of the demoiselle-type that occurs earlier in the book. Since Fabo has represented himself in both the pose of the dying slave and the demoiselle, these final portraits are not only representations of the model but potential portraits of Fabo himself. The degree of identification between artist and model and the courage that such an identification requires preclude the use of conventional representation, which depends upon the supposed detachment of the artist.

In Fabo's work, the media's equation of 'Gays = AIDS = Death' is rejected as not only oppressive but as a negation of the experience of gay men who have to a great extent imaginatively re-conceived a world in which AIDS must be taken into account, a world that the media's mythical 'general' population appears to be unwilling to contemplate. As Fabo presents it, the world in which AIDS exists is a world of immense contradictions, not the least of which is the rupture that the syndrome has caused in the sense of self in those of us who remember a distinct before and after. But Fabo refuses to simplify these contradictions with paradoxical dualities. It is in his resistance to these dualities that his 'dialogue' with the art of the Italian Renaissance can be viewed. Like Michelangelo and Raphael, Fabo views the body with a degree of confidence and hope, for his work is nothing if not an expression of an angry and defiant optimism in the midst of the plague. But at the same time, he 'exploits' and 'defaces' their images, stripping them of their Neoplatonic certainties that ultimately render the body as the site of 'pathos.' And if Fabo 'dreams' of a new Renaissance, it is a Renaissance of the transient and the uncertain, a Renaissance that has little concern for the 'masterpiece' because it is too busy celebrating the unknowable body.

In the ninth year (officially) of the epidemic, confronted with a science that raises the average rate of progression from initial infection to recognizable symptoms annually (usually coinciding with the

International AIDS conference), all gay men who were sexually active prior to 1981 face a world that is inexplicable and inhabit bodies that have become unknowable when we compare them to the bodies we inhabited a decade ago. If we are now seropositive, we were probably infected before there was any significant warning of the existence of AIDS. If we are not seropositive, then, as friends are dying, the world makes no sense at all for there is no reason for the absence of the virus in our blood. In this, we are most at odds with the media and medical establishments who express in their privileged discourses the supposed 'logic' of disease. Although I have not been able to articulate accurately the sense of inhabiting a world of irreconcilable contradictions that overwhelms me when I look through Fabo's books, I believe more strongly now than when I first set eyes on them that it is only through the activist response he represents so powerfully that we will be able to live in this world. It is only through our continued activism that our friends and our loved ones with whom we cannot help but identify may continue to live with us as we face this world of contradictions together, for activism is also our angry celebration of our uncertain bodies.

NOTES

1 Michel Foucault 'Nietzsche, Genealogy, History' in *Language, Counter-Memory, Practice* ed Donald F. Bouchard (Ithaca, NY: Cornell University Press 1977) 153
2 Gerald Hannon 'Raids, Rage, and Bawdyhouses' in *Flaunting It!* ed Ed Jackson and Stan Persky (Toronto: Pink Triangle Press 1982) 286
3 Richard Rhodes 'Catalogue Essay' *ChromoZone / Chromatique* (Regina, Sask.: Norman Mackenzie Art Gallery 1983) 5
4 Andy Fabo, letter to James Miller, 1988
5 Jan Zita Grover 'Introduction' *AIDS: The Artists' Response* (Columbus, OH: Hoyt L. Sherman Gallery 1989) 3
6 Richard Rhodes 'Catalogue Essay' 11. A reproduction of Fabo's *The Wall* can also be found in the exhibition catalogue.
7 David Kaufman 'AIDS: The Creative Response' *Horizon* 30:9 (Nov 1987) 16
8 Edmund White 'Esthetics and Loss' *Artforum* 25:5 (Jan 1987) 68–71
9 Jamelie Hassan, interview in *Songs of Experience* ed Jessica Bradley and Diana Nemiroff (Ottawa: National Gallery of Canada 1986) 104
10 Janson *History of Art* 425–6
11 Larry Kramer *The Normal Heart* (New York: New American Library 1985)

12 The Gauguin painting was the subject of a witty pastiche in Fabo's collaboration with Jim Anderson and Oliver Girling in the 1982 exhibition, 'Collaborations: Mythologies; Aesthetics in the Modern World' (Mercer Union, Toronto).

13 Sander Gilman 'AIDS and Syphilis: The Iconography of Disease' in *AIDS: Cultural Analysis / Cultural Activism* ed Douglas Crimp (Cambridge: MIT Press 1988) 88

14 David Graham 'AIDS in the Arts' Toronto *Sunday Sun* 22 Oct 1988, 35

15 Leo Bersani 'Is the Rectum a Grave?' in Crimp, *AIDS: Cultural Analysis* 222

16 Ibid

17 Gilman 'AIDS and Syphilis' 99

18 Ibid 100

19 Bersani 'Is the Rectum a Grave?' 211

20 Janson *History of Art* 653

21 Albert Gleizes and Jean Metzinger 'Du Cubisme' in *Theories of Modern Art* ed Herschel B. Chipp (Berkeley: University of California Press 1968) 209

22 Michel Foucault *The Order of Things* (New York: Random House 1973) 240

23 Timothy Hilton *Picasso* (London: Thames and Hudson 1975) 79

24 Sander Gilman 'Jack the Ripper: Race and Gender in Victorian London' University of Western Ontario, 23 March 1989

25 Michel Foucault *The Birth of the Clinic* (New York: Random House 1975) 135–6

26 Guillaume Apollinaire 'The Cubist Painters' in Chipp *Theories of Modern Art* 222

27 Hannon 'Raids, Rage, and Bawdyhouses' 286

28 Bersani 'Is the Rectum a Grave?' 218

29 Paul Joannides *The Drawings of Raphael* (Berkeley: University of California Press 1983) 38

30 Foucault *Discipline and Punish* 29

31 Ovid *The Metamorphosis* trans Mary M. Innes (Harmondsworth: Penguin Books 1955) 227

32 Cindy Patton *Sex and Germs* (Boston: South End Press 1985). Throughout this work Patton explores the combined impact of erotophobia and germophobia on media representations of AIDS.

25

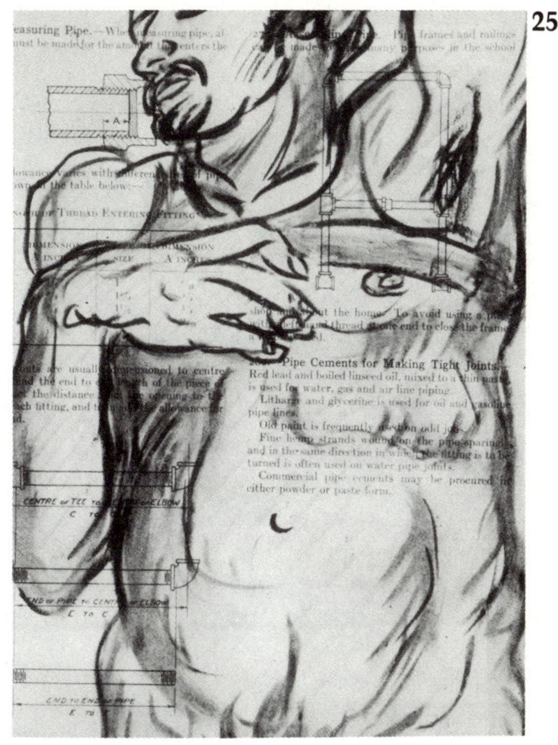

25 Andy Fabo,
Rubenesque self-portrait
from *dying slave / desiring machine* (bookwork 1988)

26

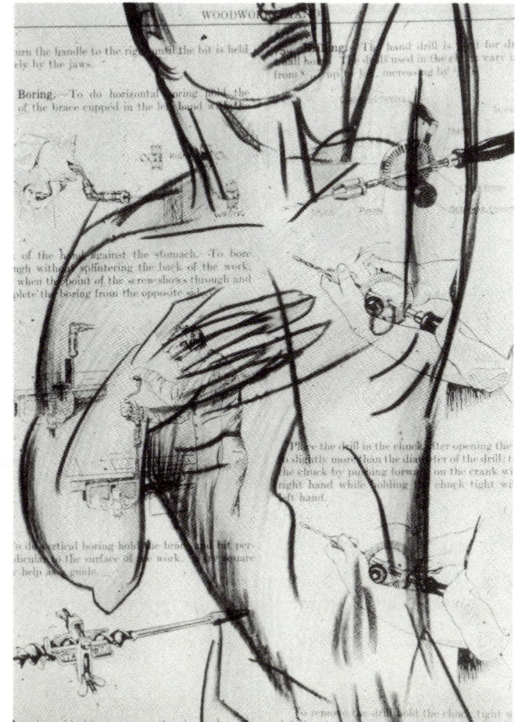

26
Fabo, dying slave as
St Sebastian with drills on
woodworking text, *dying slave / desiring machine*

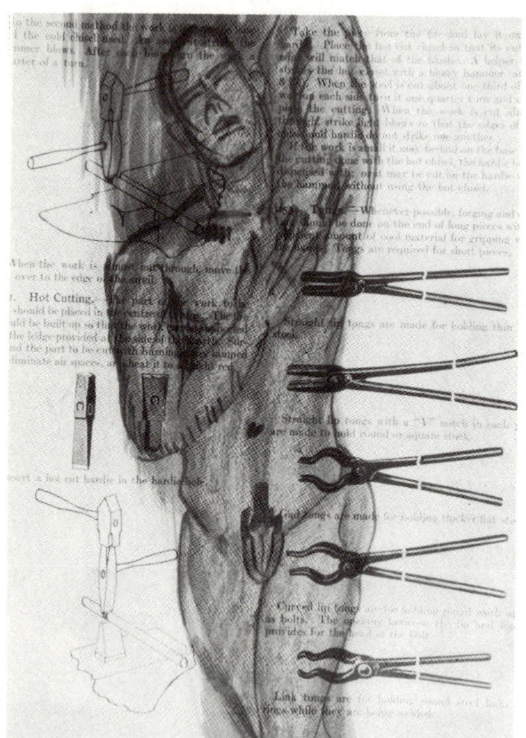

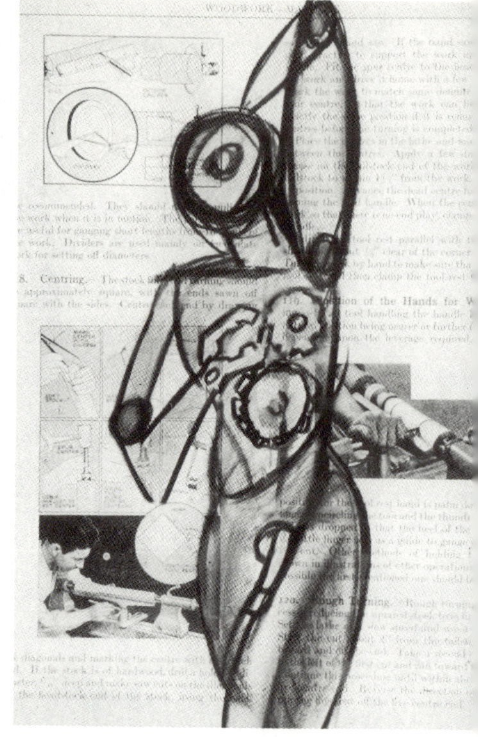

27 28

27 Fabo, dying slave as St Sebastian with tongs, *dying slave / desiring machine*

28 Fabo, dying slave as St Sebastian with gears, *dying slave / desiring machine*

29 Fabo, Demoiselle with ACT UP sign, on an anatomical study by Raphael, *Conduct Sheet* (bookwork 1988)

30 Fabo, Gauguin figure as St Sebastian with suction-cup arrows, *A Catalogue of Accusations and Counter-Actions* (bookwork 1988)

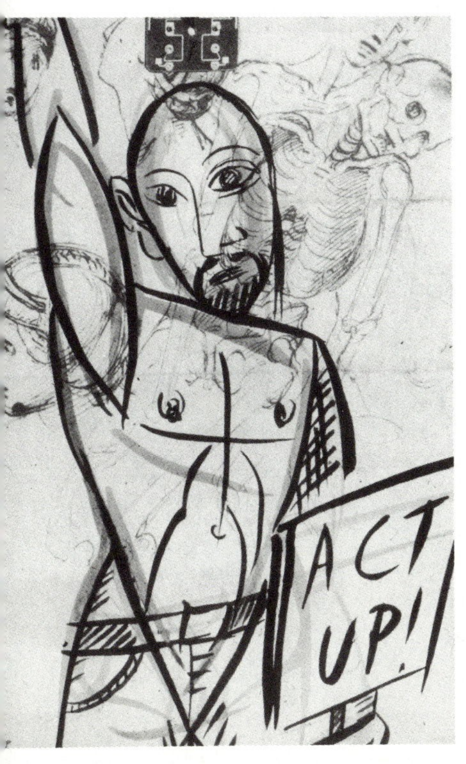
ACT
UP!

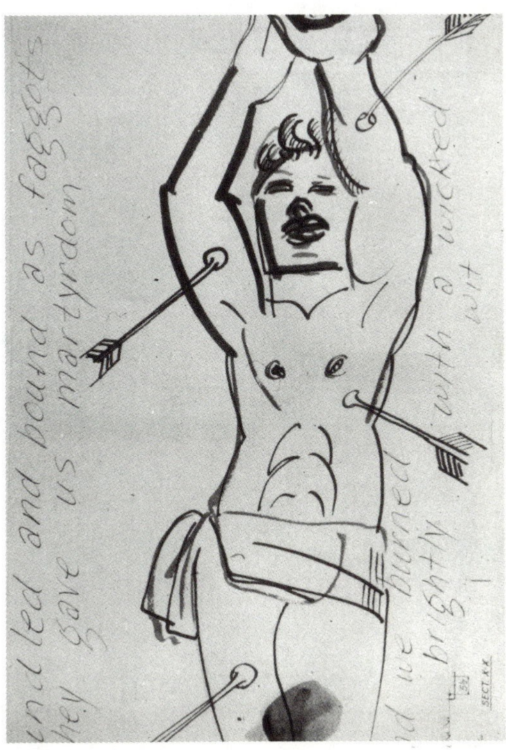
nd led and bound as faggots
hey gave us martyrdom
d we burned
brightly with a wicked
wit

29 30

31

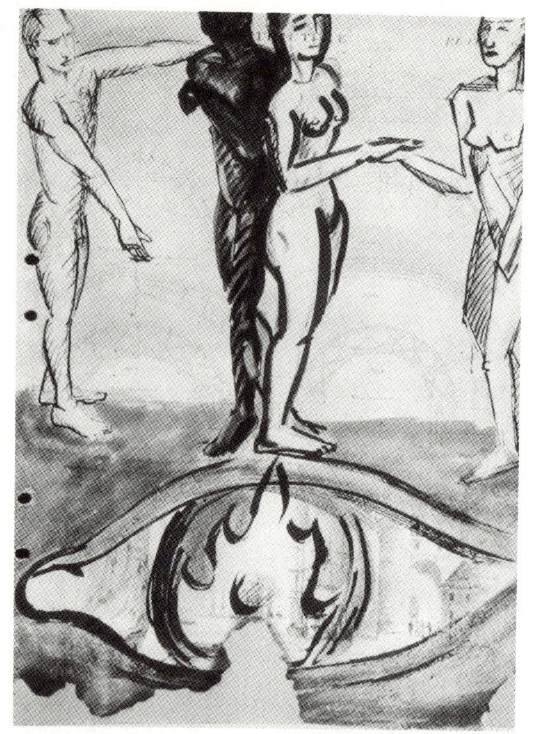

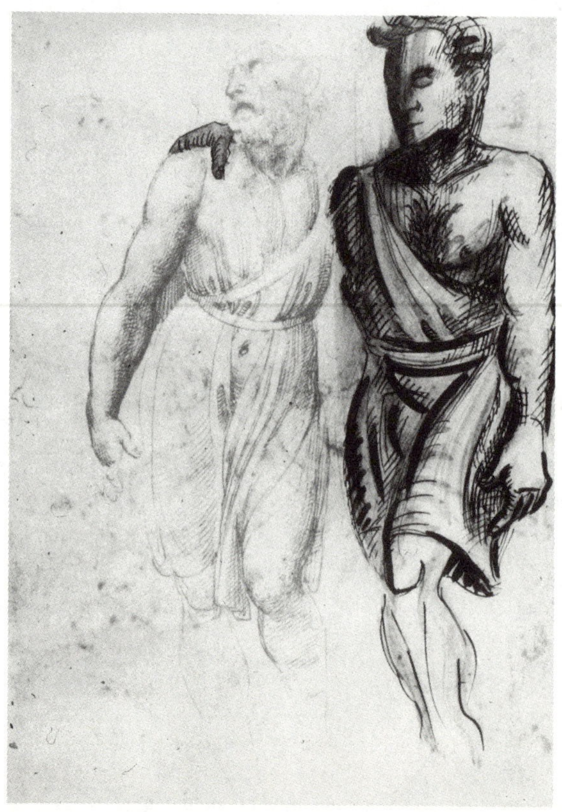

32

31 Fabo, Philia represented by same-sex couples triumphantly embracing over eye of state surveillance, *Conduct Sheet*

32 Fabo, Philia Homo or 'same-sex love,' revision of a Raphael drawing after Michelangelo, *Conduct Sheet*

33 Fabo, woodcut of artist at his drawing board, reproduced in *Mandate* (May 1987)

34 Fabo, coiled spirit-bodies flanking 'noose of representation,' *Conduct Sheet*

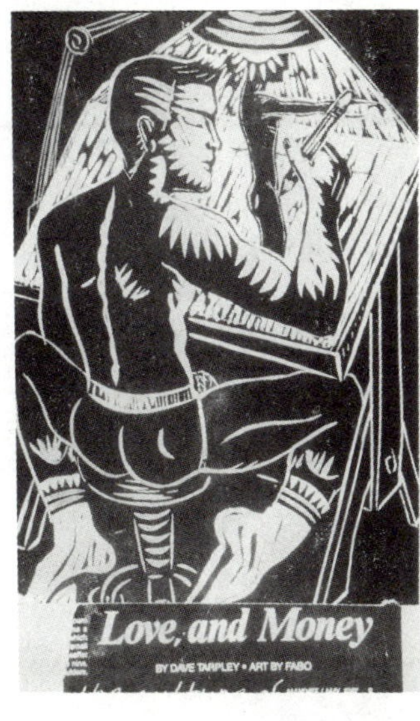

33

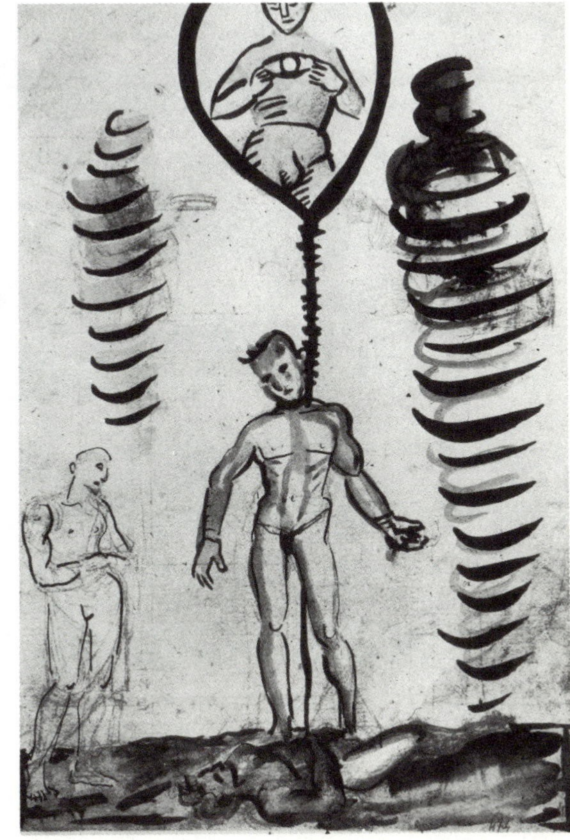

34

35

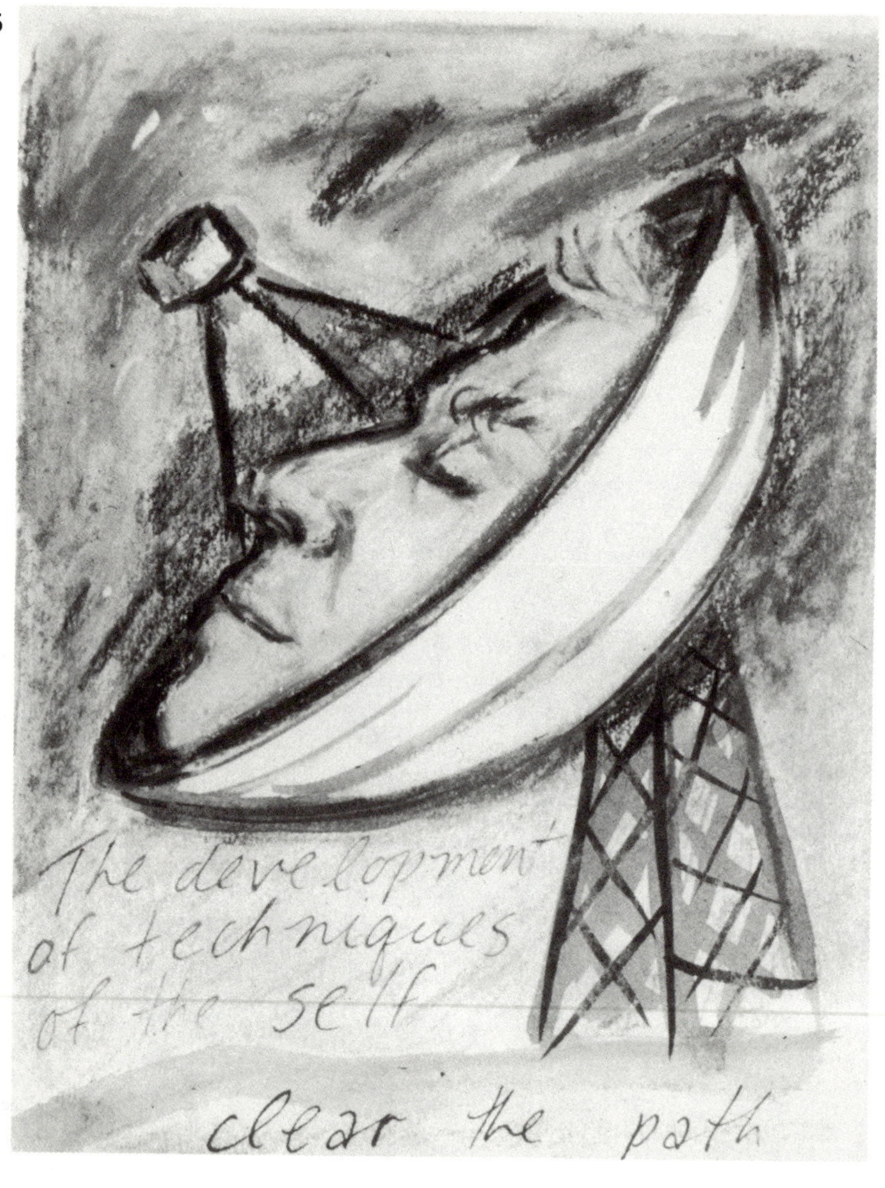
The development
of techniques
of the self
clear the path

35 Fabo, head of Orpheus on satellite dish, *The Body Under Duress: A Manual for Those Who Suffer the Syndrome* (bookwork 1988)

36 Fabo, fluid exchanges as communication flow between satellite-dish phalluses, *The Body Under Duress*

36

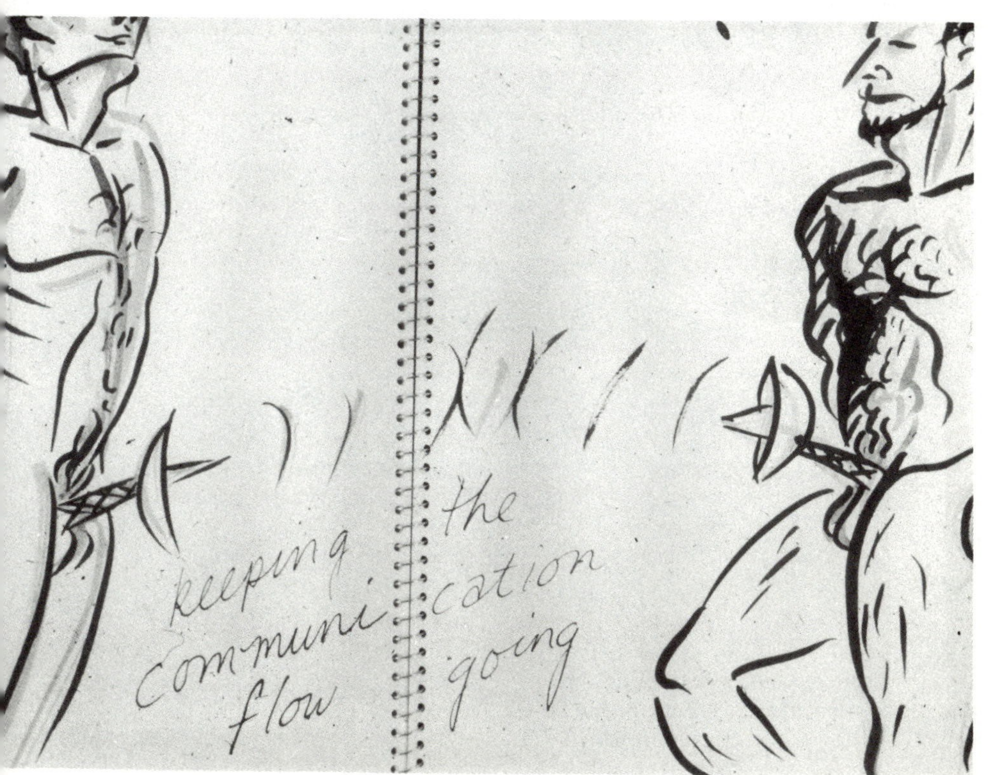

37

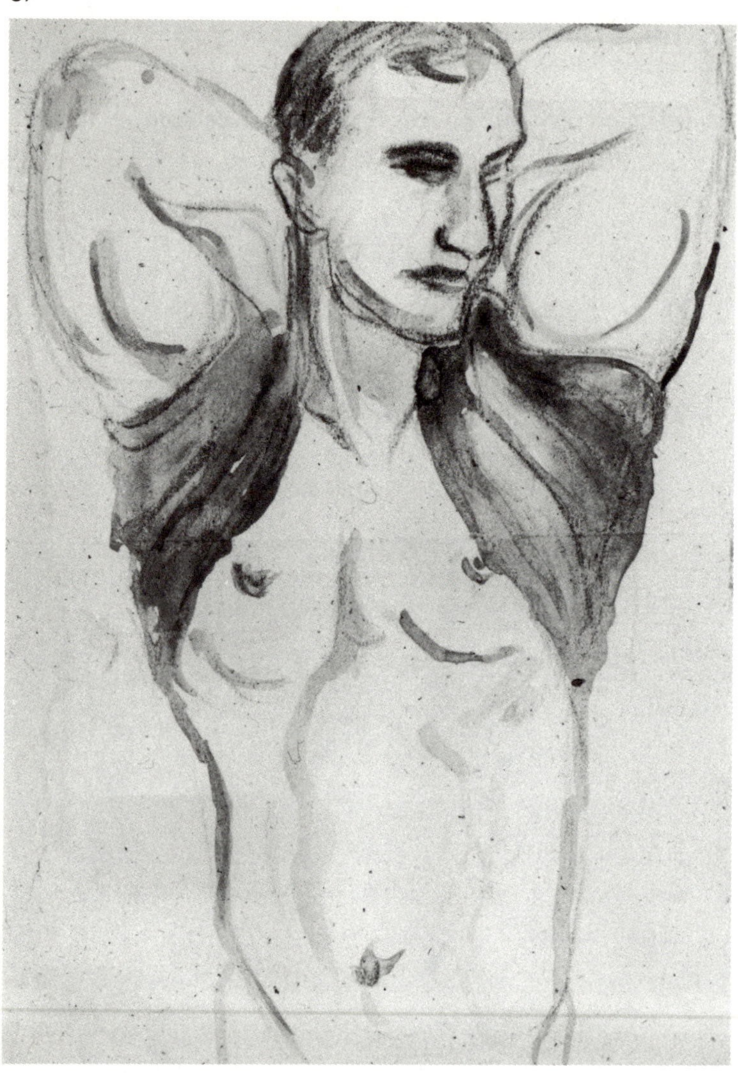

37 Fabo, classic pose of seduction representing erotic life of gay PWA anticipating return to health, *dying slave / desiring machine*

38 Photo-diptych of Sunnye Sherman and unidentified black soldier in *Life* (July 1985)

38

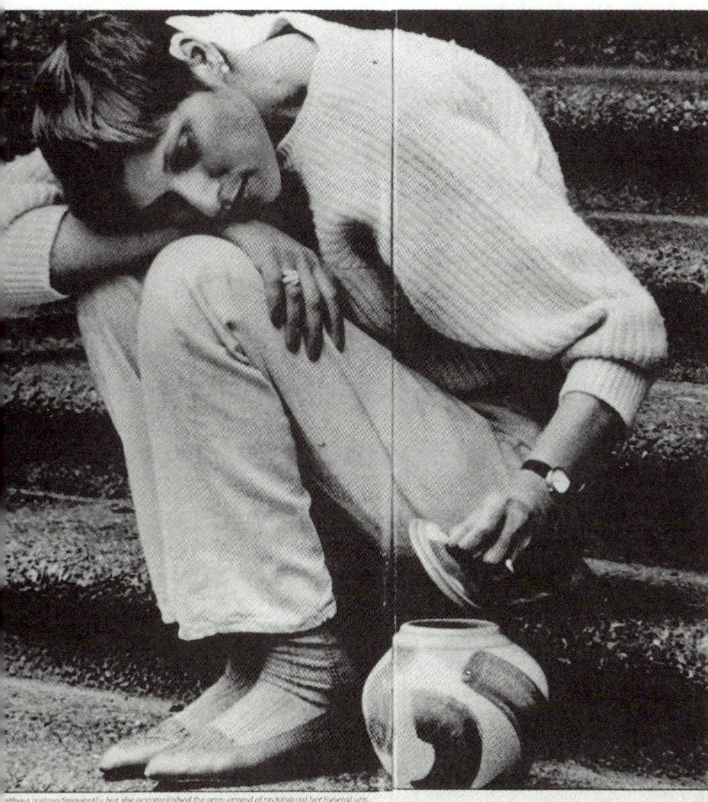

ithout resting frequently, but she accomplished the grim errand of picking out her funeral urn.

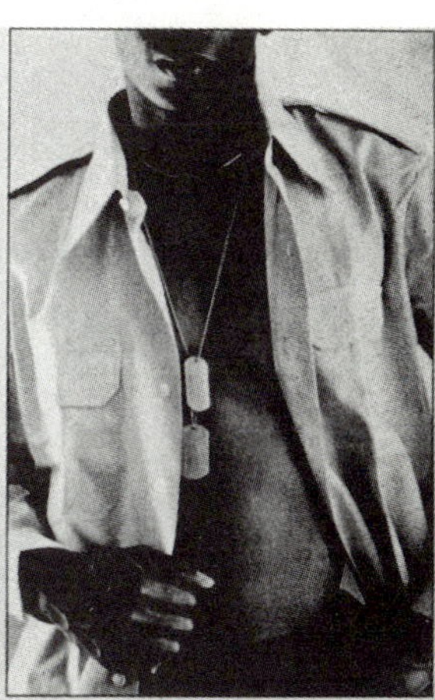

This infected soldier has had to put away his uniform for good.

In adults AIDS is slow to develop. It is not contagious through casual contact, like the flu, but the virus can take hold if it manages to get into the bloodstream by needle or sexual intercourse. It may be as long as five years before full symptoms appear. As a heterosexual venereal disease, AIDS seems to pass more readily from men to women than from infected women back to men. Sonya Sherman, a 34-year-old legal secretary from Washington, D.C. (*left*), had a year-long relationship with a man she says was bisexual. In 1983, long after they broke up, she got a rash that wouldn't go away. Her immune system gradually weakened; AIDS was diagnosed that fall. Sonya has so far survived four major infections, including two bouts of pneumonia, which for an AIDS patient is something of a record. Doctors have tried a desperate battery of drugs, one of which left her with severe hearing loss. Two members of her support group of AIDS patients died this spring. Serenely, Sonya has written a will and planned her funeral, even selecting her own burial urn. "My mother hopes that one day we'll use it for flowers," she says, "but I have to be more realistic."

Although a cure or vaccine is not yet in sight, since the epidemic began four years ago researchers have isolated the virus and devised a test for it in the blood. The test is already screening the nation's donor supply to prevent cases like Patrick Burk's. But it has also allowed ominous projections: From one to three million Americans may be harboring—and passing on—the virus without having symptoms. Predominant in this group are those with active sex lives, such as young men in the military. One study done by the Army has found that a third of 41 AIDS cases can be traced to heterosexual contact. For instance, the soldier above—not gay, not a drug abuser—admits to scores of sexual partners during his 12-year military career. Now 29 and twice hospitalized, the man was recently forced to leave the service. He is about to start a civilian job. He has not told anybody about his potentially terminal illness.

39

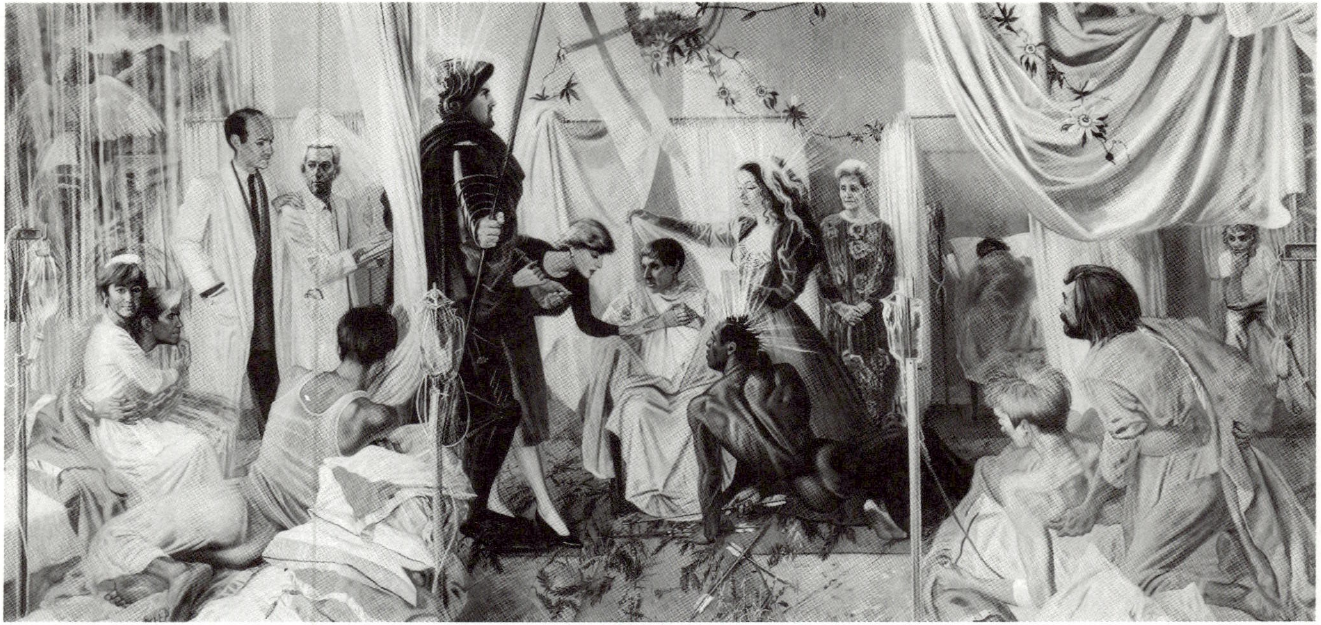

39 André Durand, *Votive Offering* (oil on canvas, 72″ × 144″) 1987

Our Lady of AIDS: The Occult Design of André Durand's *Votive Offering*

JAMES MILLER

When I first set eyes on the photograph of Sonya Sherman in the July 1985 issue of *Life* magazine (see plate 38, following p 88) – the same photograph that moved André Durand to paint *Votive Offering* two years later – I was struck by the massive erotic energy of the pent-up figure. There was no 'lust in action' in this shot, no 'expense of spirit in a waste of shame'; it was all potential eros, love constrained, desire under pressure. I couldn't tell whether the woman's violent stillness would suddenly explode and set her libido free, or implode and suck it down into the urn at her feet like a genie into a bottle.[1]

Though her legs were demurely closed and her feet primly set together, Sonya Sherman did not look like a coy mistress. Her figure was too large and leggy to fit on just one glossy page. It had to stretch over two, like a celebrity centrefold, with a staple through her navel. Another figure, that of a young black soldier removing his shirt, appeared beside her in a smaller photo cropped to reveal no more of his face than a strong chin and sensuous lips. Who was this man? And why was he stripping for the camera? His image, like the photos of androgynous young men in cologne ads, invited erotic investigation. It could almost be a still from a military stag film, or a turn-on shot from a gay porn magazine, the sort that tempts the viewer to turn the page and see more of the forbidden body in full-frontal 'spreads.'

Had Sonya and the Unknown Soldier ever been lovers? Together in *Life* magazine, if not in life itself, they formed a strange lopsided diptych advertising the polymorphous pleasures of the Flesh.

Or so it seemed at first glance. Closer inspection revealed quite a different sort of advertisement: a subliminal command to keep this particular man and woman apart, to lock them away forever in the solitary confinement of their photographic cells. Sonya, who called herself 'Sunnye' in sunnier days, was definitely not being presented here as a love object, though she was gracefully posed and lithely beautiful. Nor was the Unknown Soldier really meant to be lusted after, for all his male-modelly charms. I'm sure I wasn't the only viewer to do a double take on discovering that both of them were dying of AIDS.

Their photographs had tempted me into desiring (feebly) what was and still is socially beyond desire – Sex with the Dead. That verboten act includes, of course, Sex with the Living Dead. I was appalled at myself for momentarily confusing Eros with Thanatos, for indulging in what amounted to mental necrophilia.

Among the stranger psychological consequences of the AIDS crisis is a shuddering collapse of traditional dichotomies pertaining to the body and its multiple social constructions. What I shuddered to see collapse before Sunnye's photo was the West's age-old distinction between the sensual Flesh and its discarded shell, the senseless Corpse, a distinction most strongly expressed in our deeply rooted taboo against intercourse with cadavers. Since the Western media have insistently focused on cadaverous bodies in representing persons with AIDS, I was not prepared, in 1985 at least, to imagine the bodies of PWAs as sexually existent or valuable. Their living bodies were effectively dead and buried in the popular mind, and in 1985 even their dead bodies were such worthless trash that few undertakers (who normally know the value of a good corpse) would care to bury them.

The diptych of Sunnye and the Unknown Soldier was not designed to correct this popular misconception of the bodies of PWAs. Its effect, rather, was to reinforce the very taboo it so casually denied and so playfully offended. The caption underlying the black man's photo set me straight about his social value: 'This infected soldier has had to put away his uniform for good.' His uniform clearly signified his once sensual flesh, now no better than a senseless corpse. His body was really what he was going to put away – for good – when his true identity as an AIDS cadaver was publicly exposed in *Life* magazine. His arrested striptease, a private spectacle for the erotic imagination, turned out to be a public court martial, a defrocking ceremony, a flaying of his corporeal dignity.

I was horrified at the trick that had been played on me by the wily disease, for at the time I naïvely supposed that it was the disease (and not these particular photos or the media in general) that had played the trick on me. Was AIDS really so powerful that it could transform lovers into corpses right before my eyes? Apparently, for here was radiant Sunnye, stooped with disease, contemplating her own funeral urn: an emblem of fleshly frailty if ever there was one. Death and the Maiden in modern dress, I thought, though the Maiden hadn't been one for some time and Death was an absent presence in the moral tableau.

Perhaps Sunnye was a postmodern Pandora casually lifting the lid on all the horrors of the Age of AIDS. After all, had she not had a year-long affair with a male bisexual, the new bogey man of our era, and therefore deserved to be regarded as the female cause of all our woe? So the gossipy text beside her photo suggested:

> Sonya Sherman, a 34-year-old legal secretary from Washington, D.C., had a year-long relationship with a man she says was bisexual. In 1983, long after they broke up, she got a rash that wouldn't go away. Her immune system gradually weakened: AIDS was diagnosed that fall. Sonya has so far survived four major infections, including two bouts of pneumonia, which for an AIDS patient is something of a record. Doctors have tried a desperate battery of drugs, one of which left her with severe hearing loss. Two members of her support group of AIDS patients died this spring. Serenely, Sonya has written a will and planned her funeral, even selecting her own burial urn. 'My mother hopes that one day we'll use it for flowers,' she says, 'but I have to be more realistic.'

Yet, like Pandora and her biblical counterpart Eve, Sunnye was still alluringly lovely after the Great Mishap – that was the strange part. The hideous reality of her disease and the haunting loveliness of her figure were paradoxically fused in the shot so that the dying model and her deathless image were inseparable in the hyper-reality of mediated 'Life.'

Sunnye Sherman was not a frail person living with AIDS at the time this shot was taken. She was a forceful symbol of American Womanhood dying, impossibly dying, of what had been known up until then as 'gay plague.' So impossible did her fatal diagnosis seem, in 1985, that it had to be a case of trick photography! After all, as anyone who watched American TV commercials well knew, American Womanhood was protected from dirt and germs and all nasty things by the disinfectant daimones of Western capitalism.

But it wasn't a trick photograph, at least not in a mechanical sense. She really was infected with the virus. My initial impression that her image had been forced to fit a space too small to contain its symbolic implications was enhanced by Sunnye's disconcerting pose: she seemed to be straining heroically against the top and bottom of the magazine, as if her body had been painfully folded into a narrow cell, the black-and-white coffin of the photo itself, in grim anticipation of being squeezed by AIDS into the claustrophobic confines of the urn. Like the Coy Mistress's imagined grave, the urn's a fine and private place, but none, I think, do there embrace.

Here was no candid shot of an ordinary American consumer resting after a hard day's shop, though the snatch of Dickensian narrative beneath the photo bleakly evoked the fatiguing world of the working woman. 'Sonya Sherman can't walk without resting frequently,' read the caption, 'but she accomplished the grim errand of picking out her funeral urn.' As slices of life go, this one was hard to swallow. It seemed too dramatic, too allegorical an image for a woman who in real life (which of course should not be confused with *Life* magazine) was only a legal secretary from Washington, DC, with fairly bourgeois tastes, to judge from her taste in pottery, and with fairly ordinary Jewish-American parents, Ina and Murray Sherman, who were no doubt deeply distressed to see their daughter catapulted to fame by a 'social disease' – a disease, screamed the magazine cover in red capitals, from which 'NO ONE IS SAFE' these days, not even a humorous girl-next-door with a steady job whose Dad sells real estate.

So what had gone so wrong in her life? How had she ended up dying for love in *Life* magazine? A tabloid-style headline centred in the margin to the left of her photo supplied the answer: she had been 'BETRAYED BY A STEALTHY INVADER.'

This dramatic gloss translates her from the steps of the capital of middle-class America onto the raked stage of an imaginary grand opera. The opera might be called 'Amore Traditore' (Traitor Love). In its final act Sunnye has become a tragic heroine – La Tradita Amorosa – betrayed by an invasive lothario who has secretly poisoned her blood while stealing her heart. The Invader was not simply an operatic version of her bisexual lover, the nameless man who had stealthily carried his poisonous bodily fluids from the underworld sewers of homosexuality into the heterosexual theatre. He was the poison itself, the Human Immunodeficiency Virus, a villain evidently endowed with devious intelligence and icy charm. The unwritten libretto for Sunnye's swooning-unto-death scene is easy to read as political allegory: it plays upon a lingering McCarthy-era fear that America the Beautiful has been invaded and violated by the secret agents of a body-snatching, soul-destroying foreign government.

When I considered Sunnye's photo from an iconographic angle, its artful composition and allegorical contents reminded me of various Renaissance paintings in the 'memento mori' or 'vanitas mundi' tradition. The profound impact of the Black Death on pre-Enlightenment European culture can be sensed, even today, in the remarkable body of religious paintings designed to provoke pious meditations on the vanity of the world and the inevitability of death. In such art the living confront the dead or the dying or touch concrete symbols of mortality in an effort to make sense of the Plague, to render its seemingly senseless outbreaks culturally significant, to conceptualize and hence to contain the expansive horror of pestilential death within a restrictive religious or philosophical context.

I can't think of a more compelling example of 'vanitas' art than Mantegna's third and last portrait of St Sebastian, which was completed around 1480: here we see the patron saint of plague victims straining at head and foot to pass through the narrow frame of this life, to step out of his own picture as it were, to escape the conventional icon of the tormented Flesh and the transient World (symbolized by the gutted candle at his feet) through a heroic burst of anagogic energy. A quieter but no less provocative image of saintly transcendence is Georges de La Tour's chiaroscuro portraits of Mary Magdalen contemplating symbols of earthly transience. No arrows prick the Magdalen's conscience or goad her into meditations on her own mortality: a skull or a candle is all she needs to stimulate her penitent thoughts on the postlapsarian frailty of woman's flesh. As Thomas Nashe lamented in 1590 in his 'Litany in Time of Plague,' beauty is but a flower which wrinkles will devour.

So might we all piously lament on viewing the allegorically composed photo of Sunnye Sherman. Like Mantegna's Sebastian, Sunnye is a martyr for the plague years – a celebrity victim straining to transcend fleshly agony and yearning for a return to original innocence. And like de La Tour's Magdalen, she is a solitary daughter of Eve contemplating the utter worthlessness of worldly beauty as she fixes her gaze on a traditional symbol of inexorable death. Martyr and Meretrix: she is both. Escape from either role is impossible within the implicitly moralistic narrative of her erotic 'betrayal.' As her urn is to her, so she is to us: a stimulus for fatalistic meditations on the ultimate powerlessness of the Fallen Flesh.

Whether we see her vainly struggling to escape the fatal frame of her photo or folding herself into a fetal position as she prepares for death, the photographer has ironically forced her to serve moralizing Christian ends that cannot have been her own. She was not a Christian. Nor was she, so far as I know, a Jewish businesswoman like Mary Magdalen who saw the light of Christ and repented in the darkness of Sin before it was too late. Yet to be visually accepted – and socially valued – by the moral majority of *Life*'s mainstream American Christian readers during the conservative 1980s, Sunnye had to be 'converted' by the camera into a paradigm of the Fallen Woman betrayed by Lust and punished by Death.

I would like now to consider Sunnye Sherman's surprising rebirth as the central figure in André Durand's massive plague-icon *Votive Offering* (see plate 39) and to contrast its politically and spiritually provocative imagery with the photo that provoked it. Let me start by suggesting how the painting reverses the psychological strategies of the photo. The *Life* magazine diptych, as we noted, presents Sunnye and the Unknown Soldier first as erotic stimuli and then as moral advertisements of death – Thanatos triumphing in the end over Eros. *Votive Offering* with its seven PWAs in various physical states (from asymptomatic robustness to deathbed frailty) looks at first like an elaborate illustration for the *Morbidity and Mortality Weekly Report*; but then, without denying the potent presence of death in the imaginary ward occupied by Sunnye and her fellow patients, it counters this initially morbid impression by visibly asserting the dignity of their sexual natures and the beauty of their still sensual flesh in the face of terrible suffering. For Durand, it seems, Eros must triumph in the end over Thanatos.

My feeling that the *Life* photographer had been influenced (perhaps at a conscious level) by painterly conventions established centuries ago in the wake of the Black Death – conventions that not only shaped the composition of Sunnye's portrait but also determined the erotophobic significance of its moral subtext – was shared by Durand himself, who, as I was intrigued to discover during our first conversation about his work, had also been struck by the resemblance of the photo to a Renaissance painting.

Where I had seen St Sebastian and Mary Magdalen behind Sunnye's tragic figure, Durand saw *La Derelitta* – the pathetic figure of an outcast weeping in solitude on the cold hard steps outside a locked palace gate. This tempera painting, originally a side panel from one of a pair of Florentine marriage chests, was attributed to Botticelli by Venturi in the late nineteenth century, but it is now generally believed to have been the work of one of Botticelli's studio assistants, perhaps the young Filippino Lippi, who may well have based it on a cartoon by his master. Despite the outcast's long hair, flowing robe, and tragic diva pose, the popular nineteenth-century nickname 'La Derelitta' (meaning 'the Abandoned Woman') is historically inappropriate. She is really a he. Il Derelitto, as he should be called, has been conclusively identified as Mordecai the Jew weeping before the palace gate of the Persian king Ahasuerus – an identification based on the scenes from the Book of Esther featured on the other panels of the marriage chests.[2]

This iconographic correction by no means undermines Durand's intuitive association of the Florentine painting with Sunnye's photo, though what originally reminded him of *La Derelitta* was the way Sunnye looked like Esther – an archetypal Jewish heroine. Overlooking the sexual difference between Sunnye and Mordecai, we can still see a clear visual parallel between their respective representations as well as a strong political resemblance between their perilous situations. Both figures were posed on stairways, their faces inclined downwards, as if misfortune had suddenly halted their expected progress up the social scale. In both cases, it had. Mordecai and Sunnye both knew what it was like to come down in the world: he because of political suppression, she because of immunosuppression. After seeing his cousin Esther happily married off to the king, Mordecai thought himself safe from social harm until the wicked vizier Haman decreed that all the Jews in the kingdom were to be slaughtered. On the cassone panel, as in Esther 4:1, Mordecai protests this imminent pogrom by weeping and rending his clothes outside the palace. Sunnye's public appearance in *Life*, despite its fatalistic Christian gloss, is also a heroic Jewish protest against an impending holocaust: she has bravely 'come out' in public – onto the street – as a physically and socially condemned PWA to rally public opinion against a blatantly discriminatory government that in 1985 had barely acknowledged the existence of the epidemic. If Reagan was to play Haman the wicked vizier in the Book of AIDS, Sunnye would save the day by assuming the double role of Esther and Mordecai.

Her public appearance (which amounted to a confession of uncleanness) did not save the day, of course, either for herself or for her despised 'people,' the legions of PWAs who would put their uniforms away for good because of America's Darwinian public-health policies. Sunnye died in 1986, and her ashes are now stored in the very urn she opened in her fetal-fatal pose for *Life*.

Why did Durand remake this picture in High Renaissance style? Surely not just because it reminded him of a particular Renaissance painting: he could have remade *La Derelitta* in the raging primitivistic style of the late Picasso (as Picasso remade *Las Meninas*) if he had wanted to modernize its fatalistic or latent anti-feminist implications. Clearly that was not his intent. As a depiction of salvation and sanctification through martyrdom, *Votive Offering* implicitly protests the existential fatalism and dispiriting nihilism that have darkened much modern art since the Second World War. It is a piece of defiantly un-modern art, perhaps even anti-modern art, in its enthusiastic homage to Renaissance figuralism.

'Homage' is perhaps too weak a word for Durand's bold appropriation of Renaissance imagery in his painting. So too is 'allusion,' since *Votive Offering* not only alludes to votive offerings and altar pieces by a host of Renaissance artists but also reflects deeper aspects of their densely symbolic designs such as triptych structure and sacred symmetry. Perhaps 'return' is the best word to describe Durand's approach to his Quattrocento sources. He has returned to them in a spiritual as well as visual sense ('epistrophically' as a Neoplatonist would say) in order to re-create something divinely powerful, something harmoniously healing, in the pristine yet archaic art of idealized forms.

For all its School-of-Botticelli formalism, *Votive Offering* is more than an imitation of the glowing surfaces of Quattrocento art. To see it as *only* that is to perceive it as a parodic *démontage* of Pre-Raphaelite painting, which is surely a reductive reading of its ambitious therapeutic design. Pre-Raphaelite painting may have been very Renaissance in style, but it was thoroughly Victorian in ethos. *Votive Offering*, as I shall argue, is 'rinascimentale' in ethos as well as in style.

Sunnye for all her 'incredible beauty' (as Durand has called it) is not a tragic heroine dying prettily like Ophelia in Millais' bathtub; nor is Diana, Princess of Wales, an imaginary intercessor leaning out from the 'gold bar of heaven' like Rossetti's Blessed Damozel. Sunnye really was dying when Durand sketched her in hospital, and Diana really did visit an AIDS ward to touch society's new untouchables. Their meeting in the renascent world of Durand's icon is imaginary, to be sure, but that does not mean that it will have purely imaginary effects on spectators (those on *our* side of the canvas as well as on *theirs*) who regard the visionary possibility of such a conjunction as more than the quaint aesthetic fancy of a nostalgic pietist.

Durand has painted *Votive Offering* in a Renaissance style because it is ideologically as well as iconographically appropriate to the mystery of rebirth celebrated in its central panel. What he envisions here is not just the symbolic rebirth of Sunnye as Our Lady of AIDS, but the actual resurrection – in paint – of a particular kind of Renaissance style. That style is part of a magical agenda for imitating and improving life that the Neoplatonists originally called 'theourgia' or 'the art of divine works,' and reborn with their theurgic art is an active faith in the mystical thinking that justified it in the days of Ficino and Botticelli.

That kind of thinking is now commonly dismissed as a lunatic offshoot of Christian Neoplatonism, but throughout the Renaissance it was known in quite respectable academic circles as 'occulta philosophia.' Ficino's occult philosophy was a kind of cultural activism, an application of high-flown Neoplatonic theory to the humble practical problems of health, politics, and social survival. It entailed the magical participation of academic philosophers in the wisdom and power of the divinity that shapes our ends.

Participation was effected mainly through talismans invested with elaborate cosmological, numerological, and mythopoetic significance. Ficino, who was the teacher of Botticelli's patron Lorenzo di Pierfrancesco de' Medici, described the construction and manipulation of such talismans in the third book of his medical treatise 'On Life' (*De vita*), and it is clear from this influential text that talismanic images were not primitive signs scratched on stones, as we might suppose, but highly complex 'devices' involving painted or sculpted forms of the gods, magical incantations of divine names, astrological arrangements of medicinal plants, choral rituals imitating the cosmic dance, and even architectural re-creations of the cosmic mysterion. Talismanic images do not merely represent things. They actively contact and influence the things they represent, serving both as receivers of celestial energy and as transmitters of divine power to the theurgists who create their concord-inducing designs for the benefit of discordant humanity.[3]

If Durand was striving to be a theurgist when he painted *Votive Offering*, as I think he was, he could have found no greater artist to follow along this magical route than Botticelli. According to Frances Yates and Edgar Wind, Botticelli's *Primavera*, which Lorenzo di Pierfrancesco commissioned for a private study in his family palace in

Florence, was constructed and originally construed as an elaborate charm according to Neoplatonic principles of harmony.[4]

Durand, who is familiar with these principles through the writings of Yates and Wind, returns epistrophically to the *Primavera* at several points in the design of *Votive Offering*. Its oracular focus on a central female figure; its choral disposition of figures within an imaginary idealized space; its triadic division of that space into a visual triptych; the occult presence of a winged Cupid above the ritual action of the scene; and the subtle hint of transcendence beyond the veil of phenomena in the upper-left corner – all these aspects of Durand's icon of rebirth are notably reborn from Botticelli. Even the red bus in *Votive Offering* (a surrealist image also used by C.S. Lewis in his allegories of transportation to the afterlife[5]) is a symbolic vehicle of transcendence corresponding in function and position to Mercury's Caduceus in Botticelli, a magical device for leading souls towards the clouds of unknowing beyond the visible world.

Theurgical paintings typically hide a divine mystery from the eyes of 'somatikoi' or carnal people, while revealing it in all its paradoxical glory to the eyes of the 'pneumatikoi' or spiritual initiates in a mystic cult. In the *Primavera* Botticelli revealed to Neoplatonic initiates the paradoxical nature of Venus as archetypal 'virgo et procreatrix.' In the Ficinian cult of beauty, which was founded on the Plotinian doctrine that all beautiful things in the natural world participated in the aesthetic unity of the Primal Soul, Venus was worshipped as both the eternally inviolate source of virginal loveliness and the temporal or planetary cause of natural fecundity. Hence her bizarre Botticellian guise as a pregnant virgin, which is of course a syncretistic visual allusion to her Christian counterpart the Virgin Mary. Venus' mysterious nature as the beautifully voluptuous virgin is unfolded for the initiated eye in the harmonious triad of the Graces, who represent the enchanting powers of Pulchritudo, Castitas, and Voluptas – that is to say, Beauty, Chastity, and Marilyn Monroesque Sex Appeal.

If *Votive Offering* is a theurgical painting in a full Renaissance sense, as I've been suggesting, then it too will conceal and reveal a divine mystery. But whose? Certainly not Venus', though eroticism is darkly present in its design. Considering the triad of saints in the painting, we might be tempted to say that it is obviously a Christian mystery that Durand celebrates in his quasi-altarpiece. But the obvious, at least to a narrowly Christian eye, is what *conceals* the mysterious in a theurgical design: we've seen how the obvious Virgin Mary in *Primavera* turns out to be the mysterious Virgin Venus.

I don't mean to imply that the conspicuous Christian significance of the healing rite conducted around Sunnye must be ruled out in our meditation on what *Votive Offering* has to offer the initiated eye. It certainly should not. Still, I would argue that the painting does not imprison Sunnye (who, we should recall, was not a Christian) in a narrowly Christian frame of reference – as did her moralizing photograph in *Life* magazine. As a stand-in for the Virgin Mary, particularly for the Maestà or Virgin in Majesty, Sunnye is perhaps even more preposterous than Botticelli's Venus: she's sick, childless, unmajestic, and by puritanical standards scandalously, promiscuously 'unclean.'

It is her very absurdity in this Marian role, however, that forces us to look beyond a strictly Christian interpretation of Sunnye's rebirth if we are to succeed in making sense of it. We should not let the saintly surfaces of the painting blind us to other levels of meaning in Durand's allegory of the Flesh and the Spirit, levels that might lead us back to pre-Christian mysteries, archetypal visions, pagan paradoxes.

The key to Durand's mystic design is not the other-worldly chorus of saints but the very worldly princess who joins them at Sunnye's bizarre apotheosis. Where Botticelli revealed the mysteries of Venus, Durand, I believe, reveals the mysteries of Diana.

In classical antiquity the elegant goddess of the chase and the chaste was often hailed as 'Diana Triformis' – literally, the 'three-formed or three-personed Diana' – which the Florentine Neoplatonists inevitably interpreted as a reference to the Christian Trinity prophetically veiled in a pagan epithet.[6] Like Venus, whose nature was triadically unfolded in the Graces, Diana could be viewed as a mysterious unity of three seemingly disparate and even discordant deities. In the heavens she was Selene or Luna, goddess of the moon; on earth Artemis, goddess of virgin huntresses; and in the underworld Hecate, goddess of witchcraft. As Hecate she was often identified with Persephone, Queen of the Dead, and like Demeter's daughter, was worshipped in nocturnal fertility rites as the source of potent sexual charms and vital springtime energies.

In the central panel of *Votive Offering* the Diana Triformis is unfolded anew in the three persons of the priestess, the princess, and the PWA. The celestial priestess, appearing in the Christian guise of Catherine of Genoa, holds the white veil of purity over Sunnye's head like an Eleusinian mystagogue in the temple of Demeter dramatically veiling – or unveiling – the reborn Queen of the Dead. The pearls adorning the priestess's bodice are traditional 'lunaria,' gems of the moon, and her lunar aspect is further suggested in the silvery strands of hair radiating down from her halo. Within Catherine the 'Pure' gleams the archetypally pure form of Selene, Diana's heavenly self.

Her earthly self is revealed in the instantly recognizable figure of the Princess of Wales, whose slender form and dauntlessly sure foot recall the athletic figure of Artemis. From her ear hangs another cluster of lunaria, a pearl-and-diamond earring, in which is reflected the splendour of her planetary counterpart. Three arrows near her foot suggest not only the torments of martyrdom but also the delights of the hunt, the worldly sport Diana has temporarily abandoned as she bows to her underworldly incarnation. Can the princess's Christian name be a mere coincidence? Not to a theurgic initiate. From a mystical perspective Diana of the Mead lives again in Diana of the Media.

Even though the princess we all know through television and countless magazine covers is a married woman with two children – and so hardly seems like a suitable person to embody the perpetual virginity of her pagan namesake – Durand perceives her mystique as essentially virginal. He has represented her elsewhere (in a painting provocatively entitled *Mystic Marriage*) in her famous wedding gown as the bride of an infant boy whose cult, like hers, has little to do with orthodox Christianity. In this strange wedding portrait, which may be read as an occult foreshadowing of *Votive Offering*, Durand literally drives orthodox Christianity out to sea – in the satiric guise of an ox and a donkey heaving-ho on a slave-pushed galley – while a veiled Diana enters into her cultic union on the strand beside a hermetic Egyptian barge. Like *Votive Offering*, *Mystic Marriage* has to be seen to be believed.

Unveiled in *Votive Offering*, this same adventurous Diana transcends her media cult to initiate a new medical cult. She will be the immortal virgin-healer of the lazar-houses, touching the sick with her invincible royal hand, as the Virgin Queen once did in the plague-ridden London of the poet Spenser's day. Like the great Spenserian heroine Una, who was also a healing virgin at home in the satyr-haunted woods of Diana, the former Lady Diana (née Spencer) retains the virtuous essence of her classical identity as she steps before us on the hand of her mystical Renaissance fiancé, the Redcross Knight.

The Diana Triformis needs only a Hecate to complete her triad in *Votive Offering*, and we find her in the patient at the painting's controversial heart. Who better than Sunnye, ravaged by an infernal illness, to play the princess's dark under-self? Durand himself has remarked to me that it was the remarkable similarity of the princess and the PWA that led him to imagine them face-to-face in the temple-hospital of his painting. Like Diana, Sunnye was a tall, slender, rather long-nosed yet serenely beautiful young woman whom fate had thrust from total obscurity into the celebrity spotlight as a media heroine. Both women have been in a sense victimized by the politics of worldly love, though Diana still lives in great wealth and health while Sunnye has been stripped of all possessions but her urn.

Initially, Durand's mirroring portraits of them might look like a study in contrasts. One can just hear the dualistic headlines in the gnostic tabloids. Perfect Health meets Terrible Sickness. Royal Wealth faces Wretched Poverty. Public Success touches Private Failure. Divine Power finds Helpless Mortal. Virgin Beauty bows to Ravaged Wanton. And of course, Glamour Girl finds Androgynous Double! Even the male saints associated with the pair encourage a polarization of their identities. While Diana clasps an armed and upstanding St George, whose upturned face seems to defy the lowly sins of the flesh, Sunnye is linked to a crouching Sebastian whose face looks passionately up at hers and whose glorified body is not only nude but voluptuously black.

Sebastian's halo is as bright as George's, however, and his strong black presence is essential to the allegorical design of the painting, not only because it restores hope in the charismatic power of the traditional patron saint of plague victims but also because it symbolizes the masses laid low by AIDS in Black Africa. I suspect there may be other reasons for his potent 'négritude.' The original Sebastian of Catholic legend was a soldier, the renowned leader of the Praetorian guard who had to put his uniform away for good when he defied the persecuting emperor Diocletian. Perhaps Durand represents him here as a black to restore to health and honour the dishonoured image of the black soldier in *Life* magazine who had to put his uniform away for good because of AIDS. Durand's Sebastian does not need to wear a uniform to be a soldier in the heavenly army: his flesh is the only uniform he needs to perform his erotic role in the mysteries of Diana.

Where the *Life* magazine diptych separated the black soldier from Sunnye, *Votive Offering* brings them into startlingly intimate contact and strips the male figure of its former porno glamour and erotophobic gloom. Embodied in this unmartyred black nude is a spiritual energy Durand recognizes as the chthonic life-force of sensuality. It was this same regenerative force, a titanic earthborn energy, that sired Hecate's magic in the ancient mysteries.

As Diana's shadow, Sunnye sits on her occult throne as Queen of the Dead; but under her avatar's tender touch and the pressing erotic influence of her male consort she will rise Persephone-like from the hall of death – a virgin once more, like her unfallen sisters, but one to whom the fallen flesh will be no stranger. Standing in the background is Ina Sherman, who attends her daughter's rebirth and re-chastening with the grave dignity of Demeter.

A healing concord, a binding together of sexually disparate and even socially discordant figures within a therapeutic space, dominates Durand's composition even as it dominated Botticelli's. The graceful triadic imagery of the *Primavera* was designed not only to imitate the imagined concord of Venus' enchanting domain but also to instil such concord in the erotically enchanted souls of its noble beholders, who, as divinely guided leaders, would be magically empowered to bring harmony down from the cloudy realm of their élite contemplative life into the commonly discordant domain of physical life and political action. That domain has never seemed more discordant than now, in the Age of AIDS, when political action (or inaction) more often harms than helps the millions of people whose physical, mental, and social life has been threatened or devastated by the new plague.

Magical thinking traditionally flourishes in plague times, especially when mainstream health practices and medical techniques seem powerless on their own to stem the tide of death. So they seemed in the mid-fifteenth century with each new outbreak of black death, and so they seem now with the discovery of each new strain of HIV. Panic drives the afflicted towards the remotest sources of potential healing power, towards any technique however obscure or inexplicable that holds out the slightest promise of recovery, regeneration, rebirth.

I am not surprised these days to find perfectly down-to-earth people, even college graduates normally contemptuous of any form of superstition, reverting to arcane talismanic beliefs in response to the AIDS crisis. John Gordon, an acquaintance of mine who learned he was seropositive during his last year of college, now carries a small quartz crystal around with him in his pocket (see p 225 of this volume). He calls it his 'security stone' and rubs it whenever he feels insecure about his future, believing with intrepid certainty that quartz has the power to concentrate 'positive energies' in his body. How it does this he does not know, or care to know, though Ficino would tell him (if he ventured to read the *De vita*) that crystals grow in the earth under direct astral influence and thus have an innate sympathy with celestial sources of creative power. John would probably laugh at this unscientific lore, for it is physical results he wants for his magical efforts – not abstruse explanations.

His lithomancy is a relatively primitive example of AIDS theurgy compared with a talismanic ritual I recently read about, and as a reader unconsciously helped to conduct, in the diary of New York translator Emmanuel Dreuilhe. Dreuilhe, who lost his lover and many friends to AIDS, was himself fighting the disease with every weapon he could muster, including words, until his death in 1989. His stirring memoirs as a soldier in the War against AIDS came out in 1988 under the French title *Corps à Corps* and in English as *Mortal Embrace*. In its penultimate chapter ('A Farewell to AIDS') he fantasizes that each phrase, each metaphor he writes will stand in for one of his lost lymphocytes. 'In my world turned upside down,' he explains with shamanistic conviction,

> writing is not only a form of therapy but also a magical exercise. By confronting the epidemic through its reflection in my diary, I can hope to decapitate the Gorgon before it turns me to stone. The philtre into which I thus plunge my anguish and obsession will become all the more effective as my audience grows. Each of my readers will become a soldier in my legion. I dream of indoctrinating and enlisting all those who read my words, so that they might save me ... I will perhaps find relief from my AIDS through this verbal exorcism, these words I strive to arrange in the proper order so that they will somehow weave the thread of logic indispensable to all ritual formulas of healing. These incantations are pronounced to achieve victory.[7]

Substitute painting for writing in this incantatory passage, and it could equally apply to Durand's healing art in *Votive Offering*. Instead of exorcistic words, theurgic brushstrokes have been 'arranged in the proper order' so that they will weave the powerful spell of victorious spiritual vision indispensable to all ritual spectacles of healing.

Sensing the magical agenda behind *Votive Offering*, Brian Masters has described it as a work of 'apotropeic art' in that it was specifically designed to 'turn away' or 'ward off' the forces of Evil by invoking the forces of Good.[8] That Durand's icon is meant to ward off the plague, like the lavender and rosemary strewn on the red carpet beneath Sunnye's feet, I would certainly confirm. But I would also argue that it was meant to do far more than that, to work a stronger magic than preventive exorcism on its spectators.

In so far as Durand intended *Votive Offering* to cast a binding spell over a society plagued and riven by AIDS-phobia, it might be described as harmonic rather than simply 'apotropeic' in function. Spectators outside the canvas are encouraged by those within it to move together towards a common goal – victory over the virus – which is symbolized by the mysteries of Diana in the central panel, the healing panel towards which all sympathetic eyes turn.

I would also describe the painting as a work of 'epitropeic art,' which means one that literally 'turns towards,' 'turns over,' or 'turns on' the occult forces of the sympathetic cosmos. The epitropeic function of *Votive Offering* is first to turn towards us all the healing powers in the universe like a lens collecting the rays of the sun in a particular spot; then to turn over or yield up those powers to the spectators gathered in chorus before the icon; and finally to turn on the collective energy of cosmos and chorus so that all who believe in the efficacy of the icon and the potency of spiritual vision will be irradiated by the artist's high fantasy and moved to participate in one way or another in a universal ritual of rebirth.

The fantastic cure envisioned within the painting, in its luminous central panel, is not for Sunnye alone: if the right powers are conjured up and convened to work the miracle on our side of the canvas, who knows? Might it not happen out here 'where youth grows pale, and spectre-thin, and dies'?

Durand encourages his spectators to believe (for seeing is believing in epitropeic art) that the healing powers of his painting can penetrate the thin veil of illusions presented as reality by the media; that the white radiance of eternity can illuminate the darkest wards of time like the light streaming off the heads of the saints; and that the erotic glow of divine life can emanate from Sunnye's mediating presence into a world where death will have no dominion. Rather than proclaiming the power of positive thinking like the various holistic healing books published for PWAs, *Votive Offering* imaginatively collects and channels the positive energies in the interpenetrating worlds of the Flesh and the Spirit as if it were the central power station in an emergent system of defences against the invasion of the demon virus.

This station, as the cruciform carpet and resurrection banner suggest, is a new Station of the Cross. Collected here are all the ancient and modern powers Durand could think of as 'crucial' in the struggle to defeat the virus: the charismatic power of the saints; the militant power of the martyrs; the charitable power of the churches; the political power of the nations; the economic power of the cities; the miraculous power of the royal healers; the celebrity power of the media princess; the lobbying power of the activists; the emotional power of the families; the technological power of the doctors; the intellectual power of the researchers; the empathetic power of the nurses; the erotic power of the patients and lovers; the talismanic power of the strewn herbs; the idealizing power of the artist; and the all-encompassing energies of the magical cosmos represented by the pastoral firmament glimpsed through the round window. These vital energies are gracefully introduced into the station, along with the ultimate regenerative power of the Saviour, by the rampant vine of the passion flower: a botanical detail that would have delighted the visionary soul of Ficino.

There are two ancient occult powers 'stationed' in the painting that Ficino would certainly have observed, but which are likely to escape the notice of most modern viewers. These are the interdependent powers of number and astral 'spiritus' – numinous causes scorned by contemporary scientists but still contemplated by numerologists and astrologers, whose doctrines Durand takes seriously in both his life and his art.

The numerological design of *Votive Offering* is so complex that I can only sketch its talismanic outlines here. This design, in fact, should be seen as several potently symbolic patterns integrated into the theurgic icon. Which pattern you see at any one time depends on your perception of the alignments and dispositions of the fifteen figures. Perhaps the simplest pattern divides the fifteen into three groups: seven figures on the right; one figure, Sunnye, in the middle like the Sun; and seven figures on the left. Seven is of course the number of the planets aligned in the old astrological heavens, and these celestial agents of destiny have long been associated with the seven virtues or 'powers' (courage, justice, temperance, patience, faith, hope, and charity) operating throughout the Neoplatonized Christian cosmos. One, the perfect number, the number of God, stands alone outside the mathematical design of creation, yet serves through its eternal centrality to unify the sevenfold sphere of fate and time just as Sunnye (whose position recalls the unique Sun of the Intelligible Sphere) binds together the diverse people in the painting by her centring presence. They are there, after all, because she is there – and was there in the artist's imagination long before the actual genesis of the painting.

Starting with the Circle above Sunnye as the transcendent One, or with Sunnye herself as the immanent Monad, the initiated eye can move out from the icon's centre to perceive the magical generation of all the numbers in the sacred Decad or 'group of ten' worshipped by

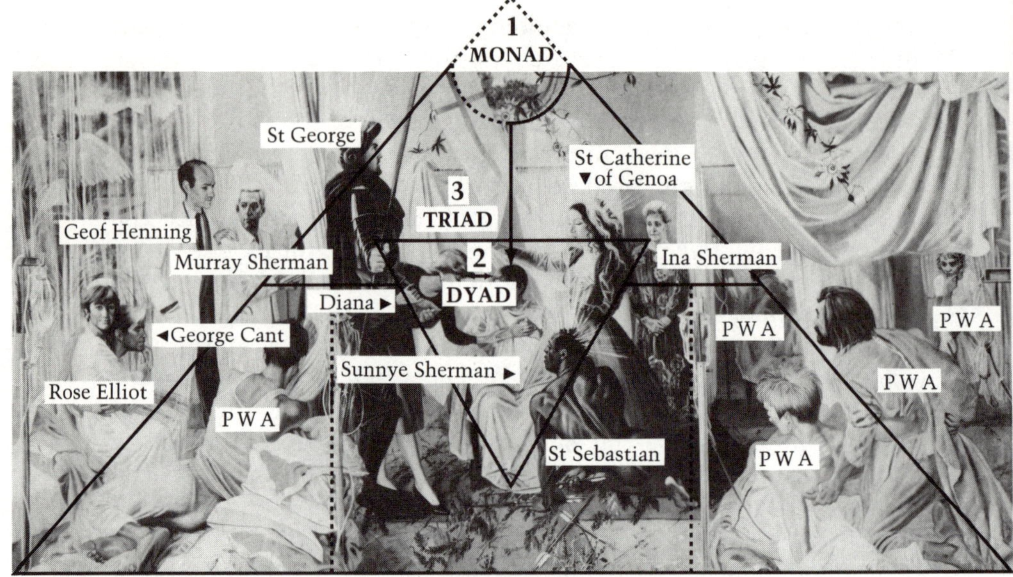

Pythagorean and Platonic mystics in antiquity and magically invoked by their theurgical successors in the Renaissance. Traditionally the Decad was represented on talismans and in manuscripts as a triangular arrangement of ten dots:

•

• •

• • •

• • • •

Hidden in the triptych structure of *Votive Offering* is a suggestion of this Pythagorean triangle, its upper apex perceptible only to the inward eye that projects the occult lines beyond the frame of the painting. With these subliminal lines the artist draws the eye down from the roundel (which represents the 'oculus Dei' or divine eye) and then out from Sunnye and Diana towards the multiplying groups of saints, relatives, healers, friends, patients. This simple ocular movement symbolically traces the complex 'pro-odos' or procession of the Many from the One. The bending of the PWAs back towards the central panel – a movement the Neoplatonists called 'ephesis' – reverses the procession so that the eye retraces the 'epistrophē' or contemplative return of the Many to the One up the pyramid of Life.

Within this pyramid Sunnye is paired with Diana to form the Dyad; the saints encircling them compose the Triad; and Sunnye's parents plus the two PWAs reclining in the foreground align themselves trapezoidally to construct the Tetrad. One plus Two plus Three plus Four equals Ten, the potent number of cosmic order and divine harmony. Mystically harmonized within the Decad are the Apollonian and Dionysian meanings of the numbers composing it. Besides divine unity, the Monad endows the design with perfective power and generative efficacy. Generated from its original integrity is the Dyad of opposition, disharmony, paradox – a perilous number that nevertheless also figures the mystical marriage celebrated in Durand's earlier icon of Diana. The saintly Triad, like the triad of the Graces, prefigures the erotic concord that will emerge from the violent discord of the Flesh and the Spirit. Like the Diana Triformis, it also prefigures the supernal concord of the Trinity. Finally, in the Tetrad, the stability of the Divine Plan is asserted as it is in the squared construction of the temple of the Heavenly City in Revelation.

Thus has Durand's theurgical vision transformed a common hospital ward into a temple of the mysteries. As a visual clue that the numerological design of the temple is intended to channel the beneficial influences of the stars into the hospital ward, the artist has placed a portrait of noted British astrologer Rose Elliot at the extreme left of the procession of figures. She is the nurse who looks out at us in order to draw us in by ocular 'fascination' – the enchanter's fixating gaze – towards the mysteries of Diana.

With all this enchantment going on inside the painting, we may well wonder whether it has had any constructive effect on the *real* world outside the fantasy. It has certainly had an effect on the hyperreal world of the media, for Durand's double portrait of Sunnye and Diana has frequently appeared in the British press. There has been a procession of many 'Votive Offerings' from the One, as it were, replicating the original projection of unity into the multiple spheres of time and life; and this vast multiplication of the painting has fixed the Princess of Wales in a benevolent iconographic role she can hardly renounce without damaging her public image. And to date she has not renounced it.

The mediated procession of the painting (not to mention its actual procession from church to church throughout Britain) has brought the British public face-to-face with a beatific vision of the epidemic and its martyrs that forcefully counters the pessimistic, discriminatory, narrowly moralistic, hysteria-inducing images of PWAs normally promulgated by the media. Durand has used the press not only as a means to counteract the media's hideously spellbinding representations of the crisis, but also as a worldly channel to conduct the other-worldly powers collected and activated in his visionary talisman. No one can deny that the talisman has activated a certain amount of economic power in the form of donations to the British AIDS charity CRUSAID.

Left-wing AIDS activists, die-hard Foucauldian theorists, practical scientific realists, and other worldly-wise outsiders are likely to be disenchanted with Durand's conservative depiction of PWAs as powerless victims within a nested sequence of institutionalized hierarchies – family, hospital, church, state, monarchy. Whose interests are these PWAs really serving in the painting? Not God's, some would argue, because of course there is no God. And not their own, since as martyrs they are rendered powerless by their 'deadly disease' and by the oppressive social institutions that construct it as such to promote their privileged political agendas. ACT UP should have an iconoclastic field-day protesting the exhibition of *Votive Offering* if Durand ever finds a church brave enough to show it in New York. Durand's conciliatory monarchist design is the exact opposite of the confrontational aesthetic practices of ACT UP, though like the cultural activists of that group the occult activists in the painting have formed an 'AIDS Coalition To Unleash Power.'

The painting has already proved politically controversial because it provokes a clash of world-views between those who deeply want to believe, and those who strongly refuse to believe, in the supra-political mysteries it discloses. Durand's pictorial stratagem for avoiding controversy – for discord is never the goal of a theurgist – is to disarm the sceptical critics of the icon by including them figuratively in its design: they are collectively 'present' in the Rodin-like thinker sitting apart from the epistrophic chorus and looking left on the extreme right in the direction of the recessed deathbed scene. There is room for puzzled inquiry as well as profound wonder in Durand's hospital-temple. From a theological angle the painting can be seen to counter modern political criticism of old martyrological miracles by illustrating the simple point that in a Renaissance Christian world-view (even a radically idealized one) the martyrs are potent forces for change in the secular world. They are victors in the end, not victims.

As a work of epitropeic art, *Votive Offering* was intended to have a miraculous effect on the mental and even physical health of PWAs brought before it. One PWA brought before it is also a spectator in it. He is George Cant, whom Durand portrayed with a rapt expression on his face in the centre of the left panel. On Sunday 1 November 1987, Cant was annointed before the painting after it was unveiled and blessed by the dean of St Paul's in St James's Church, Piccadilly. Though neither the unveiling nor the annointing was expressly performed by the Anglican clergy as a healing ceremony in a shamanistic sense, it would not have surprised Durand then (nor would it surprise him now) to learn that these transient reflections of the archetypal healing scene in the painting have had a positive therapeutic effect on Sunnye's annointed surrogate. 'Since Sunday,' wrote Cant in a letter to the artist, 'I have had an understanding and peace that I had previously thought un-understandable. I feel that your painting played an instrumental role in helping me achieve this grace ... You helped me see something truly wondrous.'[9] Cant was not cured before the unveiled image of Our Lady of AIDS, and as far as I know, the first miracle cure achieved through Sunnye's or Diana's gracious intercessions has yet to be recorded in the annals of the painting. Yet by his own account Cant perceived something 'truly wondrous' – some other sort of miracle – in the painting's presence, which seems to attest if not to Durand's efficacy as a theurgist then at least to his wizardry as a painter.

What was this wonder? St Augustine, whose Neoplatonic psychology was incorporated by Ficino into Renaissance theurgy, would have explained what Cant had experienced in these terms: his 'visio corporalis' or physical glimpse of the painting had stimulated his 'visio spiritualis' or visual imagination to illuminate his 'visio intellectualis' or mind's eye so that it might pierce the veil of sensibilia and attain a blessed understanding of the 'invisible things of God.' In its mediations between eyesight and insight, the 'visio spiritualis' (if properly stimulated by concordant images) can actually exert a healthful influence over the soul and body of the Neoplatonic Spectator.[10]

So claimed Augustine and Ficino ages ago. So, in different terms, claim modern doctors and therapists who have studied the positive effects of 'imaging' on terminally ill cancer patients. Anyone who finds it difficult to view *Votive Offering* as a theurgic talisman may find it easier in the end to perceive it as a stimulus for therapeutic imaging. In the end, I think, it amounts to the same thing.

NOTES

1 'The New Victims' *Life* (July 1985) 12–21. The photograph of Sunnye and her urn is on pp 14–15.

2 On *La Derelitta*, see Ronald Lightbown *Sandro Botticelli* (Berkeley and Los Angeles: University of California Press 1978) 2:208–9. This painting is now catalogued under the title 'Mordecai Weeping before the Palace-Gate of Ahasuerus.'

3 Marsilio Ficino *De vita* III.xviii–xix, in *Opera omnia* (Torino: Bottega d'Erasmo 1962) 1:586–90

4 See Edgar Wind *Pagan Mysteries in the Renaissance* (New York: Norton 1968) 113–27; also Frances Yates *Giordano Bruno and the Hermetic Tradition* (London: Routledge and Kegan Paul 1964) and *The Occult Philosophy in the Elizabethan Age* (London: Routledge and Kegan Paul 1979).

5 See C.S. Lewis *The Great Divorce: A Dream* (London: G. Bles 1946).

6 On the classical sources for the 'Diana Triformis' (eg Horace *Carmina* III.xxii), see Wind *Pagan Mysteries in the Renaissance* 249, 251.

7 Emmanuel Dreuilhe *Mortal Embrace: Living with AIDS* trans Linda Coverdale (New York: Hill and Wang 1988) 139–40

8 The following statement by Brian Masters (dated June 1987) appeared on the printed invitation to a 'Service of Receiving for VOTIVE OFFERING' held at St Mary's Episcopal Cathedral, Palmerston Place, Edinburgh, on 12 August 1988: 'With this painting, André Durand has revived the notion of apotropeic art, wherein the artist invokes the forces of Good, through the medium of the Church and with the intercession of the saints, to turn away evil. The tradition of the artist as supplicator to the Deity ascends to the pre-Christian era, when the artist's work was the fulfilment of a vow, or *votum*, the petition for a specific favour accompanied by the promise of a specific due. Durand made such a vow. Hence the title of his painting.'

9 This letter, undated and hitherto unpublished, remains in the personal archive of André Durand.

10 On the three kinds of vision, see St Augustine *The Literal Meaning of Genesis* vol II, bk 12, ch 6–7, trans John Hammond Taylor (New York, NY, and Ramsey, NJ: Newman Press 1982) 185–8. On the theology of martyrdom in relation to Durand's painting, see my article 'Acquired Immanent Divinity Syndrome' in *Perspectives on AIDS: Ethical and Social Issues* ed Christine Overall and William P. Zion (Toronto, Oxford, New York: Oxford University Press 1991) 65–6.

The Syndrome is the System: A Political Reading of *Longtime Companion*

BART BEATY

'The personal is political!' was a rallying cry of the Women's Movement in the early 1970s. What this slogan sought to impress upon women was the notion that politics was not an abstract system operating in the 'public' world of business and government but a pervasive system of privileges and practices shaping all personal relationships in the 'private' world of everyday life. In response to the then radical equation of the personal and the political, a few Hollywood films made a point of portraying female characters and their relationships in a clearly political light. *Klute* and *Alice Doesn't Live Here Anymore* are two notable examples of cinematic 'consciousness raising' along pro-feminist lines.

With the growing reliance of film theory on Freudian and Lacanian psychoanalysis in the mid-1970s, feminist filmmakers (especially in Europe) began to reverse the terms of the original slogan so that the political was identified with the personal. In Margarethe von Trotta's *Marianne and Julianne*, for instance, political actions such as the Baader-Meinhof bombings in Germany were explained in psychological terms as the result of the oppressive inequalities experienced within personal relationships.

Exploding the old patriarchal distinction between public and private life ceased to be a popular concern with the supposed triumph of feminism in the 1980s. The radical feminism of the 1970s seemed antiquated to those who believed that all gender oppression would die as soon as the consciousness of the 'general public' was sufficiently raised and all sexual inequalities were legislated out of existence – or at least, out of fashion. What has now supplanted the counterdiscourse of seventies-style radicalism, at least in the mainstream American film market, is a feminist filmmaking that presents the personal *instead* of the political. Films like *Lianna* and *Personal Best*, for instance, focus on 'women's issues' at an exclusively family-drama level without drawing any conclusions about the need for collective action, community support, or organized resistance to the System.

Having long ago lost its political nerve, mainstream American filmmaking now tends to address all socio-political issues – including AIDS – as part of a purely personal spectrum of significance. I would argue that this retreat from political confrontation towards personal 'growth' and 'enlightenment' has also happened in gay and lesbian filmmaking, though on a smaller scale. Yet radicalization of many gay people in response to the AIDS crisis has kept the 'old' equation between the personal and the political alive through the 1980s, if only barely, so that filmmakers on the counterdiscursive margins are still fighting the Good Fight against the individuation of the public and private worlds by implicating the System in all dimensions of personal life, especially the erotic life in sickness and in health. Gay films on AIDS such as *Danny* and *A Death in the Family*, however 'underground' their character or 'specialized' their audience, have repeatedly stressed that the Syndrome cannot be understood apart from the whole system of cultural values and political relations that have constructed it for the general public. In fact, at the radical outer limits of gay cinema where liberationist pioneers of the seventies like Rosa von Praunheim make AIDS films for the eighties and nineties as bleakly political as *A Virus Has No Morals*, the Syndrome becomes the System.

So what happens to a gay-positive film on AIDS that tries to go mainstream? It assumes a markedly unpolitical title redolent of the bourgeois pieties on an obit page, and picks up an Academy Award nomination for best supporting actor (heaven forbid that the best-actor award should go to someone publicly identified with a 'gay cause'!) along the way to comfortable obscurity in local video stores across the nation. Norman René's *Longtime Companion* (1990) was advertised as the first mainstream feature film to deal 'honestly' with the epidemic from a gay perspective. It turns out to be firmly grounded in the very straight tradition of American realism.

By effacing its methods of production and denying its status as a value-laden construct or text, *Longtime Companion* betrays its realist assumption that an artistic representation of 'the Truth' (in this case the triumph of the human spirit over AIDS) will only please its viewers if they can accept it as an 'evident reality.' Central to the conception of realist filmmaking – which still underlies the vast majority of American films made for theatrical distribution – is the pleasure of the spectator. Pleasure in the cinema, as Laura Mulvey has pointed out, is primarily visual and principally aimed at the ego of the heterosexual male.[1] Visual pleasure is stimulated by fulfilling an unconscious pre-Oedipal need for cohesion: by presenting a unified male figure in the active 'masculine' role in the film, a realist filmmaker offers up to the spectator an erotically potent role-model who may be vulnerable at times to the slings and arrows of outrageous fortune but who is ultimately in control of his own destiny, which is to say, the plot. For a narcissistic ego-ideal created by a realist text and adopted by millions of heterosexual male spectators at the urging of their girlfriends, one need look no further than Tom Cruise, whose success as a screen idol has less to do with his craft as an actor than with the craftiness of his image-makers.

Building on Mulvey's theory of the male gaze in realist cinema, Christian Metz has noted that the narcissistic enjoyment of mainstream movies is enhanced by the seamless quality of the realist form.[2] Because a realist film unfolds as if it were narrated by the spectator, who, in effect, creates the 'reality' of the narrative, he or she is invited to feel omnipotent relative to the characters and events on the screen. Because realist filmmaking creates an evident (hence unchangeable and unchallengeable) reality, the audience is locked in a position of 'dominant specularity' where no action is required of the spectators or indeed possible for them.

On this account Colin McCabe has described cinematic realism as essentially reactionary, which may explain why it is the choice of most conservative and liberal filmmakers in the current political climate.[3] By inviting a strong identification with a single male character, realist films tend to emphasize the personal over the political. In fact, by working in a form that limits an audience's ability to challenge the text, realist filmmakers attempt to exclude politics from the screen. Thus René's choice of realist form for *Longtime Companion*, I would argue, is not only artistically inappropriate for an intensely political topic such as AIDS but also socially harmful.

According to McCabe, the realist form is broad enough to include at least two kinds of film texts that challenge the reactionary basis of realism itself. The 'subversive text,' as he calls the first of these self-critical forms, undercuts its *histoire* status by complicating the relationship between the visual and verbal discourses so that neither can be accepted as the authoritative basis for 'reality.' In contrast to a film like Rossellini's *Germany Year Zero*, which clearly exemplifies this counterdiscursive strategy, *Longtime Companion* can hardly be called a subversive text since its visual track is clearly constructed as an objective reality. The second option for political critique within the realist form, the 'progressive text,' presents a viewpoint conspicuously at odds with the dominant ideology: for instance, the liberal-feminist viewpoint preserved from ultraconservative extinction in *The Handmaid's Tale*. What this film 'did' for women as a historically oppressed group, *Longtime Companion* purports to do for gay men. As a progressive text, it sets out to represent the lives and destinies of individuals within the 'gay community' during the 1980s as if their collective history during the AIDS crisis was simply a virological extension of the marginalization and inferiorization of gay people since the destruction of Sodom.

Despite all the hype about its potential for raising public awareness about AIDS, I suspect that *Longtime Companion* is not as progressive as it pretends to be. First of all, it in no way seeks to challenge the tradition of narcissistic identification at the heart of realist cinema. Since the six key players in the film are all upwardly mobile white men from respectable neighbourhoods in New York, the interlacing narrative of their lives has little room to incorporate questions of class and race into its discourse. People of colour are relegated to the sidelines, appearing in bit parts (for instance, John's Indian doctor, Sean's black buddy, and the Hispanic PWA Alberto). In this way the film seeks to make the dreaded topic of homosexuality less threatening to Middle America by presenting its gay heroes as all-American boys.

The successful careers of the key players also invites narcissistic identification. All of them (with the possible exception of John) have nice apartments, well-paying jobs, and healthy social lives. The notion that their status as clean-cut white Yuppies removes them from the filthy underworld of homosexuality is driven home in the first hospital scene from the '1982' segment. The waiting room, filled with drunken bums and downwardly mobile people of colour, is shot as an eye-line match of David and Willy looking uneasily at 'Them.' We know that David and Willy occupy an elevated status among these people because the camera tracks *down* before surveying the room – a visual effect that promotes in the spectator a desire to join the superior class controlling the viewpoint. Who would want to side with the down-

and-outers, the suffering Others who are reduced to mere objects within the Foucauldian force field of the hospital? The representation of Willy and David as bright, sexy, and economically secure not only serves to elicit audience identification with them (as opposed to Them) but in so doing also fulfils the requirements of the realist form and the conservative agenda behind it by privileging a white ruling-class viewpoint.

The all-American quality of Willy and his friends is enhanced by the film's insistence on the virtues of monogamy. It is hardly coincidental that the only character not involved in monogamous longtime companionship, party-boy John Deacon, is also the first to die of AIDS. John's death is rendered tragic by his playfulness and wit – he seemed like such a nice upbeat kind of guy until his AIDS-related pneumonia laid him low in the inner-city inferno of the hospital. How the film presents John's decline and fall is a clear example of the realist text privileging its visual discourse over language in order to evoke sympathy at the personal level: while we see John being playful and witty in the '1981' beach segment, we only hear about his 'cruising' in a conversation between David and his longtime companion Sean.

Similarly, David and Sean win our sympathy as tragic (if not exactly 'innocent') victims of AIDS because they are consistently shown to us as an exemplary monogamous couple – we only hear about their pre-AIDS sexual flings in offhand remarks such as Sean's confessional aside: 'I haven't touched anyone else since Fort Lauderdale.' The visible is objective truth in a realist film; the verbal, merely subjective testimony.

What the progressive text of *Longtime Companion* fails to challenge are the moralistic concepts of 'promiscuity' and 'sexual deviance': anyone to whom these concepts apply in the film are implicitly faulted in comparison with the good gays who suffer through the bad times. For instance, while the loyally monogamous Howard remains good-humoured and even stoical in the gruelling '1985' hospital segment, the deranged punk in the bed next to him flies into a rage and rips out his IV in an effort to escape the phobic restrictions of the medical hierarchy. As his girlfriend looks on in hapless bewilderment, we can only conclude that his escape (which is swiftly prevented by strong-armed orderlies) would certainly have endangered the lives of 'innocent' bystanders less familiar with the anarchic underground than she. By suggesting through such simple juxtapositions that the deviant or the promiscuous deserve their fate as medical captives in the gloomy wards of the epidemic, the film betrays its deeply moralizing tone.

While its crypto-Christian celebration of monogamy may serve to strengthen the uneasy identification of straight spectators with the main gay characters, and hence to sell the story to the general public, *Longtime Companion* stalwartly refuses to awaken sympathy for people who for one reason or another find no fulfilment in Christian marriage or its post-Christian variations. Its earnest liberal efforts to suggest alternative lifestyles without affirming or at least exploring them, I would argue, does more harm than good in shaping the 'tolerant' attitude that Middle America is invited to adopt towards the Gay Lifestyle (as if there was only one) by its beleaguered adherents and apologists.

That Willy and Fuzzy appear to be 'saved' from AIDS by the power of monogamous love is a dangerous inference most spectators are likely to draw from *Longtime Companion* if they have not considered the health risks resulting from unquestioned allegiance to heterosexist love discourse. As Douglas Crimp has pointed out, the 'Stick to One Partner' policy advocated by the Moral Majority is potentially lethal 'since monogamy per se provides no protection whatsoever against a virus that might already have infected one partner in a relationship.'[4] Yet it is this very policy that the film unquestioningly advertises with its wholly unironic title.

If the film had been truly progressive, it surely would have countered the monogamy message (or at least opened its own romanticized moralism up to debate) by providing some safer-sex information within the paradigmatic narrative of Willy's undangerous liaison with Fuzzy. Nothing would have been easier than the introduction of a few condoms into the many 'daring' bedroom scenes – or more appropriate historically – since Willy and his friends represent the very community that invented the concept of safer sex and pioneered safer-sex techniques during the decade covered by the film. The film need not have become dourly didactic to have presented at least the possibility of non-monogamous sex as safe. Yet aside from the foregrounding of a condom manual at the Gay Men's Health Crisis scene in the '1988' segment, safer sex is never discussed in the film. Abstinence frequently is.

Roy Grundmann in his review of *Longtime Companion* for *Cinéaste* has suggested a social reason for the film's virtual silence on the subject of safer sex: any discussion of condoms and lubricants would necessarily have entailed references to anal and oral sexual practices that remain 'unmentionable in the straight world.'[5] By refusing to include dialogue pertaining to safer sex, the film inadvertently reveals its true audience. Gays, the film assumes, already know what they need to know about safer sex – while straights don't need to know anything about it because they don't have sex with gays and certainly wouldn't indulge in sexual practices popularly and incorrectly identified as gay.

The film is thus clearly not for the Gay Community but about the Gay Community. Its seemingly progressive text is designed to teach the heterosexual majority the main social 'facts' about homosexuality (namely, all good gays are white, liberal, fit, fun-loving, well-off, and if still alive, tragically sobered by the epidemic) without getting down to the messy erotic details (such as the safest and most pleasurable way to apply a condom to an erection before anal intercourse). Because the discourse of safer sex is still considered too political by many Middle Americans, its virtual absence from both the visual and the verbal narration of the film helps to maintain the filmmaker's obsessive focus on the personal and to sustain the spectator's narcissistic identification with the highly personable survivors of the Plague.

Politics, of course, is what *Longtime Companion* most ardently seeks to avoid. The early 'human-interest' reaction to the AIDS crisis presented in the film is not collective outrage against an uncaring government and a discriminatory health-care system but simply internalized homophobia on the part of gay men who fear each other as sexual partners and express panicky frustration at their own transformation into agents of infection. What politics do emerge in the film are, at best, half-hearted. In the '1983' and '1984' segments, Reagan's name is satirically connected with genocide and alien invasions, but the anti-Republican satire never really progresses beyond pop-cultural references to E.T. and the Holocaust. Moreover, the political action adopted by the central characters is mainly in the American liberal tradition of self-help and self-serving individualism. Sean, for instance, is advised to think positively and to purify his mind and body by a well-meaning (if somewhat dumb) beach buddy. It is advice earnestly followed by Fuzzy in the '1985' segment.

The possibilities of cultural activism in the civil-rights tradition are never dramatically explored by Fuzzy's set, merely hinted at in their conversations about the impact of the crisis on the City. (New York always seems light years away from the Fire Island beach house where much of the film's action is set.) Collective action to protest the city's handling of the crisis is first suggested as an alternative to paralysing depression by Fuzzy's sister Lisa, whose authority on the subject of medical politics is established early in the film by her status as its main straight character. At first Fuzzy expresses strident disapproval of the whole idea of AIDS activism. His grumbling complaint to Lisa – 'If I never hear the word AIDS again, it'll be too soon!' – seems to summarize the gay coterie's and the film's reluctance to fight the System. The good gays prefer to fight the Syndrome on an individual basis, case by case, tragedy by tragedy. The Syndrome is never identified with the System that constructs and perpetuates it.

Even the beginning of the buddying movement, represented by Willy's volunteer work with Alberto, is shown at a strictly personal level to be rooted in the myth of American pragmatism. In the '1988' segment Willy tells the listless Alberto to get up and do something – the dishes, the laundry, anything. Once again the peculiarly American notion that only the individual (not the group) can effect a change for the better is reinforced. Willy's merely nominal allegiance to the community-based ideal of social services for PWAs sounds a hollow note throughout the film, and indicates the extent to which the personal has replaced the political as a source of drama in the realist form.

The Living With AIDS benefit in the '1988' segment, the penultimate scene in the film, marks another seemingly progressive move in the direction of radical AIDS politics. A benefit concert, however, is surely the weakest form of direct action, being not so much an 'action' in the ACT UP sense as a fund-raising event to promote community-based activism such as Willy's behind-the-scenes work for Alberto. Indeed the benefit scene functions in the narrative not to relate a political agenda or to proclaim a radical viewpoint on the crisis, but to foreground the therapeutic humour of the Finger Lakes Trio, whose campy rendition of 'Down at the YMCA' provides comic relief for the plague-weary survivors. This song recalls the fun-and-games spirit of the opening sequences of the film, now forever lost in the gloom-and-doom of the epidemic. Lulled by the Trio's nostalgic strains we are instantly transported back to the beach at Fire Island for the Final Reckoning.

Here radical politics is also present, but only fleetingly in Willy's reference to a planned ACT UP demo and Fuzzy's fashionable conversion to Gay Liberation. Was it Lisa who bought her brother the 'Read My Lips' T-shirt he now bravely sports on the beach? One can hardly imagine a conservative Southern-bred lawyer like Fuzzy outing himself by investing in a shocking image of two military hunks kissing in defiance of the System! Never mind that this particular image (designed for ACT UP by Gran Fury) only existed as a poster in 1988: its strong political message against the heterosexism bedevilling American public-health agencies and American society in general was probably lost on the majority of straight people who saw the film outside New York or San Francisco.

The ACT UP demo where Fuzzy's T-shirt would have meant something political, where it would have drawn a graphic connection between homophobia and AIDS discrimination, is only planned – never shown – in the film. What is shown is the trio of survivors praying for an end to AIDS and having their prayer miraculously answered by an omnipotent off-screen spectator of their woes. Because the film's realist form privileges images over words, what remains with the audience from this final scene is not the tentative discussion of activism but the vivid impression that converts to activism are socially isolated. Their isolation on the beach is magically translated into a beach party by a bizarre fantasy sequence in which all the friends and lovers they have lost to AIDS come bounding over the boardwalk to embrace them on the strand. With its visual celebration of Hope springing eternal and Life aerobically renewed, the resurrection fantasy not only silences the discussion of activism. It denies the need for it.

How, then, can *Longtime Companion* be considered progressive? Though it tries to present the 'story of AIDS' from the viewpoint of an oppressed group, namely gay PWAs, it does so in such a politically noncommittal way that it fails to counter the dominant ideology behind the media accounts of the epidemic that provide the film's opening gloss on the crisis.

The tension between the film's pro-activist script and its ultimately transcendental vision of crisis-resolution through divine intervention can be discerned most clearly in the diptych-like contrast between its opening and closing scenes on Fire Island. In the introductory '1981' segment Fuzzy and Willy meet amid a multitude of sunbathers soaking in the rays before the storm. Fire Island is presented as an innocent pleasure-ground, a gay Eden complete with deer, beer, and pulsating disco. At the gloomy conclusion of the '1989' segment the same beach stretches before Willy, Fuzzy, and Lisa as a seascape of loss, a marginal zone between the living and the dead. Gone are the sunbathers, the dancers, the boozers, the morally unfit. A fatal silence underlies the monotonous pounding of the waves. In case you didn't get the message, Paradise has been Lost: while once the pop anthem 'The Tide is High' rang out across the dunes, now all you'll hear on the postlapsarian soundtrack are the bluesy strains of a folk ballad entitled 'The Post-Mortem Bar.' It is this pseudo-mystical song that accompanies and in a sense induces the collective dream of resurrection.

Though the fantasy sequence may be justified within the conventions of melodrama as a frail but spiritually fortifying consolation, it serves to illustrate just how far Norman René was willing to go – all the way to the Hereafter – to divest his film of its disturbing political implications for the Here and Now. In the end the film shamelessly appeals to the 'dominant specularity' of its straight audience, who merely have to wish for something good to happen (in the manner of *Peter Pan*) and instantly receive a happy ending. The fantasy of resurrection presupposes the fantasy of omnipotence. With such a closure stratagem the film can demand no political action from its spectators. The story of Willy and his friends is closed with anagogic happiness – while the tedious earthly problems created or exacerbated by the epidemic are cast for a time into the convenient abyss of oblivion. The audience has been absolved of all responsibility to end the crisis by their very presence in the theatre, their participation in the rites of cultural dominance. Like initiates in the ancient mystery cults they have learned to wish away death. Now they can go home.

Several of my friends on the liberal left have urged me to reconsider my reading of *Longtime Companion* as a reactionary film with progressive pretensions. Far from ascribing its faults to a failure of political nerve, they argue that it should be regarded as a resounding success for two reasons: first, because it was made at all (let alone distributed commercially and nominated for an Academy Award) in the repressive era of Helms and Bush; and second, because it takes a brave first step towards bringing an understanding of gay men and their lives in the Age of AIDS to the attention of Middle America. Though I would agree with the first of these reasons for valuing the film, I cannot accept the second because it ignores the complex social reality of the AIDS crisis. The very personal, anti-statistical kind of AIDS awareness the film promotes is certainly needed to offset the direly impersonal prophecies issuing routinely from the World Health Organization; but the need is long-term. Though *Longtime Companion* was moderately successful (for an independent feature) at the box office where Middle America casts its deciding votes, it would take a dozen such features a year – plus another dozen that dared to deal with the erotic refinements of safer sex – to begin to raise AIDS awareness in the straight heartland. A gradual chiselling away at ignorance and apathy is necessary and should be wholeheartedly encouraged, but as Sean notes in the '1983' segment, 'it doesn't stop them from hating you.'

An effective resolution to the AIDS crisis requires deliberate action from all sides of the social spectrum now, not later, not down the yellow brick road when Middle America is finally willing to accept its gay exiles back into the fold. Consequently, any mainstream AIDS film that seeks to end the crisis must also seek to encourage political protest, to urge a cultural change in the racist and sexist System that has stigmatized the 'high-risk groups' associated with the Syndrome. When I consider how the personal focus of *Longtime Companion* relentlessly distracts its audience from the pressing need for collective action on the political front, I can only conclude that the conventions of realist filmmaking should be avoided in bringing the epidemic to the screen if we are to find a politically engaged and engaging cinema from which there is no going home.

NOTES

1 Laura Mulvey 'Visual Pleasure and the Narrative Cinema' in *Film Theory and Criticism* ed Gerald Mast and Marshall Cohen (New York: Oxford University Press 1985) 803–16

2 Christian Metz 'The Imaginary Signifier' in *Film Theory and Criticism* ed Mast and Cohen, 782–802

3 Colin McCabe 'Realism and the Cinema: Notes on Some Brechtian Theses' *Screen* 15.2 (summer 1974) 8

4 Douglas Crimp 'How to Have Promiscuity in an Epidemic' in *AIDS: Cultural Analysis / Cultural Activism* (Cambridge: MIT Press 1988) 247

5 Roy Grundmann '*Longtime Companion*' *Cinéaste* 18.1 (1990) 48

Erotic Self-Images in the Gay Male AIDS Melodrama

THOMAS WAUGH

This essay was first presented in embryonic form at 'Pedagogy and Politics,' the Second Annual Yale University Lesbian and Gay Studies Conference in October 1988. Also on the agenda at Yale was a 'gays in the media' panel, of the kind that has become second nature to lesbians and gays over the last two decades. Three scholars in a row embarked on familiar tirades against the made-for-TV gay melodrama, focusing principally on *An Early Frost*, one of the earlier major fictional representations of AIDS on the U.S. commercial networks. It is a movie we have all come to love to hate, but one over which many of us secretly wept copious tears. The panelists were of course correct in their dissection of *An Early Frost* and I am certainly not about to defend it or the made-for-TV melodrama. Yet, in their blanket dismissal of the melodrama per se, I wonder if the panelists were involved in a somewhat careless, ahistoric, and even élitist negation of the heritage and current arsenal of gay popular culture.

In this essay I would like to defend that much-stigmatized genre, melodrama, which has in fact been the format, I would argue, for some of the most important gay male cultural responses to the epidemic. Specifically, for two or three years starting around 1984 when the first fully developed cultural responses to AIDS began to appear, melodrama was the principal vehicle in independent gay male fiction in film and video (and theatre as well, though that is beyond my territory for the moment) for our dealing culturally with the trauma, fear, bereavement, and sacrifice that AIDS has occasioned in our community.

Melodrama is the genre that popular culture has traditionally drawn on to work out the strains of the nuclear family under the patriarchy. This form that evolved for the orchestration and resolution of the conflicts of the emotional sphere and the domestic realm, constructed on the dynamics of hopeless passion and inevitable societal repression, undeserved suffering and impossible choices, has historically had special contextual relevance for the women's audience. The melodrama – the woman's film, the weepie, the tear-jerker, the soap opera – has been traditionally opposed to the male genres of effective action and rationality in the outside world, from the western to the whodunit, and, until the feminist renovation of the discipline of film studies, was unjustly stigmatized by film historians for this reason. Gay critics have often followed this pattern, batting about pejorative terms like 'sentimental,' 'maudlin,' and 'Rodgers-and-Hammerstein' to dismiss one of the special if not essential forms of gay popular culture. They follow, as Richard Dyer has pointed out, our culture's put-down of forms too closely allied to bodily responses, like horror, arousal, belly-laughs, and weeping.[1]

The 1984–6 cycle of film and video melodramas may already be familiar to the reader: William Hoffman's *As Is*, adapted in 1986 by Home Box Office for pay-TV and the home video market; the two New York indie feature films, Arthur Bressan's *Buddies* (1985) and Bill Sherwood's *Parting Glances* (1986); and Stewart Main's and Peter Wells's New Zealand television film *A Death in the Family* (1986). To this list I would like to add two safer-sex porno-melodramas that express an undeniable continuity with the 'legit' works, *Inevitable Love* (1985), produced within the U.S. sex-video milieu and directed by a man named 'Mach,' who I am told is a prolific writer of erotic fiction; and *Chance of a Lifetime* (1985), produced by the Gay Men's Health Crisis (I am speaking primarily of the third episode, 'Hank and Jerry').[2]

These works remind us, as has often been argued, that the melodrama has had a privileged relationship with gay men as well as with women, both as audience and as producers, situated as we are, like women, if not outside patriarchal power, in ambiguous and contradictory relationship to it. It is not surprising that the community that enshrined *Camille*, *Dark Victory*, *Brief Encounter*, and *A Star Is Born* in the gay pantheon (and incidentally made major artistic contributions to those films as well) should have confirmed the melodrama as the key gay film genre of the period between Stonewall and the Epidemic: think of *A Very Natural Thing*, *Sunday Bloody Sunday*, *Fox and His Friends*, *The Consequence*, *Making Love*, and even *The Times of Harvey Milk*. The pattern continues with films like *Maurice*, situated outside of the AIDS problematic (inasmuch as that is possible).[3] As the epidemic entrenched itself, it was no accident, I'm sure, that one of the first major documentary features on AIDS, Nick Sheehan's *No Sad Songs* (Toronto, 1985) – a portrait of a man with AIDS taking leave of lover and family – echoed in its title *No Sad Songs for Me*, a 1950 Hollywood melodrama in which a terminally ill Margaret Sullavan prepares her children and husband to go on without her. The melodramas *Parting Glances*, *Chance of a Lifetime*, and *Inevitable Love* may all briefly play with male-action-genre iconography in the form of fantasy interludes (cowboys, Indians, GIs, and jocks), but the effect is to accentuate all the more their hasty return to the vale of kisses and tears, their proper genre home. The melodrama became the first and foremost fictional form for independent filmmakers addressing the health crisis within a popular constituency in the mid-eighties.

My emphasis in drawing up the list of AIDS melodramas is of course on *self*-representation, gay men's images of ourselves.[4] My corpus presumes by and large, for better or worse, the context of independent cinema and video. (The examples of the New Zealand television film *Death* and HBO's adaptation of *As Is* both confirm the continuing sad necessity of our reliance on gay-controlled independent media for our representation of our lives: although in both cases, the gay point of view is maintained and gay input is determining, material relating to the gay community's political response to the crisis was deleted along the road to broadcast.)

For independent gay artists to elicit tears as a response to the crisis is a worthy aesthetic strategy, especially when the tears are accompanied by the political lucidity that is also a feature of these films (to varying degrees it can of course be argued), and perhaps most important of all, when the tears are accompanied, as I would like to demonstrate in this essay, by other bodily secretions.

Secretions and sexuality are in fact at the centre of the discourse of the AIDS melodramas, and this I would argue is one of their great merits. The framework of sexual desire and love is so essential to the generic energy of these works that they should perhaps be categorized more precisely in terms of a sub-branch, the romantic melodrama. In the romantic melodrama, the problematic is not so much the crisis within the family, the nuclear family or the alternative surrogate family, as the impediments to the sexual founding of a romantic unit, the family itself. The independent gay filmmakers who produced the collective articulation of caution, mourning, and consolation constituted by the melodrama cycle have insisted on affirmative representations of our sexuality, on its celebration. In fact they organize the dramatic structure of the works around moments of sexual union and release. As *Buddies'* person-with-AIDS hero Robert declares: 'Sex is the part that makes you in or out.' In that film, as an act of sexual comforting, David, the volunteer buddy, gets alongside Robert, the PWA, in the hospital bed and cradles him as he masturbates. The act becomes an affirmation of Robert's identity, a bond between him and the world, an assurance that he will not die alone. It is also a reversal of an earlier scene of great pain, in which Robert masturbates compulsively and without pleasure as he looks at a picture of his ex-lover. 'It was terrible,' he told David, 'I jerked off. Oh, everything worked out. I hadn't fallen apart yet. My cock came but I didn't feel it. There's more to sex than the orgasm grabbed in the dark. I started alone and I finished alone. I don't want to die.' This opposition of 'bad/solitary sex' reversed and transcended through 'good/mutual sex' provides the dramatic framework for several other works, including both *As Is* and 'Hank and Jerry.' In *As Is*, one of several works patterned on the separation and reconciliation of lovers, the first sexual encounter is derailed by the discovery of a Kaposi lesion on the protagonist Richard's back. At the end, Richard has evolved from his former anger and denial, and a final act of sexual sharing in the hospital bed between the reunited lovers signifies their serenity in the face of the crisis, and the rescue of sex from its association with disease. In 'Hank and Jerry,' the PWA's masturbatory dream, though not signified as traumatic, is supplanted by a long sequence of sexual play and consummation with his lover, orgasm dissolving into embrace, the lovers trembling and sobbing with emotion. In all three works, sexuality is a sacramental charge impelling and resolving the melodramatic moment, as well as signifying the force of renewal, healing, and comfort.

The sexualization of the person with AIDS in these films, his conception as an active sexual agent, constitutes a defiant articulation of desire and sexual identity in the face of the stereotypes, the taboos, and the death we know so well. It is also a gesture towards incorporating the point of view of the character into the discourse of AIDS, a reversal of the silencing, inoculation, and ridicule that have occulted the reality of these figures in the media. The person with AIDS is shown not only as sexual but also in several instances as downright sexy.

Characters peripheral to the key person with AIDS participate in this sustenance of an erotic narrative universe. The buddy protagonist of *Buddies* is seen more often in his underwear in this single film than

Clara Bow was in her entire career, participating in an idealized and fulfilled relationship with his lover as well as in his increasingly sexualized ministry to Robert. In *Death* also, though less explicit, a diffuse sexual camaraderie is seen as the cement holding together the group of gay male mourners. As for the safer-sex films, needless to say, they do not hesitate to follow the prescriptions of the porno genre, investing every character, line, and situation with an overstated sexual potential.

The transformational operation of sexual exchange attains a particular complexity in *Buddies* through an iconographic opposition of 'before' and 'after,' images of the previously healthy character with AIDS being inserted into the unfolding of the narrative. This is true also of Stash Kybaratas' admirable 1987 video *Danny*, and of course of the majority of the PWA documentaries. Unfortunately it is equally a gruesome feature of mainstream-media representation of AIDS, as several commentators have pointed out, the foundation of the medical pornography of the doomed homosexual and deserving victim. Bressan's orchestration of the structure, relying on both stills and home-movie images of Robert's sunny California past as a countercultural beach hunk, evokes a sexual history in the company of previous lovers that occasions no regrets, no retroactive dynamics of inevitability or morality. It is a past to be celebrated, not to be paid for. As buddy David's personal and sexual commitment to Robert grows, he begins to inhabit that flashback past; fantasizing himself as Robert's beach companion, he begins to claim it as part of his own sexual identity. His idealized and never-seen lover accepts this sharing of his lover's erotic energy with a third man who is nevertheless not felt as a rival. A further dimension is added during Robert's climactic scene of sexual re-affirmation: as he masturbates he is watching on the VCR that David has brought him the 1974 porno film *Passing Strangers* by none other than Arthur Bressan. A private self-referential conceit no doubt, but in retrospect this autobiographical insert is moving beyond words as the late artist's incorporation of *his* own past, his sexual and artistic history, even his testament, into the text. But even for the spectator unaware of this poignant extra-filmic significance, the short clip connotes *our* history through the performers' rippling hippy hairstyles and their aura of San Francisco and gay liberation, a utopian vision of sexuality reclaimed and restored from the past. An affirmation of our cultural heritage of eroticism, epidemic or no, the insert is also an exploration of the erotic component of individual and collective memory. Robert's individual home movie becomes paired with this collective home movie that Bressan's porno film represents and the gay liberationist heritage is conjured up to bolster us in the midst of crisis.

In contrast, *Parting Glances*, a film unanimously acclaimed on its release, now seems to offer by and large a sexual discourse that is somewhat less affirmative of gay sexuality than may have at first appeared. Here sexuality seems to be less transformational in both its personal and dramatic operation than a dramatic pretext and a psychic plateau to be left behind. The main protagonist, Michael, is seen emerging from a love relationship in which sex has a teasing, coercive quality. The melodramatic transformation that occurs is not the renewal of this relationship – though the open ending does not rule out this possibility – but the strengthening of his relationship with Nick, his AIDS-stricken buddy, a character for whom he has always had an unacknowledged and unrequited love deeper even than his sexual love for the *Gentlemen's Quarterly*–style heel he lives with – shades of Scarlett O'Hara's love for Ashley Wilkes. Michael's relationship with Nick, like the relationship in Bressan's *Buddies*, grows and deepens, evolving from adolescent arm-wrestling to cathartic dish-smashing, platonic embraces, and visions of open-ended voyages to be embarked on together, but it never becomes sexual in the genital sense. Though Nick maintains a kind of gaunt rock-star sexual glamour in the present (he admits to his buddy that he's a thrice-daily masturbator), and a kind of punkish friskiness in the fantasy sequences, sexual exchange seems to be out of the question. *Parting Glances*, otherwise abounding in deceitful or perverse heterosexual relationships and unconsummated gay flirtations, ultimately articulates an attitude towards sexuality that is ambiguous at the very best and at worst symptomatic of a cynical distrust of sexuality that has been reinforced by the health crisis.

Another recent gay melodrama with a not-dissimilar pattern of the abandonment of traitorous and illusory sexual passion in favour of platonic friendship is Dick Benner's Canadian sequel *Too Outrageous* (1988). Though AIDS is a minor theme in this film, Benner's profound and unresolved AIDS scars are less smoothly camouflaged than in the New York equivalent: an appealing secondary character suddenly starts a Camille-like cough and is given first the scriptwriter's trapdoor treatment, then is over-motivated retroactively through misleading and didactic fast-talking. *As Is* gives occasional evidence of a similar disturbance, though it is ultimately patched over. In addition to *As Is*'s symptomatic connotations of the first lovemaking scene privileged as the occasion for the discovery of the lesion, already mentioned, other aspects contribute to an undermining of the positive vision of sexuality that Hoffman may have been attempting. One scene offers an uncompassionate satire of a pick-up in a leather bar, retained from the play even as the health-crisis hotline scene was dropped. The secondary characterization of Chet, the most recent lover of the character with AIDS, is especially problematical. The only figure in the work constructed in terms of conventional erotic codes of nudity, Chet is seen splitting up the originally happy couple and deserting his new lover after the diagnosis; then he himself gets the AIDS trapdoor treatment in the next act, implicated by simple inference as the adulterous source of the hero's infection.

Inevitable Love, one of the two safer-sex videos that are part of this melodrama corpus, is successful in almost entirely avoiding the naming of AIDS (there is a single reference).[5] Nevertheless, AIDS is a structuring absence, accentuated by the conspicuous emphasis on safer sex and condoms and the occasional passing lecture on condom use. It deploys very much the same transformational structure of sexual meanings and positive perspective of sexuality as *Buddies* and *Chance*. Two closeted room-mates, unaware of each other's love, must suffer an ordeal of separation and bad sex (safe and hot, but bad) before finally being reunited, sexually this time, with the line 'Forget about the past.' The melodrama of unspoken passion has always been a basic formula for the porno industry, with *Navy Blue*, Francis Ellie's mid-seventies classic, providing the basic plot formula for this variation that substitutes college jocks for sailors. The final sex scene risks being anticlimactic, given the intensity of the various 'ordeals' and adventures along the road to the lovers' reunion. The editor comes to the rescue with an interpolated flashback of the lovers' original crotch-grabbing wrestling scene from their innocent sublimated past. The effect, in its endearingly trashy way, lacks neither erotic power nor melodramatic transcendence.

A Death in the Family is the only one of the AIDS melodramas to confront through full dramatic representation the death of a major character with AIDS. Surrounded by his alternative gay 'family,' Andrew lapses in and out of consciousness as the last sixteen days of his life parade by. The transformational sexual structure of the other melodramas is nevertheless still recognizable, now however altered by the circumstances of the plot. After his death the ritual of sexual renewal is taken over by two of the mourners who have been brought together by the death. The two men, who have been seen exchanging meaningful looks throughout, are shown kissing, tentatively at first, as much out of mutual consolation as desire, and their eventual sexual union is only implied.

As for the PWA, like the characters with AIDS in *Buddies*, *As Is*, and *Parting Glances*, Andrew's moribund figure is still eroticized in his way. I am speaking on one level of a certain element in his visual conception that consigns an almost ethereal beauty to his face, body, and limbs.[6] At the same time, through the mise-en-scène of non-verbal communication, Andrew's body is constantly maintained in sensuous tactile contact with his grieving friends. Comfort is implicitly shared back and forth through caresses, touching, looks, and smiles. The bathing scene, a traditional format for the erotic representation of the body, is particularly eloquent in this regard, luxuriating in the textures of skin and fabric, in the light reflected in the movement of water, and above all in the simple child-like pleasure registered on Andrew's face. At another point, Andrew plays with his doctor's baby, enriching the atmosphere of pansexuality (as well as inserting an important didactic message about contagion). Even after his death, Andrew's corpse continues to be an erotic icon, like the bodies of martyrs in the Baroque painterly traditions evoked continuously by the filmmakers' composition and lighting; his body continues to be touched, even caressed, with the classical imagery of candle flame, flowers, and sky now adding to the sensuous luminosity.

It is Wells's and Main's insight into the erotic nature of comforting and receiving comfort, of the human body even in abject humiliation and pain, of the sexual dimensions of the act of mourning itself, whether solitary or communal, that particularly distinguishes *A Death in the Family*. This insight is present in a more diffuse way in all the melodramas under discussion, by the very nature of their generic construction and address: all melodramas invoke after all the contradictory beauty and pleasure of suffering. In *Danny*, the videomaker's grieving voice makes this point explicitly as his camera lovingly scans in tight close-up both of Danny's bodies, before and after AIDS-related chemotherapy. Eroticism is clearly a potentially creative phase in the trajectory of the responses to dying and death, an embodiment of acceptance and affirmation of the body. As Michael Bronski has argued in his moving personal reflection on this unconventional association of sex and death, eroticism is, for the mourner, as in this context for the artist and the spectator, 'a constructive way to regain a sense of self and strength in a world that is too difficult to bear at the moment ... The primal act of sex seems to mock death by reaffirming the feeling of being alive.'[7]

What about safer sex? The space remains only briefly to inventory and reflect on the discourse of nuts-and-bolts sexual behaviours within the framework of the melodrama genre, and in reference to the political imperative of the films' context. The 'legit' films (that is, non-explicit ones) tend to privilege relationship sex, as the current fashion and the generic demands of the melodrama would have it, though they do not close the door on what the lovers of *As Is* nostalgically call 'non-committed sex.' Masturbation is acknowledged to exist and to be a valid dimension of the sexual spectrum, as is group sex, but ultimately the couple is the locus of the positive incarnations of sexuality that are envisioned. Except for *Buddies*, none of the legit films depicts orgasm directly, and this may testify to an evolving conception of sexual behaviour in our community, the dispersal of the cult of cum. The safer-sex videos support this hypothesis, not only through the almost total banishment of the close-up 'money shot' from the iconographic register (the de-fetishization of the infested discharge?), but also in the opening up of the spectrum of sexual behaviours. Of particular interest is the legitimation of a sexual union in which one or even both partners may not come. Otherwise, heavy scrotal licking and on-the-belly and between-the-legs *frottage* are on the ascendent. Condoms are surprisingly rare, except in *Inevitable Love*, where they are everyone's 'favourite thing to wear' (to quote John Greyson's safer-sex rock video *The ADS Epidemic*). *Chance* eschews anal fucking, even protected, but *Inevitable* goes all out. It is ironic that kissing rather than fucking remains the litmus test of sexual politics, as it was before AIDS: its absence from *As Is* calls into question the good faith of the Home Box Office apparatus and the straight-identified actor in the lead role, just as its delirious presence throughout the safer-sex films and *Parting Glances*, and of course its climactic function in *Death*, *My Beautiful Laundrette*, *Maurice*, *Torch Song Trilogy*, and even *Kiss of the Spider Woman* indicate a new maturity in our sexual self-representation. Kissing, with the romantic even transcendental semiotic baggage it has acquired in our culture, returns us to the subject of melodrama, where the nitty-gritty of condoms unfortunately seems ill-suited to the spiritual union of two hearts. Did Rock Hudson wear a condom in *Magnificent Obsession*?[8]

The mechanics of love and orgasm are thus evolving in the domain of our self-representation. Our melodramas have reflected this to a greater or lesser degree. Perhaps more important, their resurgence in the mid-eighties may have helped keep in view a certain continuity of cultural tradition and sex-positive erotic energy, mingling the 'positive image' ideology of seventies gay-lib aesthetics with the cathartic function of narrative fiction, to help us in the crisis of the eighties and nineties to communally mourn the dead, comfort the living, and imagine the future. None of the films or videos I have discussed is without ideological tensions and elisions, yet they have participated in a kind of cultural healing process within the framework of gay popular culture. In so far as they have succeeded in flowing through the channels of ghetto distribution, they have been at the centre of our evolving political and cultural consciousness.

Nevertheless, the melodrama cycle may now have spent most of its force and its mythic concerns may be resurfacing within other generic forms. A possible indication of future directions is the German filmmaker Rosa von Praunheim's *A Virus Has No Morals* (1986), a film that replaces the aesthetics of comfort and eroticism with one of assault. Towards the end of the film, the principal character (played by the filmmaker himself), an unscrupulous gay sauna owner who thinks safe sex is bad for business, is wandering amid the flower beds of a cemetery, thinking about the epidemic, his sex life, and a departed employee, organ music sobbing in the background. 'This disease makes me horny ...,' goes his voice-over soliloquy. 'Sex is life and I believe in life.'

One might think out of context that this is a conventional scene of the melodrama genre: von Praunheim might have been Shirley MacLaine at the end of *Terms of Endearment*. Yet the context in *Virus* disallows this reading: elsewhere, this 'black comedy' (as it is tactfully labelled by distributors to ward off audience uprisings) is a bleak nihilistic dystopian farce in which every possible implicated constituency is scornfully satirized – medical researchers, health-care workers, tabloid reporters, people with AIDS, AIDS activists, Christian celibates, gay profiteers, AIDS therapists, bureaucrats, mothers, widows, and babies. Everyone gets AIDS and ends up in a concentration camp called 'Hellgayland.' In short, *Virus* is an anti-melodrama. A long series of melodramatic situations is shredded with gleeful Brechtian savagery: in addition to the hospital-bed suffering scene exploding in a murderous assault with an infected syringe, there is also a tearful reunion with a mother figure that degenerates into a raucous screaming match, and a poignant diagnosis that quickly slides into slapstick.

What about sex? Sex is a half-hearted ritual in an empty sauna littered with shit, in a cruising park where condoms dangle from the trees and used kleenexes cover the earth. It is hesitatingly approached by naked young innocents wandering around at the end of the world.

Sex becomes what Arthur Kroker would call cynical and parodic, panic sex, sex without secretions by bodies in ruins at the postmodern end of the simulacrum of the world, the pleasure of catastrophe. Eroticism is as impossible as is melodrama itself. Is von Praunheim engaged in a clever political tactic for stirring up our profoundest cultural response by turning the melodrama upside down, or is his work simply a way of dealing culturally with the epidemic, an artistic embodiment of the stage of mingled rage, paranoia, and suicidal self-pity that many of us have gone through or shall go through? It is only our knowledge of the context of *A Virus Has No Morals*, and its use within its author's tireless AIDS activism in Germany, that allows us to infer some level of sincere commitment from the graveyard credo. It is interesting that the film, despite a few enthusiastic reviews, has to my knowledge not really struck a responsive chord outside of Germany.

The anti-melodrama is not the only alternative: Canadian video-maker John Greyson has evolved from a 1985 coming-out melodrama *The Jungle Boy* to a new feature film *Urinal* (1988), a political sci-fi parlour mystery, as playfully sex-positive and studiously camp as it is lucid and angry, situating the health crisis on a spectrum of other gay political issues and beyond. This hopefully may be part of a larger pattern. Will the gay melodrama expand its role of conscience, consolation, pillow-book and elegy, cross-fertilizing with those other resilient cultural forms of our heritage, comedy and camp, as they adjust to the imperatives of the current political emergency? Can the deconstructive froth of the camp response and the visionary anger of the activist documentaries absorb the depth of feeling and affirmation of desire that the AIDS melodramas articulated?[9] Should we ask for both the moon and the stars?

NOTES

1 Two book-length historical studies of the film melodrama that appeared in 1987 are Mary Ann Doane *The Desire to Desire: The Woman's Film of the 1940s* (Bloomington: Indiana University Press) and Christine Gledhill, ed, *Home Is Where the Heart Is: Studies in Melodrama and the Woman's Film* (London: BFI), which includes several of the pioneering individual articles on the subject that have appeared since 1970. A similar re-estimation of the importance of the melodrama is taking place in literary studies, as Geoffrey Rans mentioned to me at Western, pointing me to such works as Philip Fisher *Hard Facts: Setting and Form in the American Novel* (New York:

Oxford 1985) and Jane P. Tompkins *Sensational Designs: The Cultural Work of American Fiction* (New York: Oxford 1985). Dyer's comment is in 'Male Gay Porn: Coming to Terms,' special section on 'Sexual Representation,' *Jump Cut* (Chicago and Berkeley) 30 (March 1985) 27–9.

2 The 1988 French film by Paul Vecchiali, *Encore* (*Once More*), may also be added to this list, but I will not come back to it since I have not ascertained its cultural context and cannot say whether the producers are merchandising AIDS to the dominant culture as yet another morbid metaphor or whether this problematical and disturbing work can be situated as an authentic utterance from within the gay community. Outside the purview of my audiovisual corpus, Larry Kramer's theatrical play *The Normal Heart*, it may be noted, also has a strong melodramatic line, involving a traditional teeter-totter between the demands of love and vocation, and culminating in a deathbed marriage ceremony.

3 Mark Finch and Richard Kwietniowski have commented on the melodramatic affinity of *Maurice* in an astute and acerbic article ('Melodrama and *Maurice*: Homo Is Where the Het Is' *Screen* 29, no. 3 [Summer 1988] 72–83), but it is a film that I am not ashamed to admire. *Maurice* belongs to an impulse towards literary adaptations from the pre-AIDS universe that admittedly signifies in some ways an escape from the demands of the present, but, notwithstanding its Masterpiece Theatre class aura, Ivory's work has importance in terms of a popular project of the restoration of gay historical memory.

4 For this reason I do not consider such made-for-television melodramas as *An Early Frost*, regardless of how much gay input may have been present, since their emphasis on the heterosexual point of view moves this work over into the problematic of media representation of AIDS, a topic that is currently receiving the lion's share of gay cultural analysis.

5 There is no space here for a tirade about the thriving porno industry's avoidance of the epidemic (except for a few exemplary figures like Richard Locke). It's unfathomable to me why there has been so little debate about the industry's utter bad faith in its masking of whatever safe sex the performers are fortunate enough to be allowed to practise on the set, and above all in its abundant glamourization of risk behaviours. Apart from perfunctory printed guidelines scrolling here and there, and some producers' self-righteously pronounced avoidance of internal ejaculation (when did the cum-shot trade *ever* show internal ejaculation?), the industry's culpability in this matter is a baldly stated matter of record. Nor is there space to savour the irony that our arguments about the difference between individual consumer fantasy and the collective politics of sexual practices, advanced in the porn

and censorship wars of the early eighties, are now coming back to haunt those of us who are very disturbed about the foot-dragging of the porno sector.

6 Of course, this has left *Death in the Family* open to the criticism (not long in coming in today's vigilant climate) that the ugliness of AIDS deaths is thereby trivialized, a criticism that if valid is equally applicable to all the works under study. However, unless we insist that fiction's aims are to provide medical documentation, rather than to operate mythically on some level, this criticism does not invalidate the films.

7 'Death, AIDS and the Transfiguration of Grief: Thoughts on the Sexualization of Mourning' *Gay Community News* (Boston) 24–30 July 1988, 20, 13

8 Cindy Patton is developing some interesting analysis of the representation of sexual intercourse in mainstream material, heterosexual as well as lesbian/gay, since the onset of the epidemic. A promising instalment is 'The Cum Shot: 3 Takes on Lesbian and Gay Sexuality' *Outlook* (San Francisco) 1, no. 3 (Fall 1988) 72–7.

9 One listener's response at the London conference reminded me that my discussion is open to the misreading that I am arguing an 'unproblematical return to the melodrama' as a useful activist cultural strategy. This is certainly not the intent of this historical assessment of various works within gay popular culture of the mid-1980s. If there is any implied tactical prescription in this analysis, it would simply be that activist artistic initiatives need to harness positive erotic energies, as well as incorporate existing momentum from within gay popular culture(s), as opposed to some of the inaccessibly avant-gardist and deconstructive efforts in which our community resources have been invested (which fortunately remain in the minority). It would also seem appropriate for the activists who have surfaced during the crisis to profit from the lessons learned by the earlier 1970s generation of cultural activists, on the left as well as within the gay/lesbian movements: namely, that a wide range of cultural responses (pleasure, humour, eroticism, fantasy, and pathos) is important within a broad-based culture of resistance; and that anger, denunciation, and reactive media critique cannot be the sole cultural diet of a community in for a long haul.

Parma Violets for Wayland Flowers

JOHN GREYSON

Many well-meaning souls (including even Richard Goldstein, an otherwise thoughtful gay writer for the *Village Voice*) have claimed that the AIDS crisis is resulting in a cultural renaissance – that old 'great art is born of suffering' line. Well, thanks but no thanks. Concepts of 'great art' ultimately benefit only those collectors who want hefty returns on their investments, rarely the communities that originate such production. Renaissances are usually identified after the fact, claimed by bystanders who have achieved a safe, contemplative distance. The romance of suffering is affordable only to the bourgeoisie, who vicariously consume it, but by definition never do it.

For us artists in the midst of the maelstrom, it's a matter of supreme indifference to us to learn, as another critic has suggested, that our collective body of work from this last decade will one day be studied with the same reverence and fascination currently reserved for the literature of the Second World War. Our motivations for making art about AIDS are as diverse as our sexual, regional, racial, and political identities, but they are all rooted in the absolute terms of this very present moment. We make AIDS art to heal, to mourn, to rage, to engage, to change. It is often as much for ourselves, our friends and lovers, as it is for our communities and our publics. It is hardly a surprise that our cultural production is addressing our experience of AIDS. Indeed, it would be truly shocking if our response were any less urgent, vital, and voluminous.

What is also not surprising is that an urgent, vital, and voluminous critical debate has accompanied this production, on the one hand dissecting mass cultural constructions of AIDS and its effects and, on the other hand, interrogating the various expressions of artists addressing the crisis.

The following fake video script was written as a contribution to a particular debate among gay male artists that reached a head (so to speak) with an exhibition called 'Against Nature,' sponsored by the Los Angeles artists' space, LACE, in January 1989 (an adapted version of this script constituted my catalogue essay). The curatorial concept was inspired by Joris-Karl Huysmans' *Against Nature*, a satirical nineteenth-century French novel that celebrated artifice and dandyism. With tongue firmly in cheek, Huysmans recorded the self-imposed aesthetic exile of Des Esseintes, an aesthete languishing from an (unnamed) malady that suspiciously resembled ennui. Like other closety classics that metaphorically conflate disease with desire (*Death in Venice*, *The Picture of Dorian Gray*, the collected works of Denton Welch), *Against Nature* has been virtually re-written (or rather, re-read) into a fable about the health crisis.

Rather than resisting such re-reading, the curators sought to reclaim, seeking work that referenced AIDS from the ironic, campy perspective of latter-day dandies. They looked for stuff that was biting, bitchy, irreverent, self-consciously decorative, elegiac, impolite, bad boy, and certainly not 'politically correct,' whatever that insidious phrase means. In part, they said the show was a response to the emergence in 1987 of activist AIDS art, as typified by artists' collectives in New York like Gran Fury, Testing the Limits, and various ACT UP (AIDS Coalition To Unleash Power) artists, among others. Unfortunately, this intention was never spelled out in the catalogue, only discussed orally on several occasions.

'Against Nature' intended to insist on the relevance of a particular fag sensibility in combating the AIDS crisis. Whether it succeeded or not is a matter of opinion. Like any group theme show, there was a disjunction between the curatorial intentions and the diverse work gathered, which didn't always neatly fit the organizing premise. Within the LA art scene, there was heated debate before the show opened. Some were appalled because it was an all-boys show – others were outraged at the almost total lack of artists of colour. Rumours that ACT UP was going to picket the opening because the show allegedly lacked 'activist art' proved to be totally unfounded. Though agitprop artists were notoriously absent, the show did end up including works that certainly referenced the political and social experience of gay men and AIDS (Doug Ischar's photo-text works and Michael Tidmus' computer piece being two examples).

My own responses to these arguments were complicated (I was in town for the pre-show debates but not the show itself). I certainly welcomed the curatorial premise (especially with its promise of humour) since such a fag sensibility in culture is too often woefully undertheorized or simply denied, and the show seemed to offer an opportunity for exploring the subjective experiences of gay men living in the AIDies. Just as there is a need at times to have lesbian-only shows (what an understatement!), likewise it's sometimes appropriate for gay men to get together and find out where we're at. Still, fags have always been somewhat privileged members of the white-boy art scene, as long as we didn't get too outrageous, while dykes have always suffered the systematic exclusion shared by most women artists. This was the first 'gay' show, and the first 'AIDS' show, in Los Angeles – and for lesbians, out-PLWAs, and AIDS activists to be excluded (and for fags of colour to be represented in such token numbers) seemed inexcusable, given that the art scene is notorious for never returning to an uncomfortable subject: 'We did a gay/AIDS show last year – it's time for something else.' At the same time, no one show can correct the injustices of history, nor can it answer everyone's agendas. Certainly LACE's track record around such issues of representation in the past has hardly been exemplary; yet other previous group theme shows (like the Surveillance show) didn't spark the outrage that this one engendered. On reflection, this is not surprising – AIDS, by personally affecting so many of us so deeply, demands a vehemence that few other issues can approach.

For the catalogue, I chose to take up in fictive form the debate that posited 'activist' art against 'dandy' art, a particular debate that is occurring among gay artists in many cities in North America and Europe. Fags everywhere feel the absolute necessity of responding to this viral holocaust, but we disagree about the aesthetic and political strategies that are appropriate. We especially disagree about what we variously mean by aesthetics and politics. During a war (which this most definitely is), should we adopt conventional forms (for video artists, the documentary or the music video) to reach large audiences who mistrust artsy experimentation, or should we develop a critical deconstructive vocabulary that stands in sharp contrast to the smug distortions of the mass media? During a war, should we put our personal voices (with their ambivalences and doubts) aside in favour of collective calls-to-action that empower? During a war, should we prefer elegies or agitprops? During a war, should we abandon our campy sensibilities and adopt the ideological uniform of the 'fighting man'?

Metaphors of war inevitably invoke those very constructions of masculinity that gays and lesbians have struggled for so long to reject. Indeed, Susan Sontag has similarly noted how militaristic metaphors are continually trotted out to describe AIDS, and pleaded for an end to 'the metaphors of AIDS.' Yet metaphors have always been weapons that fags and dykes have used to advantage, even as they were used against us. Persecuted by languages that transformed love into perversion, we were forced to build our illegal culture with the same tricks of language – it was with the double entendres, the allusions, the code words, and the metaphors of our slang that we invented ourselves, and dared to speak our names. Such an armoury should obviously not be abandoned in the face of this crisis, but rather pressed into active duty.

Nearly a year has passed since 'Against Nature,' and the dandy vs. the activist debate has continued on other fronts and in other contexts. Most people seem to agree now (perhaps I'm being optimistic) that the debate sets up a false opposition – that indeed the dandy and the activist can sometimes be one and the same. Artists are continuing the dialogue, listening to the subtleties, the surprising points where our disparate aspirations and practices mesh – and appreciating critically the places where they contradict. We seem to be beyond a point where narrow manifestos are called for, prescribing that propaganda (or, alternatively, personal expression) is the only correct artistic response. 'Against Nature' (not despite of but because of the debates it triggered) certainly contributed constructively to this process.

This dialogue among artists is occurring in the fringes and shadows of what has become a sprawling AIDS cultural industry. Worldwide, millions upon millions of dollars are now spent annually spewing forth books, films, tapes, pamphlets, posters, plays, and even limited-edition art objects that claim to address the subject. Some of the work is wonderful. Most of it is reactionary, opportunistic dreck. Within both academia and the art scene, careers are being built on the backs of the AIDS crisis, often on the backs of people living with AIDS. Too often during the 'Representing AIDS: Crisis and Criticism' conference, I noticed the voices of activists and dandies being dismissed by the 'more authoritative' discourses of medicine, social science, philosophy, law. I hope that people who read this volume won't be satisfied with simply consuming AIDS as a theoretical paradigm of the postmodern condition. Instead, readers should also search out those harder-to-hear voices (the fags, the dykes, the activists, especially the PLWAs) in the alternative magazines, the grass-roots AIDS organizations, the gay bookstores, at the rallies and demonstrations that demand direct action. To quote Gran Fury from their 1989 catalogue insert for another AIDS and the Arts conference: 'WITH 2962* DEAD, ART IS NOT ENOUGH. Our culture gives artists permission to name oppression, a permission denied to those oppressed. Outside the pages of this catalogue, permission is being seized by many communities to save their own lives. We urge you to take collective direct action to end the AIDS crisis.'

*I changed this number to record the number of Canadians who are known to have died from AIDS, as close to the date of publication as possible (3 June 1991). Sadly, this number is out of date. Sadly, by the time you finish reading this fake video script, it will be out of date again.

A Fake Video Script

Scene One

[Medium shot of Venice Beach in winter, with a few gulls and fewer bathers. An AFRICAN GREEN MONKEY strolls toward the camera. His movements are awkward, since he has been killed, stuffed, and then mechanized.]

GREEN MONKEY (*sounding like Alistair Cooke*): Good evening. Tonight on *The Wonderful World of Human Nature*, we examine the bizarre and often misunderstood habits of the *dandy*. This sub-group of the Homosexual species used to proliferate in 19th-century European artistic milieux, but its numbers have sharply decreased in the last few decades with the ascendancy of the more aggressive *clone*. The *dandy* can be identified by its eccentric clothing, its erratic wrist movements, and its predilection for Parma violets in lieu of a cravat.

[Camera cuts to medium shot of man in a beach chair.]

GREEN MONKEY (*sotto voce*): Let us quietly observe the typical behaviour of the dandy in its habitat. Our scientists have learned that this one goes by the name of Gustav Aschenbach.

[ASCHENBACH is dressed from head to toe in a white suit and boating hat, just like Dirk Bogarde in that Visconti film. After adjusting his pillow and pince-nez, he petulantly turns the page of his book. Mahler plays mournfully in the background. A flowery script, the colour of Parma violets, begins to roll over the screen.]

ROLLING TEXT: Dandies are a special breed of nature lovers, searching for those corners of the urban where the rural erupts. Dandies seek out those bridges that traverse polluted rivers, with deep shadows over the water. They embrace the stench of tea-room sewers, casting their pollution into the drains that lead to the sea.

GREEN MONKEY: Like many of the Dandy sub-species, he is sick with a peculiar malady that causes him to imagine things that aren't really there.

[Medium shot: ASCHENBACH looks up and out to sea. Cut to: long shot of an 18th-century cargo vessel in the fog. Its sailors (all naked) are leaping from the decks into the cold grey water.]

ROLLING TEXT: In 1721, the plague swept across Europe from the east and reached Marseilles. The Dutch imposed a strict quarantine on all shipping from the east – even burning cargoes and making sailors swim ashore naked.

[Series of close-ups of the men's bodies, shot from underwater, their thighs and forearms getting tangled with one another as they desperately battle the cold, polluted waters of Santa Monica bay.]

Scene Two

[Later in the afternoon on the beach. Medium shot: ASCHENBACH has set up a writing table and is sorting through piles of correspondence. He dips a quill in ink the colour of Parma violets and begins to write.]

ASCHENBACH (*very faggy and affected*): 'Dear CBC: I am thrilled to be able to participate in your exquisite TV special, *AIDS: Culture and Nature*. What a divine concept! An entire show devoted to our languid reveries, our elegiac *ennui*, our plaintive sighs of capitulation in the face of mortality! We decorative dandies have been marginalized too long by those puerile politicos, those righteous gay libbers, those dykes and feminists who *on principle* disdain both soufflés and sequins! It's time to reclaim our rightful place as the arbiters of aesthetic transcendence! At last, a space of our own, where we may celebrate dilettantism as the penultimate expression of art's true mission! A chance to spill our glorious seed, to let it go forth and multiply, to let it breed with disease and desire, so that we can wallow in our truly bitter harvest! A chance to finally, fully, go camping ...'

[SFX: Phone ringing. Tight shot of answering machine and phone at ASCHENBACH'S feet in the sand. Reaction shots of ASCHENBACH listening as people leave messages.]

VOICE ON MACHINE: It's Paul, calling from the hospital ...

[SFX: Beep.]

ANOTHER MESSAGE: It's Bill, I'm just on my way to the hospital ...

ANOTHER: It's Bev, we're planning the memorial and we hoped ...

ANOTHER: Please call Dr Simian about your test results ...

[ASCHENBACH reaches for the phone and falls back, his listless hand falling to the sand. A delicate tear drops onto the letter, mixing with the wet ink, blurring the word, reveries ...]

Scene Three

[Split screen of two maps of Africa – one negative (black), one positive (white). The head of the GREEN MONKEY appears in the middle of each and simultaneously reads the following texts:]

'If art is to confront AIDS more honestly than the media have done, it must begin in tact, avoid humour, and end in anger. Begin in tact, I say, because humour seems grotesquely inappropriate to the occasion. Humour puts the public (indifferent when not uneasy) on cosy terms with what is an unspeakable scandal: death.'

Edmund White *Artforum* 1987

'Art does have the power to save lives, and it is this very power that must be recognized, fostered, and supported in every way possible. But if we are to do this, we will have to abandon the idealist conception of art. We don't need a cultural renaissance; we need cultural practices actively participating in the struggle against AIDS. We don't need to transcend the epidemic; we need to end it.'

Douglas Crimp *October* 1987

[The two maps and two monkey heads begin to superimpose.]

GREEN MONKEYS (*speaking in unison*): This juxtaposition, brought to you courtesy of the CBC, should be mistrusted. These two quotes, taken out of their contexts, plucked from their sources, are symbolic of two opposing polemics, two prescriptions for cultural practices concerning AIDS: the art of the dandy vs. the art of the activist. This roughly parallels a similar division that some claim has polarized AIDS organizations: on the one hand, the conservative service organizations, like the AIDS Committee of Toronto, which are characterized as being uncritical beneficiaries of conservative state funding; and on the other hand, the newer, radical AIDS activist groups like AIDS ACTION NOW!, which use direct-action strategies to fight for the rights of people living with AIDS.

Of course, such simplistic oppositions quickly become inflexible, didactic, exclusionary, defensive, ignoring contradictions and erasing common points of allegiance. The reciprocal (and certainly uneasy) *developing* relationship between service and activist groups is far too complicated to reduce to dogmatic disavowals. In a similar way, the work that gay men are producing about AIDS cannot be reduced to a false opposition between *propaganda* and *personal expression*. As Crimp and others have pointed out many times, the complex intertwinings of political and aesthetic agendas in cultural productions are far too subtle (and vital) to reduce to expedient dichotomies. Under careful scrutiny, the dandy and the activist may turn out (in some cases) to be one and the same.

Scene Four

[Tracking shot follows the GREEN MONKEY *wandering through a toy store, past rows and rows of stuffed animals.]*

GREEN MONKEY: Dandies express their relation to nature in peculiar ways. For instance, King Ludwig II of Bavaria created an artificial forest and filled it with mechanical animals that he killed, stuffed, and then animated with wind-up clock-work mechanisms. That's how I ended up this way. *[He gestures to his mechanical limbs.]* Sir Richard Burton, that brilliant dandy and close friend of Ludwig, similarly loved African animals and was an infamous adventurer. He translated the unexpurgated *Arabian Nights* and developed a theory of sexuality based upon what he identified as the 'sotadic zones.' He claimed that warm tropical climates encouraged the proliferation of homosexuality, while colder temperatures tended to produce heterosexual behaviour. However, when he sketched out a map illustrating his theory, it proved to be wildly indifferent to actual equatorial temperatures, conforming instead to the moral and legal geography of the time. His sotadic zones, in fact, consisted of those countries uncolonized by Christianity, where homosexual acts were tolerated.

[Shot of Sir Richard Burton's sotadic-zone map, which is then superimposed over a map illustrating the prevalence of AIDS *around the globe. They do not correspond.]*

Scene Five

[Long shot of SIR RICHARD BURTON *walking along Hollywood Boulevard. He enters a sex shop. Interior: He gives the guy at the cash register a dollar. Camera follows them both as the guy unlocks a door and leads* BURTON *down into The Sex Museum, pausing to switch on an audio cassette tape-loop of passionate groans and clanking chains. Camera surveys various dioramas, lit by spotlights. Each illustrates a category of sexual perversion, as identified and isolated by scientific study. Pedophilia is a young mannequin boy in shorts on a square of astroturf. Necrophilia is a blonde mannequin woman lying in a coffin wearing a see-through negligee. All the mannequins are from the sixties – the women have flips and beehives, the men have Rock Hudson haircuts, parted on the left side.* BURTON *moves towards a pool of light depicting bestiality. A mannequin man is on his back, pink plastic legs in the air, being mounted by a huge, stuffed toy dog – the sort you win at the fair playing Racetrack with squirtguns.]*

SIR RICHARD BURTON (*sitting at a table in the Pioneer Chicken on Hollywood Boulevard. He is writing a letter with ink the colour of Parma violets.):* 'Dear CBC: I regret I can't participate in your documentary about AIDS and artists entitled *AIDS: Culture and Nature*. I'm afraid I disagree with your editorial premise, which suggests that our artistic response to this health crisis has been nothing more than an ineffectually morbid flap of the wrist. We dandies may be obsessed with aesthetics, but that doesn't mean we're also immune to responsibility. Just because we don't produce works that engage actual agendas of social change doesn't mean we're ultimately vulnerable to being recuperated by the very system we seek to disrupt. Your program seems to exclude artists of colour, women artists, activist artists, focusing exclusively on us 'white fags.' I suspect you want to perpetuate the portrait of the self-hating queer, resigned to his fate, who produces transcendent objects for consumption as he lies gasping on his lonely garret death-bed ...'

[SFX: Phone rings. Tight shot of BURTON answering.]

ASCHENBACH (VO): Mary dear, what's this tripe about not being in the TV show?

BURTON: Trust you to jump on the gossip. Let's meet at the Natural History Museum in New York – we can talk about it there.

Scene Six

[Long shot of BURTON and ASCHENBACH embracing in the vaulted entrance (discreet European cheek pecks) and wandering up the stairs. Leisurely tracking shot follows them as they wander past the dioramas, where herds of mammals and flocks of birds have been frozen for a century. They pause to admire the marsupials, the leopards, the buffalo, the African green monkeys, paying special attention to those species that have become extinct. A crane shot follows their heated argument around and under the giant blue whale.]

[Just off the blue whale is a hallway filled with pictures and captions. A history of epidemics. From the black plague to AIDS. They try to picture the curator who pulled it off: someone young, well-meaning, who had read Sander Gilman's Disease and Representation *but not really understood it, someone who had probably lost a friend seven months earlier after protracted bouts with pneumocystis. They proceed through the woodcuts, the engravings, the stigmata of syphilis, leprosy, bubonic plague.]*

[They reach AIDS. It's a rear-projected slide show of photos of PWAs from Miami, Brazil, and New Jersey: men in hospitals, wrapped in IV tubes instead of leather straps, with lesions instead of bruises. The new S/M. Real kinky. A grade-school class in search of the African dioramas accidentally enters the exhibit. A little boy glances, freezes. In a split second, without the aid of captions, he can 'read' the image. Nine years old and he has mastered the visual semiotics of a purple splotch on a forearm. It takes him two seconds. 'AIDS!' he screams. The others, the same age, freeze, glance and get it. They too can read. They scream 'AIDS!' They stampede, their terror cut with giggles: a herd of unstuffed little animals fleeing from visual contagion, half-convinced the KS lesions could leap from the projected image onto their pre-pubescent bodies. Perhaps they are not so sophisticated – perhaps they think the slides are front-projected, that they could interrupt the beam of light and cause the image to spill over their faces.]

[Cut to: scene from biblical film by Cecil B. DeMille where St Veronica wipes Christ's face on Calvary and the cloth is imprinted with his image.]

[Cut to: clip from Star Trek *episode, where alien woman cures Spock and Kirk by transferring their lesions onto her own arms.]*

Scene Seven

[Panoramic view of Black Sand Beach, a gay nude beach just across the Golden Gate Bridge from San Francisco.]

GREEN MONKEY: Aschenbach the dandy turned to nature for a cure and was betrayed. Sir Richard Burton the dandy turned to nature for an explanation and was deceived. As representatives of a species facing extinction, they have turned against nature. At the same time, the sea wind sharpens their senses. They are less cynical, more critical. They are beginning to turn against culture.

[Long shot of ASCHENBACH and BURTON standing on cliff, looking out to sea. Their POV: the 18th-century cargo vessel reappears in the bay, with the naked sailors leaping from the deck into the water, attempting to escape the plague. Cut to: tight shot of ASCHENBACH and BURTON, transfixed (slipping into a reverie), unconsciously stepping nearer the edge. Mahler. The waves pound below.]

GREEN MONKEY: That peculiar species, the dandy, flourished in societies of unquestioned privilege and inflexible stratification. In this moment of turmoil and crisis, the dandy is threatened with extinction. Like all species, it must adapt or perish.

ROLLING TEXT: The ritual plunge, leaping from the cliff into the brine, recurs again and again in diverse cultures. For some, it could cleanse the body and soul. For others, it could appease wrathful gods and fend off earthly demons. Sappho, the most famous of divers, was claimed by Pliny to have been reborn as an androgyne through her leap.

Possible Conclusions:

One: BURTON and ASCHENBACH join hands and leap into the frothy waves. Swimming out past the treacherous rocks, they join the naked sailors in the bay and commence with some impromptu water ballet. A helicopter shot reveals their complicated formation of intertwined limbs, which spell out: *SILENCE EQUALS DEATH – AIDS ACTION NOW*!

Two: They pause on the cliff, undecided. After much hemming and hawing, they pull out sketch-books and begin to draw the drowning sailors, with ink the colour of Parma violets.

Three: BURTON leaps while ASCHENBACH sketches.

Four: They debate their options. ASCHENBACH argues that the leap is a cop-out, romantically embracing the utopian image of collective action while denying their own subjective experiences of AIDS *and* art. BURTON concedes that ASCHENBACH may have a point but argues that sketching the death throes of anonymous *victims* is hardly a viable (let alone an aesthetic) alternative. Achieving no satisfactory solution, they appropriate the helicopter (which has been waiting around all day on the off-chance that the Esther Williams shot might happen) and commence with an air rescue of the sailors.

Having nowhere better to go, BURTON and ASCHENBACH fly downtown to the secret pirate TV headquarters of AIDS ACTION NOW! in Toronto. Plans are being laid there to disrupt the CBC broadcast of the special, *AIDS: Culture and Nature*. Naturally, the arrival of two dozen naked men on the set causes quite a stir, but the show must go on. The pirate transmission by AIDS ACTION NOW! goes out nationwide, successfully wiping out the CBC documentary.

Shocked viewers are treated to an hour of anarchic antics.

BURTON and ASCHENBACH continue their debate with the cast and crew from AIDS ACTION NOW!, while the sailors perform *impromptu* demonstrations of safer-sex techniques ...

The Scythe, the Scales, and the Palette: AIDS and the Rupture of Representational Strategies

MONIQUE BRUNET-WEINMANN

Translated by Judith Berman

> Discourse on such topics as the economy, medicine, grammar and the science of living things leads to certain organizations of concepts, certain groupings of objects, certain kinds of statements which, depending on their degree of coherence, stringency and stability, form themes or theories ... Whatever their level of formality, these themes and theories are conventionally called 'strategies.'
>
> Rupture is the term given to those transformations concerning the general functioning of one or several discursive formations.
>
> Michel Foucault *Archaeology of Knowledge*

Michel Foucault's *Archaeology of Knowledge* was written during the urgency and upheaval of May 1968. Now, only a few decades later, we are living through the early stages of an even more widespread rupture, an upending of our discursive strategies and systems of representation. The new link with death created by AIDS (a philosophical issue, if ever there was one) is revolutionizing the connections between the disease and medicine, and consequently those between science and art. This rupture in representational strategies is the subject of the present article.

The Scythe: The Return of the Death of the Individual

In explaining the classifications put forward by Edgar Morin in *L'Homme et la mort*,[1] in which he made the distinction between the death of an individual and the death of the species, Heinz Weinmann, speaking at a conference on 'the death of the species' held in Montreal in October 1987, concluded: 'Today, we are surrounded by all kinds of death: the death of individuals, death between peoples (in war), the death of the human race, genocide.' He remarked that nuclear death was a kind of annihilation that could not be represented, for its images are unimaginable: 'At the end of the Middle Ages, death evoked images of death ... Dances of Death ... A rather joyous and idyllic affair, as compared to our idea of it. What makes death by atomic vaporization so horrible is that it leaves us nothing, no images to contemplate. It is thus unimaginable, unrepresentable death.'[2] It is total nothingness, a return to the original cosmic state of 'star dust,'[3] an utterly 'dead' kind of death.[4]

Alain Resnais' film *Hiroshima mon amour* puts into images this failure to provide an idea or representation of the nuclear experience. 'You saw nothing at Hiroshima. Nothing,' repeats the French woman's Japanese lover. The rest is but a news story about what was left: archival documents, photographs of those who survived radiation, strips of skin preserved in formaldehyde, reconstructions and eyewitness accounts of the disaster of 6 August 1945. 'I saw everything. Everything,' she replies. But a juxtaposition of fragments of the horror is not really a representation of it; it is barely a museum: 'Four visits to the museum in Hiroshima.'

Death between peoples, as in war, is graphically brought into our homes through the cold medium of television, with 'live' reports and images devoid of the imaginary.

But what about the death of individuals? We don't teach our children about that anymore. In fact, it was after one of his three young children asked him about AIDS that James Miller, organizer of the travelling exhibit of international posters about AIDS, called 'Visual AIDS,'[5] felt involved and *committed*: 'I suddenly found myself being an AIDS activist on the domestic front. As a parent, I found myself dealing with sex and death simultaneously.'[6] (See plate 40, following p 161.)

The adults of his generation – my generation – we enlightened university graduates find ourselves innocents, struck dumb as death snatches away our loved ones, leaving us orphaned for life. For illness, old age, and death have become taboo, hidden away, shut up in hospitals, in the chronic and palliative-care units. For a long time, cancer has been a calamity whose name is never mentioned, its victims dying 'following a lengthy illness.' We were led to believe (and how we wanted to!) that this was a disease to respect, controlled by flasks, test tubes, X-rays, radiation, and other neutralizing treatments, by the powers of surgery, medicine, and hospitals.

When death occurs, it is, or has been until now, clinically separated from family life, socially quarantined. In fact, Sander Gilman writes that 'it is in the world of representation that we manage our fear of disease, isolating it as surely as if we had placed it in quarantine.'[7] It brings to mind the glass bubbles of Hieronymus Bosch in which our most terrible fantasies are isolated. They are the iconographic symbols that make it possible for us to keep intolerable realities at a distance, realities that are so unacceptable in their true form that we must use representation to falsify the evidence.

However, AIDS is breaking down our lines of defence; it is attacking our immune system against representing the death of the individual that we have laboriously, ideologically, and scientifically built up through our positivist faith in the indefinite progress of modern medicine. The mask has been pulled away. But unlike the two-faced allegories sculpted on Renaissance tombs, the face uncovered is not the wrinkled and ravaged one of old age. As our comforting illusions are shattered, we are forced to deal with the unbearable death of *young people*, something we had generally believed to have disappeared (not counting accidental deaths) in the West since the conquest of tuberculosis. The entropy is revealed: the healthy, supple, well-maintained, and celebrated body is reduced to miserable, skeletal emaciation.

The tragic irony of it all, which is also the complex embrace of opposites, is that AIDS entered our consciousness in the early 1980s, at the time of the great return to individualism.[8] This return was primarily manifested by the stifling of ideologies, the demobilization of liberation movements, and the narcissistic cult of the body, of which body-building is the most extreme form. And as the cultivation of muscle masses replaced the different kind of mass culture born in 1968, the *subject* became no more than an *individual*, the *object* of the Vanities as portrayed by art: Liberace was rich, Rock Hudson was handsome, René Payant was always up on the latest fashions.[9] But the pampered body began to rediscover the mortality beneath the yuppie disguise; it is eminently fragile, no matter how thick the muscled armour. Visible beyond the well-oiled machinery is the figure that haunted medieval dances of Death: the skeleton with his scythe, the allegorical representation of the abstract idea of Death.

He can be found once again in the iconography of posters designed to make people aware of the danger of AIDS and encourage regular condom use. Among the 'Visual AIDS' posters exhibited at the Galerie John A. Schweitzer, at least two displayed links with medieval themes, telescoping five centuries of history into one image. One from Australia (plate 41) was reminiscent of a striking Klaus Staeck poster. Staeck's work, which decried the pollution of the Rhine River, showed a likeness of Goethe dominating the skyline of Frankfurt, the city of his birth; his forearm is unwisely dipped in the water and the flesh is eaten away to the bone. James Miller says about this Australian poster: 'As a reenactment of the age of the Black Death, the Age of AIDS evokes many "memento-mori" images, like this one, which is reminiscent of the art created for medieval knights. The traditional image of Death touching people, parodying their social habits, brandishing the objects that define their occupations [the object here is a hypodermic syringe], all this is incorporated in this postmodern remake of the Dance of Death.'[10]

The other work is a Danish poster that uses a comic strip by Jerslid (plate 42). In it, an honourable fellow, 'without reproach,' if not 'without fear,' stands drinking at a bar; he is covered in armour from head to toe, with a straw sticking out of his visor, and he stands apart from the heterosexuals who are busy flirting and 'cruising.' The artist uses irony to attack false information and fearful fantasies, and to jeer at our ludicrous efforts to protect ourselves.

It would seem that the multiple meanings and connotations evoked by the suit of armour give it a promising career as an image in this resurgence of the Middle Ages in our memory, our conscience, and our imagination. It isolates the individual within a steel 'bubble,' defending him against any insidious attack. It also sticks to the skin, like a condom. It is the warrior's instrument, an incarnation of courage, determination in battle, and the will to overcome the enemy, whether he be the English for Joan of Arc, the Spaniard for Bayard, the 'knight without fear and without reproach,' or the human immunodeficiency virus that has yet to be conquered.[11] It brings to mind the Crusades and the 'cours d'amour,' that is (as James Miller puts it) 'the neo-feudalization of social relations in the Age of AIDS.' Prudence leads to Purity, to borrow the allegorical language of the 'carte de tendre.' James Miller calls up the 'modern-day Galahad, the purest of the pure, defender of chastity itself.' The prudence in question is, of course, a condition of survival, if not immortality. Since the death of individuals has made its sudden reappearance in our daily lives, on the 'home front,' as it were, there has been a parallel resurgence in fiction of the theme of immortality and the quest for the Holy Grail.

I can think of three recent examples, each at a different level of language and designed for a different audience, proving that this transhistorical dream covers the entire spectrum of the social imagination. Indiana Jones's latest adventures are once again drawing huge summer crowds; this time, rather than seeking the Ark, he is after a popular version of the Holy Grail (*Indiana Jones and the Last Crusade*). As usual, our hero comes up against a variety of skeletons, but the snakes of his first adventure have been replaced by rats, notorious carriers of the Plague. The first part of the plot leads Indy to an armour-clad knight who has been guarding the hall of sacred vases since the last Crusade and has been waiting for the new valiant knight for centuries.

The Navigator, an Australian film, is a tale that links the Middle Ages to the present as two opposite points on the earth might be linked by a fault line. It tells the story of the spread of an epidemic resembling the Plague over which man can triumph in the imagination through a dangerous climb to the top of a church spire, that is, the positive reversal of the dream of falling. A Gothic spire in the same medieval flashback vein and with the same connotation of salvation appears in a poster produced by the AIDS-Hilfe Schweiz and the Swiss Ministry of Health. Rising above the night-time skyline of a city (Bern), it is associated with the peace of mind that a spare condom affords: the condom appears in place of a full moon, implying that if you're *dans la lune* ('in the moon,' that is, not on the ball) you're not dealing with reality. We know that Switzerland, the only country in the world with an organized network of underground atomic shelters, doesn't fool around when it comes to the survival of its people.

Last, but not least, I would present the example of *Progeria Longaevus*, a fictional biography dealing with the fantasy of immortality, by Canadian Richard Purdy. Like *The Navigator*, this work falls into that in-between zone, the stream-of-consciousness of daydreams. 'In the morning when I awake,' says the artist, 'I let myself fall into a kind of hypnotic state, somewhere between dream and reality. The entire project comes from my morning dreams, which I control with different readings.'

The creation of the fictional character and of the project itself was closely linked to the issue of AIDS: '*Progeria Longaevus* was begun three years ago. When I started working with the *Comité Sida-Montréal*, I asked a doctor what would happen in the case of a disease that strengthened the immune system [the opposite of AIDS]. He said it would cause hyperstimulation of the pituitary gland, which might slow the aging process. He told me of a disease called "progeria simplicus" under the effects of which children age ten times more quickly than normal. So I proposed a disease that would do the reverse. I made 992 my character's year of birth so that he would be a thousand years old in 1992' (the five hundredth anniversary of Columbus's 'discovery' of America).[12] Note also, by the way, that the city of Ptolemaïs fell to the Turks in 1291, marking the end of the eighth and last Crusade. This date does not appear in the biography of the character as currently described in the exhibit catalogue. However, it does say that in 1290, 'succumbing to passion, he made himself the Prince of Death.'

To go back to Purdy's enlightening comments: 'There are three main ideas running through the work. The first is the idea of death. While he doesn't die, everyone around him does. He is constantly being confronted by death.' The others disappear: he remains the sole, chronic survivor. The slaughter is widespread in 1300, at the time of the Great Plague, during which the 'Prince' founds his death cult. At this point, the illuminated manuscript roll (365 feet long) shows skeletons performing the dance of death, as well as the invasion of the rats (see plate 43). Purdy's narrator speaks to us from the third millennium, that is, he talks about *us* in the past: 'We know that prior to the third millennium catastrophes and disasters had already given the people a tremendous desire for *change*. The never-ending famine in Africa, Third World debt, troubles in Central America and the Middle East, the spiritual decadence of Japan and industrialized Asia, the financial crashes of the late 21st century, *the worldwide AIDS epidemic* [italics mine], all this crushed humanity with despair. Around 1980, a consensus began to be formed that all that could be hoped for was an *inversion of the world.'* This is representing 'the world upside down' to a T; it gives a real form to the semantic expression of absolute rupture and total revolution foreshadowed in the medieval theme of world-inversion studied by E.R. Curtius.[13] We are thus placed in a post-apocalyptic context: since the catastrophe has already occurred, it can be re-presented in the true sense of the term.

Our detour through the Middle Ages leans towards this vivid, imaginary re-presentation of AIDS, death, and life with AIDS. In closing this section, I'd like to go back to my opening remarks on death of the species and death of the individual. I'll get some help from Jean Baudrillard who, in a fascinating interview in the *Magazine littéraire*, says:

> It would be better to take this presumed end, the future, the catastrophe, and turn it into a kind of past, an already existing state of affairs; we should tell ourselves that this is a brand new deal and seek out the rules of the game. **This is the problem AIDS presents**. It can be seen as a protective kind of epidemic, possibly affecting the species as a whole, defending it from something even worse. If you accept the notion that we are experiencing a real catastrophe, then you can't view things in the same way; you don't necessarily see AIDS as a thing of pure evil. Perhaps it is already the reversal of something, a homeopathic epidemic against a kind of total, sexual dilapidation of the species which could be even more dangerous, who knows. At this point, there is a kind of shutdown, a failure, a breakdown which indicates that we really must give AIDS a meaning other than the one currently attributed to it.[14]

The Apothecary's Scales: Weighing Diseases against Each Other

Perhaps we will know what that other meaning is when we meet the narrator of *Progeria Longaevus* in the third millennium. In the meantime, we must convince ourselves that the old models are only images, references, and points of comparison; faced with the challenge of HIV, we must *invent* new responses based on new models. According to Charles E. Rosenberg, 'AIDS has shown itself both a very traditional and a very modern sort of epidemic, evoking novel patterns of response and at the same time eliciting – and thus reminding us of – some very old ones.'[15]

Science, medicine, and etiology also use analogy: they define the disease and discuss its treatment and possible causes in reference to existing models. The known is weighed against the unknown. Sander Gilman provides an enlightening parallel between the representation of syphilis from the time of its first appearance in Europe (beginning with a Dürer engraving dated 1496) and the way AIDS is now represented.

The name 'AIDS' was officially adopted in the fall of 1982, although it was first called GRID, for 'gay-related immunodeficiency.' The sexual connotation has persisted, despite the fact that, since the end of 1982, we know that the disease is also common among intravenous drug users and haemophiliacs. 'AIDS was characterized not as a viral disease, such as Hepatitis B, but as a sexually transmitted disease, such as syphilis.'[16] J. Seale compared AIDS to hepatitis B in the *Journal of the*

Canadian Medical Association in 1984: 'AIDS and Hepatitis B cannot be Venereal Diseases.'[17] Charles Rosenberg, a sociology and history professor at the University of Pennsylvania, revised the definition of the epidemic by comparing AIDS to Camus' idea of the plague, and to the cholera epidemic of 1832.[18] Finally, after the Fifth International Conference on AIDS (Montreal, 4–9 June 1989), the 13 June *New York Times* published an article under the headline: 'A New Therapy Approach: Cancer as a Model for AIDS.' It was a return to square one: the disease first presented itself as Kaposi's sarcoma, a rare form of cancer, back in 1979.

That headline triggered a shock reaction within me that sent the thoughts I had intended to pursue in this article onto another path altogether. I was dumbfounded: after some 5000 speeches, papers, and so on, it was announced as a 'result' that cancer treatments should be used as a model; not only that, but such an approach to AIDS should be considered something new. I felt sick to my stomach – a nausea that Lawrence K. Altman's report did nothing to relieve: 'Many experts spoke of managing AIDS like cancer and other chronic diseases, with "cocktails" of several new and existing drugs.' This was one cocktail I could not swallow.

And then there were the inevitable comparisons: AIDS on one side of the scale, infantile leukemia on the other. 'Many people "predicted with a certainty that is exasperating that there would be no progress with leukemia," Dr Broder said: "They were as wrong then as those who say that we will not make progress against AIDS are wrong now." In using the word cure, Dr Broder said he did not necessarily mean ridding the body of the human immunodeficiency virus. Rather, he said he used the term in a statistical sense, the way doctors speak of people who are free of cancer for five years as being cured.'

Oh, the attempts to find euphemisms, to make it banal and ordinary! AIDS is being set up alongside cancer as the Grim Reaper's second scythe, a chronically fatal condition that we had better learn to live with. 'If AIDS comes to be seen as just another routine killer like cancer or coronary disease, professionals and Government will lose one of the few weapons they have for the mobilization of support: fear.'[19]

And so we return to the threat of the death of the human race, the shadow of which has faded in the light of the recent East–West détente and nuclear-arms-reduction talks. 'Today we live with AIDS in much the same way as we live with thermonuclear weapons. Neither is likely soon to disappear from the scene. The question, then, becomes one of determining how the disease can be lived with.'[20]

This time, however, the analogy strikes me as false. For while atomic holocaust has remained but a spectre since Hiroshima (and despite Chernobyl), the situation is altogether different with the death of individuals with a disease that, we are suddenly realizing, is seriously ravaging our 'medically guaranteed' societies. Because we are now identifying as 'AIDS victims' not only those who are known to be seropositive but also those who unknowingly 'carry' the virus, statistically predictable deaths are suddenly appearing in the news. As if in reaction, the same is happening to heretofore taboo cancer statistics that have been hushed up by scientists or ignored by the media. The numbers are weighty, not only in terms of dollars and hospital costs. In the United States, 'reported AIDS cases now exceed 90,000, of which more than 50,000 have died, and the Federal Centers for Disease Control estimates that the disease will kill 35,000 this year. Of the $2.2 billion in Federal spending on AIDS in 1989, $1.3 billion will be for research and prevention. By comparison, the report said, the Government will spend $1.5 billion on research and prevention of cancer, which will kill 500,000 people this year, and $1 billion for heart disease, which will kill 777,000 Americans.'[21]

In 1989 there were around 2,500 people with AIDS in Canada, 743 of whom were in Quebec. In France, 'one person in four has, has had, or will develop cancer,' according to Professor Christian-Jacques Larsen, and 250,000 new cases are reported in that country every year;[22] in Canada, the statistics for cancer increase to more than one person in three, with 52,000 deaths a year.

The arithmetic is sinisterly simple: given the annual number of deaths and the number of decades during which cancer has been the subject of intensive scientific research, how likely is it that 'the AIDS crisis' will soon be resolved? What kind of budget should be granted for AIDS research? What kind of figures can be forecast for AIDS, given that it took eighteen years to develop a vaccine against hepatitis B?

If we are bold enough today to ask these questions, it is precisely because of the impatient revolt of those affected by AIDS, as demonstrated by the PWAs who organized themselves and protested in Montreal at the Fifth International Conference, where for the first time they were allowed in, along with people from fields other than biomedical research.

'While scientists boast of having learned more about the AIDS virus in the six years since it was discovered than they have ever learned about any virus, ... some protesters called them arrogant and misleading.'[23] Many researchers reacted to these interruptions by calling for a return, at future conferences, to the old concept of separating political debate from scientific debate; a return to the peace and tranquillity of the laboratory, where scientists are safe among themselves in the glass bubble that keeps them at a distance from the sick.

Dr Luc Montagnier of the Pasteur Institute, one of those who discovered HIV, was right to point out to these people that many patients know as much about AIDS as their physicians. In fact, we are correct in thinking that the pressure exerted by the sick upon the powerful has undoubtedly had a positive effect on the apparently exceptional speed with which results are being achieved.

In any case, there is no going back. Collaboration between scientists and the sick is the first major victory for PWAs and their organizations: they are demanding explanations and accountability, not waiting around passively. The moral immunity of medicine and science has been attacked; people no longer have blind confidence in them. Patients are growing impatient, rejecting their role as *objects* of treatment, as *consumers* of therapeutic 'cocktails'; instead, they are becoming *subjects* – people who assume their own illness and face their own death. They are no longer PWAs ('Persons with AIDS'), but PLWAs ('Persons Living with AIDS'). In the United States, 'physicians became increasingly prominent advocates for making out-of-hospital services available for persons with HIV infection.'[24]

We must hope that this attitude will have an impact on cancer patients, particularly since the tendency there also is to return people to their homes, to families totally unequipped to handle such a situation: 'Cancer comes home.'[25] You can't take the terminally ill out of medical institutions and expect them, or their loved ones who must deal with the calvary of 'secondary effects,' to remain in a state of passive dependence.

From now on, whatever science does is likely to be weighed against results and consequences. 'Many advocates also demanded more public accountability from scientists who use tax dollars.'[26] The issue is no longer one of simply demanding more funds for research, education, and prevention; there is also the issue of controlling how those funds are used, particularly when they come from private donations or voluntary contributions. After all, such a right to know is firmly established in the art world and no one is offended by it.

The Artist's Palette as Laboratory Aid

On the triple front of the fight against AIDS – research, education, and prevention – Quebec has displayed a specific identity, inherited from its Catholic past. The first case of AIDS recognized in Canada was treated at the Hôtel-Dieu Hospital in Montreal, where 27 per cent of all Canadian AIDS patients are treated; 80 per cent of women and 85 per cent of children with AIDS in Canada live in Quebec, where 22 per cent of patients are heterosexual, as opposed to 1.6 per cent outside the province; Montreal's Convention Centre hosted the Fifth International Conference on AIDS, a mammoth affair with the theme 'AIDS, the Scientific and Social Challenge' that included 180 sessions, 993 meetings, 10,000 delegates from 77 countries, 1,000 exhibitors, and as many journalists ... And yet, Quebec is the only Canadian province that still has no prevention program in its schools, nor any televised information campaign.

Dr Norman Lapointe, AIDS research director at the University of Montreal, expressed his indignation at this state of affairs:

> Canada has set up the Federal AIDS Centre, an agency that coordinates programs and channels funds. Canada is also the first country to have a national advisory committee to help the public service and federal departments to develop policy and handle critical problems.
>
> By comparison, Quebec is seriously lagging behind. Until 1984, Quebec did nothing about AIDS-related issues. Nothing at all; zero. Fortunately, the province was forced to inject half a million dollars to test blood in the Red Cross blood banks, it invested $2 million over two years in the *Fonds de recherche en santé du Québec* and it created three clinical research units at the University of Montreal, McGill and the Laval University Hospital Centre. But it could have done more ...
>
> All these ministers have had a right-wing, traditional, élitist Catholic upbringing and education, and they are slow to change. They don't understand that it takes very particular approaches to reach the target groups we have defined. They work according to principles. We all believe in virtue, but go preach that at the corner of St Catherine and St Lawrence [a downtown street corner famous for its prostitutes] ...
>
> Professionals should be given the contract for a national advertising campaign, and Radio-Canada [the French CBC network] should be forced to broadcast it ...
>
> AIDS is a cultural and religious problem. The CECM [Catholic School Commission] decides that the program can't be taught in

> its schools because it encourages sexual activity or drug use. It's hard to make people aware when you're dealing with this kind of information control. National information campaigns are extremely important. People are ready to be informed; the élites are the ones who are having a hard time dealing with this.[27]

The powers that be are leaving things in the hands of patients' families and volunteer organizations. And the public at large, raised on the same 'God helps those who help themselves' culture and morality of charity and good Samaritanism, answers the calls, makes donations, and tries to make up for the inadequacies of the system.

The best example of this is that in Canada, the first art auction to raise private funds for AIDS was held at the Galerie John A. Schweitzer in Montreal, on Sunday, 16 November 1986. James Miller remarks, with some humour, that 'many Americans (and not a few Canadians) suppose that the first extensive art auction to benefit AIDS research and support groups in North America was the [June] 1987 *Art Against Aids* auction in New York City. Predating the Liz Taylored gala by several months, however, was the 1986 *L'Art contre le Sida / Art Against AIDS* benefit at Montreal's Galerie John A. Schweitzer (plate 44). This was no local event – despite the absence of Hollywood glamour. Established artists from across Canada donated works to Schweitzer's Art SupporT committee.' A total of 127 paintings, drawings, sculptures, prints, and photographs were donated for the auction. Lise Gervais' *Soleil encerclé* (40" × 40"), a 1964 canvas inspired by Borduas, sold for the highest price ($11,000); Betty Goodwin's mixed-media *Black Arms* (18" × 22") went for $2,500, a little less than composer André Gagnon paid for *Blue Ink Corner* (16" × 11"), an ink-on-paper by Michael Snow (1956). *Tableau rouge no1* by Claude Tousignant (32" × 32") and *Interférences 3* by Louis Comptois ($8\frac{3}{4}$" × 16") sold for $3,000 and $1,200 respectively.

The auction raised $58,000. The organizers donated their time and energies, then repeated the auction in December 1987, working with Art SupporT to raise money for the Comité sida aide Montréal.

Since government was doing so little to help those with AIDS and to educate the public, something more had to be done; and we did it. The question now is whether privately organized activities like the auction should continue, thus encouraging the inertia of our elected representatives and their 'head-in-the-sand' policy. Should the art world graciously help finance scientific research in a province where the total budget allocated for culture is not even the much-touted and promised

1 per cent (it is only 0.68 per cent)? Can visual artists continue to be solicited as we deal with all our social catastrophes? 'Though New York's Act-Uppers (who want to "unleash power" through their confrontational aesthetic practices) may object that blacktie auctions for charity reduce art to a passive commodity in the crass bourgeois marketplace, money, as everyone knows, unleashes power like nothing else, and in 1986, when precious little of it was coming to AIDS organizations from national governments, few activists would have dismissed private initiatives like Schweitzer's as culturally retrograde.'

Here, James Miller is alluding (with critical irony) to Douglas Crimp's 'AIDS: Cultural Analysis / Cultural Activism.' While recognizing, as we do, that 'given the failure of government at every level to provide the funding necessary to combat the epidemic, such efforts as "Art Against AIDS" have been necessary, even crucial to our survival,'[28] Crimp denounces the concept of reducing a work of art to an object-with-market-value. Yet such a reduction is practical for fund-raising, especially when the market value of the art objects is increased (in the buyer's mind at least) by their association with the advancement of science. In a society that still cherishes a positivist belief in science as its saviour, art will be assigned the sacred duty of supporting and sustaining the Grail-like mission of scientific research.

I wonder sometimes whether here in Quebec, beyond the reification of art (and culture in general), we have not come to consider art as a donation from some luxury charity. Which, I suppose, supports Douglas Crimp's opposition ... The corporate world seems not yet ready to show such generosity. A major event had been planned at Place des Arts: the Montreal Symphony Orchestra, the Opéra de Montréal, the Grands Ballets canadiens, and many other performing artists had agreed to participate. The event did not take place, however, because no patron deemed it 'profitable' to assume the $10,000 rental fee for the hall.[29]

Similar considerations may have had something to do with the decision to organize 'A Day without Art,' 'a nationwide day of action and mourning to call attention to the AIDS crisis.' The day, held in the United States on 1 December 1989, was to be a time for action and consciousness-raising through discussions, performances, and exhibitions ... nothing terribly new. What I see as the project's originality and significance comes instead from the *non-action* it proposes: that museums, theatres, all artistic and cultural institutions be closed; that individual volunteers and volunteer organizations cease to play the role assigned to them as representatives of the system, so that the powers that be may be made aware of their importance and stop thinking only of the 'economic spinoffs' of their work. It would be nice if Quebec and the rest of Canada would participate in this event, sponsored by Visual AIDS, which describes itself as 'an organization of New York arts professionals designed to facilitate and promote AIDS-related exhibitions and events.' They clearly specify: 'Not to fund-raise.' [Editor's note: This organization is not to be confused with the 'Visual AIDS' poster exhibition, which originated independently in London, Canada, at the University of Western Ontario.]

My intention is not to belittle initiatives like *Art Against AIDS*, particularly those that are organized in a simple, unbiased, and generous way, as the Montreal gallery event was. It is my hope, rather, that the Quebec art world, ultimately through Art SupporT, will exercise its right to oversee the allocation of funds and the choice of priorities; perhaps it can do so by sitting on the advisory committee of Art SupporT, much as eminent physicians, financiers, collectors, and patrons sit on museum or art-magazine committees.

Nevertheless, such initiatives alone cannot take on the enormous task of educating the public and involving the authorities. John A. Schweitzer, James Miller, and Ken Morrison (the co-ordinator of the SIDART project at the Fifth International Conference on AIDS) have understood this well. Morrison, for instance, helped to co-ordinate a presentation of several large sections of the famous NAMES Project Quilt during the International Conference. This presentation was depoliticized and neutralized by the very places where it was shown – the Olympic velodrome, the foyer of a major convention hotel, and the display windows of a downtown department store.

It remains to be hoped that the strength and power of such exhibitions shall be multiplied tenfold, achieving through their *actions* the true effectiveness of Donald Crimp's 'cultural activism.' For watered-down messages, no matter how many of them there are; weak or complacently pornographic images (and how the topic lends itself to pornography!); literary 'tombs' and other commemorations, publications, or exhibits; the quasi-beatification of dead artists and idealizing elegies; all of these shall prove insufficient and 'normalizing.'

The challenge at hand is immensely more demanding: 'AIDS intersects with and requires a critical rethinking of all of culture: of language and representation, of science and medicine, of health and illness, of sex and death, of the public and the private realms.'[30] In this sense, AIDS is undoubtedly heralding a Renaissance, the end of one way of thinking and the need to create a new order of representation in every field. It is ushering in the third millennium.

NOTES

1 Edgar Morin *L'Homme et la mort* (Paris: Seuil, reissued 1970)
2 Heinz Weinmann 'Mort du genre, genre de mort' *La Mort du genre 2*, conference records (Montreal: Les Editions NBJ 1989) 157
3 See Hubert Reeves *Poussières d'étoiles* (Paris: Seuil 1984).
4 See also *Art contemporain* 9/10 (Summer 1984), a double issue devoted to death; in particular, 'Apocalypse Now, de la danse macabre à *The Day After*: la mort sans image' and Monique Brunet 'Morte mort.' The issue here is not yet AIDS.
5 'Visual AIDS' Galerie John A. Schweitzer, Montreal, 1–25 June 1989
6 *The Gazette* (Montreal) 4 June 1989
7 Sander Gilman 'AIDS and Syphilis: The Iconography of Disease' *October* 43 (Winter 1987) 107
8 See 'L'individualisme, le grand retour' *Le Magazine littéraire* 264 (April 1989)
9 René Payant (1949–87) was an art critic and professor of art history and theory at the University of Montreal. His articles have been published in one volume with a foreword by Louis Marin, as *Vedute: Pièces détachées sur l'art (1976–1987)* (Laval, PQ: Editions Trois 1987)
10 James Miller, analytical notes on the posters exhibited at 'Visual AIDS.' This is the same source for subsequent quotes by Professor Miller that appear without reference.
11 In *Illness as Metaphor*, Susan Sontag points out the military expressions that the 'mobilization' against cancer has produced.
12 'Je suis un empoisonneur de systèmes de réalité,' an interview with Richard Purdy by Claire Gravel, published in *Le Devoir* (Montreal) 27 May 1989, C11. This is the same source for the previous and subsequent quotes.
13 Richard Purdy 'Three Historical Fictions,' catalogue of the *Progeria Longaevus* exhibit, Galerie Christiane Chassay, Montreal, 27 May–24 June 1989. On the 'world turned upside down' theme in medieval literature, see E.R. Curtius *European Literature and the Latin Middle Ages* trans Willard R. Trask (Princeton, NJ: Princeton University Press 1953) 94–8.
14 *Le Magazine littéraire* 264 (April 1989) 23
15 Charles E. Rosenberg 'What Is an Epidemic? AIDS in Historical Perspective' *Daedalus* 118, no. 2 (Spring 1989) 3
16 Gilman 'AIDS and Syphilis'
17 J. Seale 'AIDS and Hepatitis B Cannot Be Venereal Diseases' *Journal of the Canadian Medical Association* 130 (1984) 109–10

18 Rosenberg 'What Is an Epidemic?' 3–8
19 Daniel M. Fox, Patricia Day, and Rudolf Klein 'The Power of Professionalism: Policies for AIDS in Britain, Sweden and the United States' *Daedalus* 118, no. 2 (1989) 99
20 Stephen R. Graubard, in *Daedalus* 118, no. 2 (1989)
21 Warren E. Leary 'AIDS Outlay Matching Cancer and Heart Disease' *New York Times* 15 June 1989. Two days earlier, Lawrence K. Altman reported more than 54,000 deaths.
22 Agence France Presse, *Le Devoir* 24 Apr 1989, 13
23 Lawrence K. Altman 'A New Therapy Approach: Cancer as a Model for AIDS' *New York Times* 13 June 1989, C3
24 Fox et al 'The Power of Professionalism' 107
25 Steve Fishman 'Cancer Comes Home' *New York Times Magazine* 11 June 1989, 70–1
26 Altman 'A New Therapy Approach' C3
27 'Sida, la mort aux trousses' *Voir* 3, no. 26, 25–31 May 1989, 9
28 Douglas Crimp 'AIDS: Cultural Analysis / Cultural Activism' *October* 43 (Winter 1987) 5
29 Reported by Jocelyne Lepage in 'Le sida a-t-il un faible pour les artistes!' *La Presse* (Montreal) 26 Sept 1989, E7
30 Crimp 'AIDS: Cultural Analysis' 15

40 'Visual AIDS,' international exhibition of AIDS Posters, sponsored by London Life, at Galerie John A. Schweitzer, Montreal, June 1989

41 National Advisory Council on AIDS poster (Australia 1988) recalling medieval allegorizations of death

42 AIDS-sekretariatet poster (Denmark 1987–8) using humour to fight AIDS-phobia among straights. 'Put up your visor,' says barmaid to knight. 'You don't have to be afraid of getting AIDS at a bar. So come right up.'

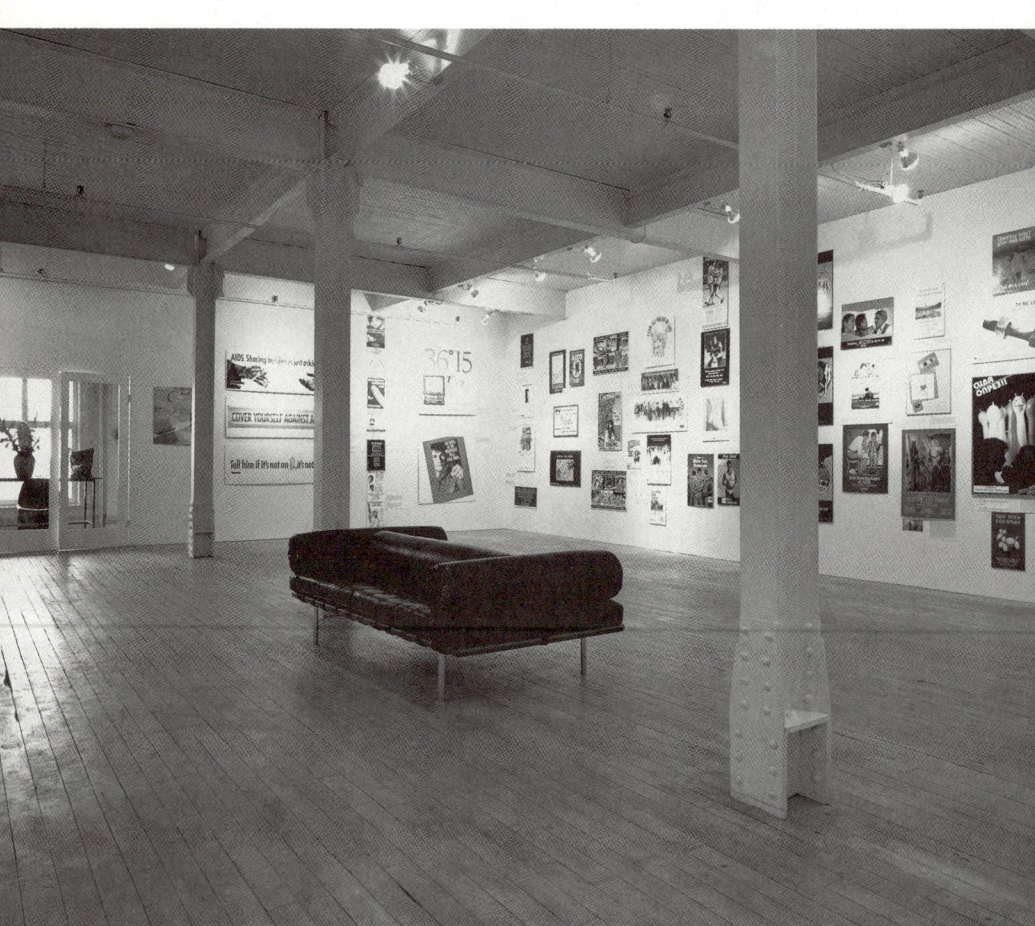

41

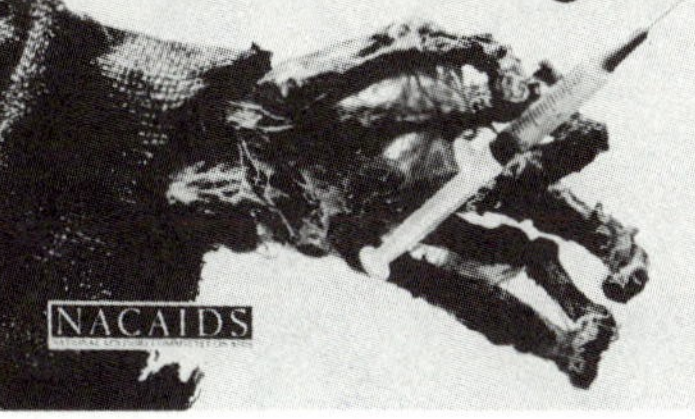

AIDS. Sharing needles is just asking for it.
NACAIDS

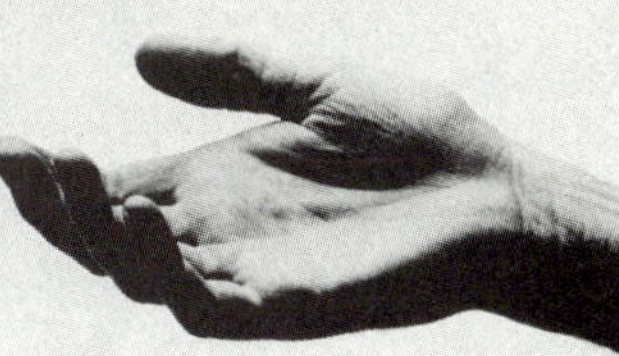

42

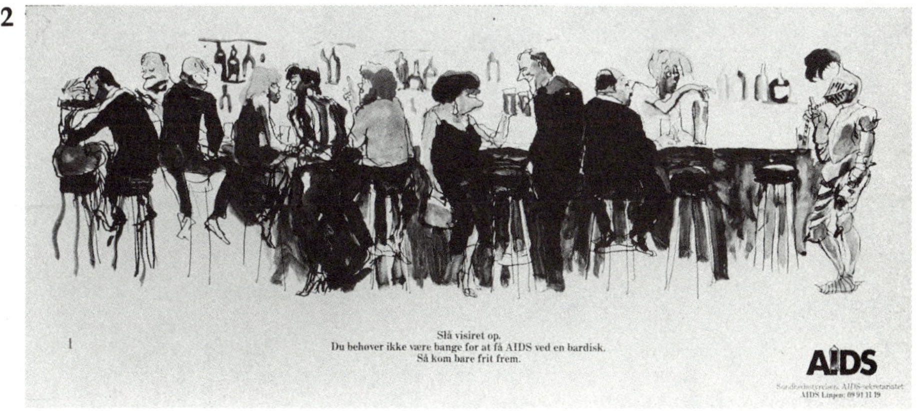

Slå visiret op.
Du behøver ikke være bange for at få AIDS ved en bardisk.
Så kom bare frit frem.

43

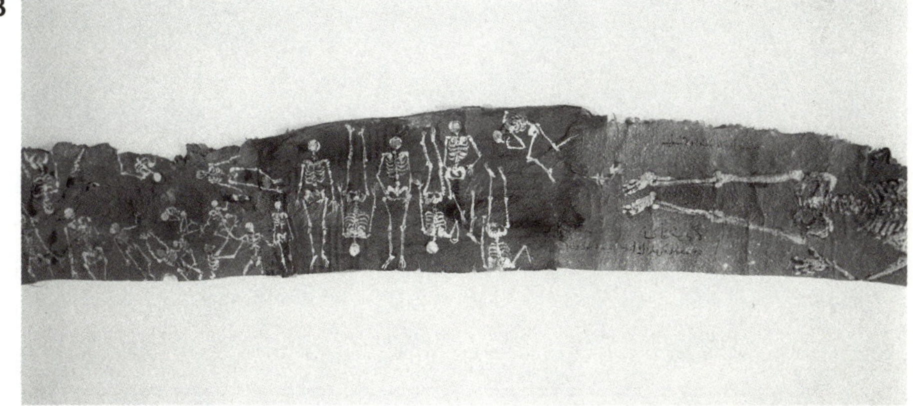

43 Richard Purdy, detail from *Progeria Longaevus* (illuminated manuscript roll, 1989)

44

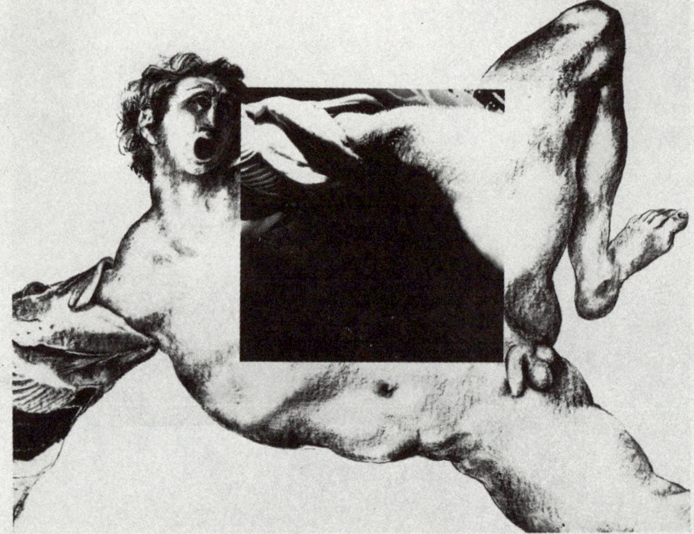

44 Brian Wood, 'Orpheus' (after Pontormo), on John A. Schweitzer's poster for 'Art against AIDS' auction, Galerie John A. Schweitzer, Montreal (1986)

45

but never one to hide his feelings. His vivid imagination and creativity fueled not only his writing but his "center of attention" behavior as well.

John is survived by his loving parents; his sister, Ann, and his birth sister, Linda; who John had the joy of meeting for the first time 1½ years ago.

We love you, John. It won't be the same not hearing you bitch and whine. We're just glad that your suffering has stopped. You will always be our favorite redhead.

A memorial celebration of John's life will be held July 29. Call 826-3329 for details. ▼

William "Bill" Wommack

April 21, 1948–July 21, 1990

Bill ended his struggle July 21 with his loving sisters and friends at his side. His wit and good humor lasted to the end.

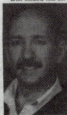

Bill arrived in San Francisco on Halloween night 1980, and adopted San Francisco as his home. He worked for the last nine years as a lab technician for I.C.I. Americas Inc. in Richmond, where he received continued support and understanding through his four-year illness.

Much credit should be given to Dr. Maureen Flaherty for her kindness and expert care. The Visiting Nurses and Hospice of San Francisco made his last days easier. His attendant, Don Hart, was especially appreciated for his big heart and caring ways.

Bill is survived by his sisters, Mary Beth Moore, Lois Wommack and Susan Wommack of Texas. His sisters, the light of Bill's life, were able to make the trip to San Francisco many times in the last year.

In lieu of flowers, please make donations to the Visiting Nurses and Hospice of San Francisco.

We love you and we miss you. — Paul, Jesse and Joe. ▼

DIGNITY

He loved so much.

Donations should go to Open Hand, Hospice/Visiting Nurses, SF AIDS Foundation, PAWS or Shanti. ▼

Mathew G. Scheiman

May 13, 1954–July 15, 1990

Wise men have said that courage is the willingness to take an action even though fear tells you not to. Matt had courage in abundance, and it impressed all who met him. As AIDS progressively narrowed his life, Matt continued to find new interests, and his zest for living never diminished. In the end he died as he lived, bravely embracing the unknown despite his fears.

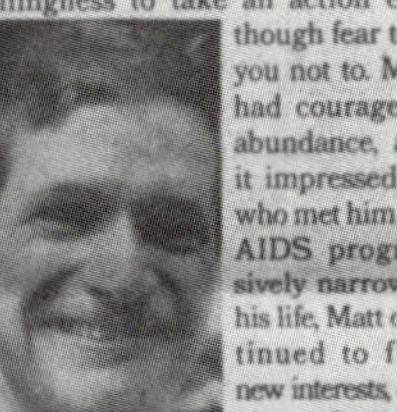

Matthew was born in New York City where he lived until he moved to San Francisco in the fall of 1987. For Matt, that move signified the beginning of an incredibly powerful period of growth and self-discovery. It was during these San Francisco years that Matt transformed himself from a frightened and dependent child into a strong and independent man. That he accomplished so much in such a short time is a blessing. That he did not long live to enjoy his hard work is a tragedy.

Matthew is survived by his lover of seven years, Aaron Percefull, and by many other loving friends in San Francisco, Los Angeles and New York.

A memorial service wil be held at Congregation Sha'ar Zahav, located at the corner of Danvers and Caselli, on July 26 at 7:30 p.m. Matthew may also be remembered by contributions in his name to the Shanti Project. ▼

Richard A. Martinez

Our dear friend Marty was granted an end to his suffering two days after Gay Pride Day. How typical of him not to want to rain on anybody's parade.

A native Californian, he grew up in Santa Maria, where he was active on his school swimming and scuba-diving teams.

He joined the Navy after high school

Michael Opal

April 1937–July 1990

Michael, a solitary gay man, a survivor of and estranged from a dysfunctional family, died at AIDS Hospice, Laguna Honda Hospital in San Francisco, in the loving care of Hospice; Paul, his longtime Shanti caregiver; and myself, July 9.

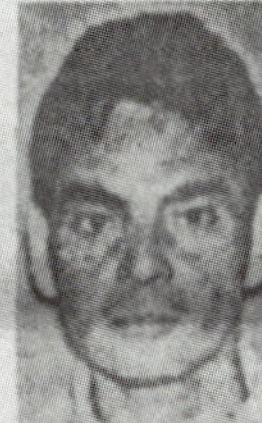

As a skilled computer professional Michael failed because of his refusal to conform to a system that denied his uniqueness. Tragically, in his failure he then found himself a victim of AIDS. With both hopelessness and quiet strength, he experienced his demise, as the disease slowly drained his body of its life.

Michael, those of us who witnessed your expression of your love with your beautiful cat, in your home and your self-crafted lifestyle are touched by your humanity.

Now that there is no more pain, I would like to think that you have found hopefulness beyond hopelessness. Love, Jeff. ▼

Obituary Policy

Due to an unfortunately large number of obituaries, Bay Area Reporter has been forced to change its obituary policy.

We must now restrict obits to 200 words. And please, no poetry. We reserve the right to edit for style, clarity, grammar, and taste.

Write name of person on back of photo. If you include an envelope to have the photo returned, please write the person's name on the inside of the envelope flap.

45 Obituary page, *Bay Area Reporter* (San Francisco, July 1990). Note 'Obituary Policy' (*lower right*): no more poetry.

46 Dr Geoffrey Foster plugging celibacy with 'Family AIDS Caring Trust' poster (Zimbabwe, 1988).

47 Jamaica Information Service poster (1988) representing AIDS as killer germ under scientific surveillance, and as murder 'clue' spotted under detective's magnifying glass

48 Kamutaza Tembo, hand-drawn 'Before-and-After' AIDS poster (Katondwe, Zambia, 1988) reflecting missionary allegorization of AIDS as shameful offspring of Sin and Death

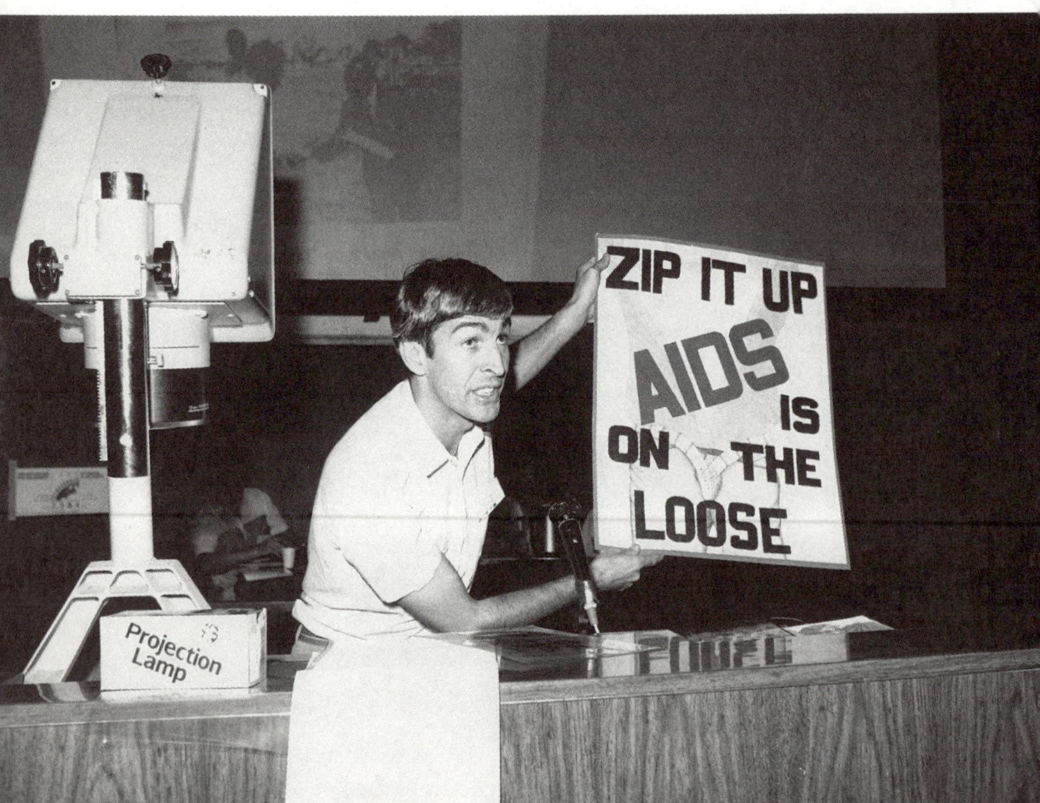
ZIP IT UP
AIDS
IS
ON THE
LOOSE
Projection
Lamp

47

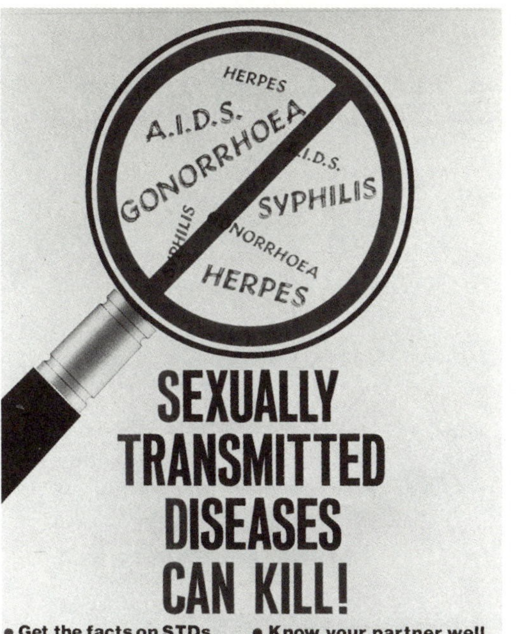
HERPES
A.I.D.S.
GONORRHOEA
A.I.D.S.
SYPHILIS
SYPHILIS
GONORRHOEA
HERPES
SEXUALLY
TRANSMITTED
DISEASES
CAN KILL!
• Get the facts on STDs
• Limit sex to one partner
• Get regular check-ups
• Know your partner well
• Use condoms
• Avoid sex with someone who has several partners

48

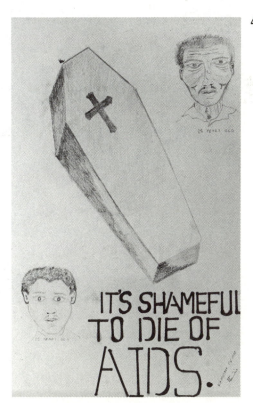
IT'S SHAMEFUL
TO DIE OF
AIDS.

49 Cover of *Beijo da rua* ('Street Kisses,' Brazil, April/May 1989). AIDS information affirms self-esteem of readers, represented by prostitute waiting in hotel door.

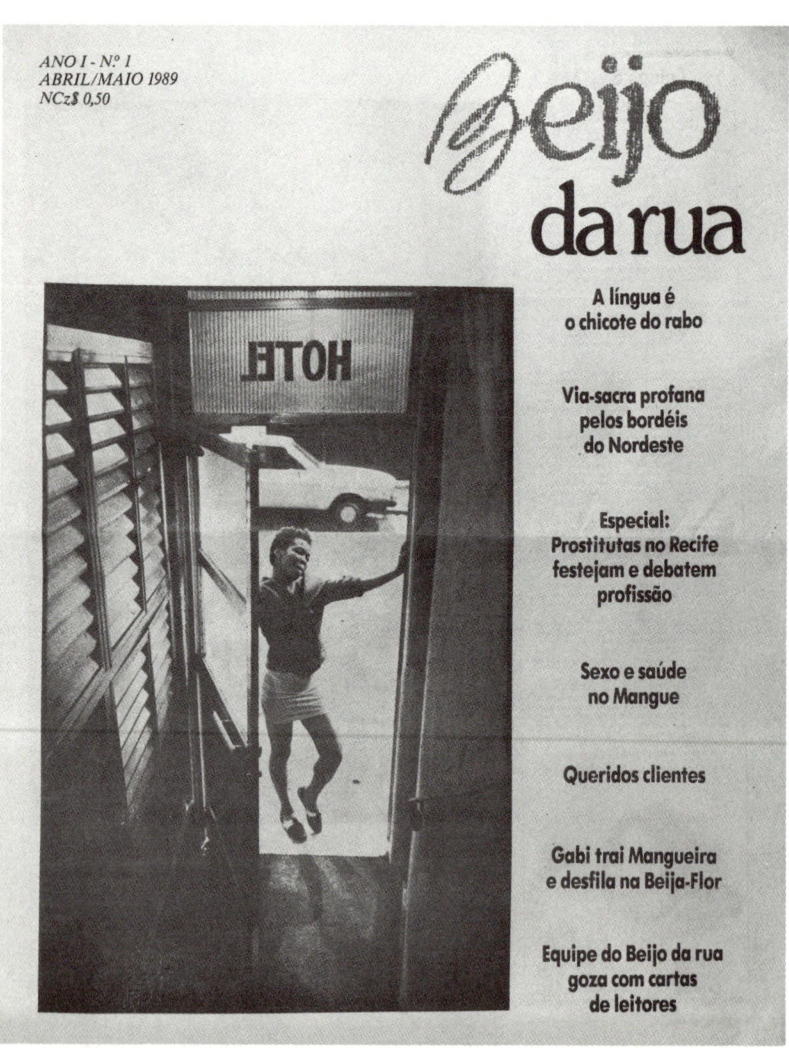

49

On Reading the Obituaries in the *Bay Area Reporter*

DANIEL HARRIS

With a disease as ideologically complex as AIDS, the act of mourning itself has been transformed from a private ceremony into a grass-roots campaign with a well-financed entourage of lobbyists and fund-raisers who vigorously pursue the new politics of grief. Mourning and militancy work profitably in tandem in things like vigils, bereavement groups, healing circles, die-ins, and, perhaps most notably, the Quilt, the shroud in which many of us have wrapped and buried the hedonism of the 1970s. Assuming unprecedentedly macabre forms, agitprop, like that staged by ACT UP, is now set in the unlikely theatre of the mausoleum, the ingenious if implausible headquarters of a fledgling political movement whose adherents have found a new and entirely original voice in the angry complaints of the bereaved.

Few examples of this sepulchral new allegiance of activism and mourning are as genuine, poignant, and unguardedly grief-stricken as the fascinating amalgam of incomprehension, camp, sentimentality, and desolation in the obituaries in the San Francisco gay newspaper *Bay Area Reporter* (see plate 45, following p 161). A weekly institution, this patchwork of bad photographs and amateurish copy written by the friends, families, and lovers of the dead men themselves is nestled like a portentous checkerboard of ashen faces among grisly advertisements for Ghia caskets, urns 'at substantial savings,' 'plain

First appeared in the *Antioch Review* 48, no. 4 (fall 1990). Copyright ©1990 by The Antioch Review, Inc. Reprinted by permission of the Editors.

wooden box' coffins, 'dignified burials at sea,' and funeral homes that promise to tell you 'everything you wanted to know about Funerals, but were afraid to ask.' Amidst the black comedy of capitalism, the incomparable world of these stark over- and under-exposed images, which bleach the individuality out of many of the snapshots or darken them into anonymous black boxes, vacillates wildly from the chintziest mortuary sentiments ('he passed from here to the stars,' one mourner laments) to comic, irreverent, and idiomatic elegies (like that written for a successful DJ, who could always be found on Sunday mornings 'dishing up the best hip-shaking boot-bopping funk anyone could find'). With no well-paid professional intervening to mitigate or blunt the grief with apt banalities, a kind of anarchy of tastelessness, humour, and sheer ineloquent misery gives us direct access to the personal consequences of the epidemic through the quavering and uncertain voices of the 'survivors.'

Full of relics, nicknames, and in-jokes, these disarmingly emotional pages create the effect of an intensely subjective space in a public setting typically reserved for the detached and unimpassioned prose of journalists. The tone is elevated and then deflated almost at random, as in this sentence from a notice in which a man hopes that his lover 'made it to Heaven, a place he looked forward to visiting even more than Hawaii, where we almost got to go.' Another writer subverts the traditional list of grieving family members and eulogizes a man who is remembered 'by his cats and a variety of potted plants,' while another speaks fondly of someone who 'got his last wish and blacked out during Bingo Thursday.' The mourners leap effortlessly from the intimate to the ceremonial, from the baroque to the laconic, from the dull rehashing of lives spent in the shadows of banks to hilarious instances of sacrilege in which the writers dump the corpses from their coffins and sling them around in their arms in an outrageous *danse macabre*. In an effort to preserve something of the uniqueness of the dead man's life in the two hundred words allotted them, they cram these notices, like drawers of keepsakes, with the names of pets ('he was alone [when he died] with his wiener dogs, Doris and Fred'); baby talk ('my little cuddlebumpkin' or 'Uncle Doug's bougumsmoudge kisses'); or admirable traits and comely features ('who valued a tanned look,' 'modern elective surgery kept him looking far younger than his years,' or 'he was much sought after for his beautiful presentations of food'). At times the obituaries are stately and pompous like epitaphs or dirges and at others they are bitterly, heartbreakingly brief: 'bye Dave' or 'tell Mickey I said hello.' Surrounded by personal 'effects' that seem too private to be exhibited so publicly, the reader often feels that he or she is wandering through a museum in which the insignificant artefacts of incomplete lives have been stuffed and mounted by a well-intentioned if somewhat careless taxidermist.

For a society that prefers to avoid death unless it has been dressed to the nines and laid in state in the parlour, we express grief in public only when we are armed to the teeth in the panoply of socially acceptable costumes and procedures. However genuine, mourning is one of the least spontaneous events in our lives, something that we censor and regulate with rigidly prescriptive rules whose reassuring formality prevents our corpses from unwinding their cerements, beating on their bone pots, and gibbering at us shrill reminders of a less cosmetic and aestheticized form of death. The *Bay Area Reporter*'s uncanny obituaries – to my knowledge the only regular forum in which friends and lovers can eulogize their dead compatriots – present mourning as we rarely see it in print: without our culture's presiding alter-ego, Emily Post, to give our grief that lustrous sheen of tactfulness and decorum. AIDS is represented here in appallingly personal terms, quite apart from politics, anonymous statistics, or the daily press's racy charnelese.

An unforeseen consequence of the epidemic is that it has permanently changed the way in which journalists discuss not only sex and the body but also grief. AIDS has led the American public on a tour through the bedrooms, bathhouses, and backroom bars of a world of quaint homosexual anachronisms, hermetically sealed in their own illicitness, which the media gleefully display like the instruments of a torture chamber: the slings for fisting, the tubs for water sports, the cells for slaves, the whips, the chains, the dildos, the amyl nitrate. From the housewife to the businessman, the uninitiated have been ushered into the privacy and esoterica of gay men's sex lives and from there right into the anus itself where, like curious tourists, they gawk at the rips in the tissue and nod knowingly at the treacherous permeability of the rectal walls.

In a similar way, it has thrown us all into the privacy of individuals' grief, which has now been liberated from the funeral homes and introduced into a forum as public as the press itself. In the aftermath of both the media's salaciousness and the gay community's theatrical new activism, mourning has lost its personal dimension and been absorbed and commodified in slick photographic essays and formulaic profiles of courageous soldiers who are portrayed less as individuals than heroic figures, the brave casualties of an honourable war.

In light of the unmitigatedly public treatment of the illness, I return to these remarkable obituaries to assign names and faces to the dehumanizing orgy of hype that has buried the intimate realities of AIDS beneath an avalanche of good intentions and political expedience. Whereas other newspapers attempt to rescue the bereaved from the intensity of their emotions and their own bad taste, mourning is uncensored in the *Bay Area Reporter*. In this defenceless moment in the survivors' lives, when their sense of the acceptable phrase and the time-honoured cliché is obscured and confused by the tin ear of grief, its editors make little effort to stand between them and their misery as they wrestle with the slippery conventions of the obituary. Like paintings on velvet, the garish colours of these elegies preserve their disturbing freshness and vibrancy within an incongruous, journalistic context. It is seldom that voices as unmediated and artless as these are allowed to speak out directly in the press in all of their startling authenticity and kitsch, unguarded and unedited. The Hereafter in particular calls forth saccharine conceits of angels hovering over billowing thunderheads – images that smack of an undertaker's unctuous condolences. 'He is free now to soar as high as the clouds and beyond,' one mourner asserts, while another evokes a 'Land of Eternal Spring' and yet another a 'world of total peace, love and light.' The act of dying is made sweetish and palatable with vertiginous euphemisms of floating, flying, and soaring that rid these Victorian deathbed scenes of cowardice and struggle, of stertorous breathing, comas, dialysis machines, life support, and panicked, last-minute triage. The image of death that emerges is the Grim Reaper of the sympathy card who bears innocuous tidings of 'new kingdoms,' 'wind-filled sails,' and 'peaceful and painless journey[s] to the other side.'

How often does one hear the voice of real lamentation in the mass media? The elaborate editorial apparatus of the press is set up precisely to suppress voices that are too loud, angry, or emotional. In an effort to bring the reality of the epidemic home to us, the *Bay Area Reporter* has broken this rule, removed an unspoken gag order, and allowed real people to speak as they choose, sometimes with waxen formality, at others with shocking directness. In the piercing keens and ornate threnodies of disconsolate AIDS widows, the epidemic takes on an immediacy that no article, TV spot, or second-hand report, no matter how impassioned, can convey. After the obligatory reduction of the dead man's life to its handful of undistinguished milestones, his grieving lover will often address him in a chilling farewell, as if, like a mourner in Jerusalem, he were slipping his words into the chinks of this wailing wall of newsprint, this slag-heap of unremarkable faces:

> Dearest Jim – my lover, my best friend, so long.
>
> My beloved Tom, my life and our home are so empty without you. I will miss you so much. I love you, as I will always love you.
>
> My dearest John, the heartbreak and anguish of your absence ...
>
> Beloved Michael, my life is empty without your presence.
>
> Thank you, sweetheart, for ... nine and a half wonderful years, and for loving me. I love you.
>
> 'Bunny,' part of me is gone now. The hurt is unbelievable but I know you are at peace and you will always be looking over my shoulder. God how I miss you!

It is this intimate voice, which is, for many, too private, too personal, too maudlin, that the media has been either unable or unwilling to represent and that the *Bay Area Reporter* has had the audacity to print unedited, heedless of the accusations of bad taste and sentimentality that the press is customarily anxious to avoid.

But perhaps the most surprising feature of this unlikely mixture of tinsel and pathos is the humour of these obituaries, the gales of affectionate hilarity that provide such a moving testament to the proverbial wit of the homosexual. Take this in memory of a baton twirler in the Gay Marching Band: 'Binkie – we love you and miss you terribly. But the good Lord must have needed another twirler, and knowing you, you probably volunteered.' Or this: 'Goodbye to the Queen Mother of All Sonoma County ...' Or this: 'We rue the passing of a mad queen. Somewhere in the Nevada desert his spirit lives on. Beware.' Often without warning, the mourners take the black crepe of these lugubrious ceremonies between their hands and rip it right in half, flouting the decorum of the genre.

As my eyes wander pruriently over this wall of faces, cheap sentiment, anguish, and linguistic bric-à-brac, I find myself disappointed with one small aspect of what has become for me my poison of choice, a way of savouring in private the magnitude and waste of the epidemic. Poring over these astonishing pages, the reader is quickly exhausted with the monotonous displays of goodness, courage, amiability, gregariousness, and integrity that are exhibited in this morgue as each mourner in turn yanks the sheet back from the cadaver he is eulogizing to reveal, not different faces but precisely the same man, an abstract and exemplary figure, a martyred innocent. Even here in these idiosyncratic and personal notices that seem to stare out at us with the hauntingly familiar eyes of Roman funeral paintings, the hagiographic conventions of portraits with which the public is more comfortable creep into these obituaries like rigor mortis. The men they honour are not just dead men but role models, tediously virtuous examples – 'footsoldier[s] in the war against AIDS,' who die after 'beautiful battle[s]' and 'long and courageous struggle[s].' This attempt to neaten up the life, to fluff it up like a pillow, and give it a classical structure with its own ennobling lesson on how to die often freezes these moving accounts into a rictus grin of optimism and forebearance which neutralizes unpleasant emotions that I would like to have faced more directly. Instead, there is a conspicuous absence of anger, rage, disappointment, and bitterness. The man who wrote his own obituary summed up this mood of unrelieved but honourable exuberance when, after thanking Rice University and the National Merit Scholarship 'for making it possible for a poor army sergeant's son to obtain a college education,' he concluded in all sincerity with a statement to which I return again and again: 'The American Dream certainly came true for me. It was fun, wasn't it?'

The Representation of AIDS in Third World Development Discourse

JEFF O'MALLEY

We saw a lot of skinny people in 1984. On the crisp white linen (freshly changed) of San Francisco hospitals or the arid plains of Eritrea in Ethiopia, 'our' moral healthiness was defined by the wasting away of sexual deviants, while 'our' sociopolitical development was absolved of recession and homelessness by a trail of corpses across the Horn of Africa – complete with moving narration from CBC anchor Barbara Frum. The crude, ignorant, and superstitious saw a righteous God withholding precipitation from black Marxists and raining disease upon white homosexuals. The thoughtful and helpful crew on 'The Journal' challenged this notion, pointing with secular assurance to civil war and epidemiology. But the discursive space was (and is) frighteningly similar.

Contemporary political theory gives us the insight that in analysing and judging the manner in which any given phenomenon is represented in social discourse, critics must not simply discuss factual accuracy and style, but must provide an archaeological analysis of the discourse. The way we talk about and understand phenomena such as AIDS and Third World underdevelopment does not simply reflect 'truth' with which we are acquainted; these discourses like all others are the product of the joining together of knowledge and power.

Only the crudest of Marxists would claim that discourse is a direct reflection of a mode of production, but only the most naïve of liberals would deny that the concepts embodied in the two words 'Third World' even exist outside of historical specificity, geopolitical relations, class, imperialism, and culture. And while HIV transmission with its attendant immune-system dysfunctions has probably been reasonably widespread for decades, our knowledge of AIDS only exists as a product not only of recent biomedical 'knowledge' but as a synthesis of 'gay cancer' (homophobia) and yet another obscure African illness (racism/underdevelopment). Given genealogy, therefore, it becomes obvious that even the most tepid social discourse is never neutral.

Simon Watney will be quoted for years for being one of the first to perceive what is now obvious: 'AIDS is not only a medical crisis on an unparalleled scale, it involves a crisis of representation itself' (*Policing Desire: Pornography, AIDS, and the Media* [Minneapolis: University of Minnesota Press 1987] 9). The words 'Third World Development' could be substituted for AIDS and the statement would remain equally cogent.

Other authors in this book and in publications such as the landmark *October 43* have clearly demonstrated that the dominant social discourse on AIDS not only militates against an effective response to the virus but also reinforces other equally dangerous infectious agents such as racism and homophobia. Similarly, since the Second World War a tightly limited discursive space has been created that restrains and defines the analytical boundaries of our understandings of exploitation, domination, and (more recently) subjection in the poor countries of the world. The 'development discourse' that has been created and propagated actually gives birth to the 'Third World.' As with AIDS in more recent times, the material conditions of illness, poverty, and abuse are reproduced in mainstream discourses to create victimization, repression, humiliation, disempowerment, and silence/ death. What a fecund breeding ground: 'AIDS and Development.'

The Northern Truths

Just as AIDS is used to reinforce homophobia and reassure the mythical North American general public of the sanctity of normalcy, the social discourse on AIDS in the Third World is a blatant construction of 'Otherness' far more effective at reinforcing prejudice than at building international solidarity.

Initial acknowledgments of the existence of AIDS in certain Third World countries are usually distinguished by most of the following misleading truisms.

1. 'Africa' is the region in question, or perhaps 'deep, dark Africa.'

Little or no geographic distinction is made between endemic and unaffected regions within the continent.

2. Heterosexual transmission is implicitly acknowledged with the use of the key words 'general population.' This is in fact often reinforced with the assertion that 'homosexuality does not exist in Africa.' But not to confuse the African 'general population' with 'the normal,' transmission is inevitably explained by African 'promiscuity' and 'polygamy' – phenomena that somehow always manage to be differentiated from North American rituals of casual relationships among young people and serial monogamy in the divorce-court set.

3. Most important, blame is imparted. Early theories of viral origins in green monkeys led to wild speculation about bestiality, and obscure references to 'ritual' practices involving blood-letting and sex not only reinforce the differences of 'Africans' from 'us,' but also allow our empathy to be dissipated by incredulity at the ignorance of the 'primitive.'

The Development Industry

Unfortunately, in a manner sadly parallel to the discourse on homosexuality and AIDS, knowledge is no guarantor of critical resistance. At a recent meeting of Canadian non-governmental organizations (NGOs) working as 'development' agents in Third World countries, a debate erupted between those who wanted to conceptualize and organize AIDS as a 'health issue' and those who saw AIDS as a 'development issue.'

'The World Health Organization sees health as more than just physical well-being. It sees psychological and social balance as part of the goal of "health for all by the year 2000,"' explained one protagonist on the health side of the debate.

'But AIDS is a development issue!' came the retort. 'The most economically active populations are being affected, valuable resources are being diverted, and prevention and care are having an impact on everything from political culture to gender relations.'

The third, unspoken position was that of silence, the discourse engaged in by the vast majority of NGOs active in the Third World – silenced, one would assume, by fear of both irate donors and unreceptive governments.

Despite seeming disagreements – and the admittedly altruistic motives of the majority of practitioners – the broad agenda of Third World development and the more narrowly defined agenda of 'health for all' tend in most instances to remarkably similar conclusions of disempowerment and the furthering of Western hegemonic control of Third World social formations. The dominant Euro-American theoretical frame for understanding Third World development since the Second World War has been modernization; the progressive erosion of traditional impediments to free markets and free elections will bring health and prosperity to the masses. The transfer of sociopolitical technologies and systems from North to South is seen as not only desirable, but inevitable. Unfortunately, even counterdiscourses of 'dependency' (in which the South has been understood to be in the process of 'underdeveloping' as a result of its relation with the North) and of 'Third World Marxism' (in which the important dynamics of class within poor countries is finally acknowledged) have failed most of the time to recognize the many kinds of oppression and the many strategies of resistance within the Third World. It is within this context of homogenizing grand theory that we can understand the emergent discourse that frames AIDS as a development/health issue.

Few aspects of life in the Third World have managed to resist problematization under the 'development' rubric. Veterans of the industry will recall the progressive incorporation of issues such as 'health and development,' 'tourism and development,' 'disarmament and development,' and 'women and development' into the terrain where developmental intervention is justifiable. Yet while 'development' casts its net wide, it has had absolute limitations based on its liberal precepts. Fundamentally economistic, developmentalism rests its legitimacy on its post-colonial nature. Its yardsticks of material advance and institutional democratization – still based on the Smithian notion of free enterprise – preclude from legitimate discussion the arena of personal morality. Development purchased its professional credentials be selling off its Christian teleology.

Developmentalism had thus traditionally met only limited success at extending control over the body, and such control (we have learned through feminism) is essential to the constitution of docility since the body is the fundamental locus of domination. In many mainstream development circles, family-planning interventions have long been in disrepute and proselytization is frowned upon. Yet the problematization of AIDS has challenged these liberal limits. HIV is usually transmitted by sex, and sex is ostensibly regulated by morals. By incorporating AIDS, therefore, the legitimated bounds of Northern discourse about the South have not simply widened into new terrain but deepened into more profound intervention.

Even where a reborn tendency to deny sexual expression is avoided,

Foucault has taught us that the humanist deployment of sexuality serves as a tool of social control as well. But what we are seeing in the Third World is not a simple Foucauldian shift from a symbolics of blood to an analytics of sexuality, but rather an emerging coexistence of different regimes of power – both traditional rights of seizure and modern rites of normalcy. Both premodern morality and contemporary normalcy are being rationalized within the narrow discourse of health promotion and the larger discourse of development.

A remarkably clear example of traditional morality interacting with the new imperative to normalcy is the work of Dr Geoffrey Foster, a British expatriate directing the 'Family AIDS Caring Trust' (FACT) in Zimbabwe. The photograph of Dr Foster displayed on FACT's posters aptly demonstrates his delight at having a legitimate – read scientific/normalizing – excuse for challenging what he must view as African immorality. 'Zip It Up,' he intones, echoing the epidemic of moralistic messages being spread across central and southern Africa (see plate 46, following p 161). While the Canadian general public is discursively protected from HIV by their self-definition as apart from threatened and threatening 'high-risk groups,' Dr Foster and many co-workers are operating in areas where seroprevalence does not necessarily vary between the pre-existing boundaries of the marginal and the mainstream. But through the formation of anti-AIDS clubs of students who promise to save themselves for marriage, the identification of single women as 'reservoirs of disease,' and the propagation of 'Zip It Up' posters, formerly blurry distinctions are becoming categorical. And the new, restrictive, and exclusionary morality is of course justifiable – for AIDS is now both a health issue and a development issue.

A contrasting example is provided by Street Kids International, a small Toronto-based NGO that has stayed within what appears to be the modernist liberal-secular frame of reference in its health promotion work. Peter Dalglish, the organization's executive director, is proud of pointing out that they have translated the word 'fuck' into thirty different languages for their new anti-AIDS video aimed at street kids. A storyboard version of the video *Survivors* was released in the autumn of 1988 to solicit feedback and build support.

On first viewing, the storyboard seemed highly problematic. In addition to more profound problems concerning the deployment of sexuality as a development issue, the narrative confused a number of key issues regarding HIV transmission, implying that the virus comes from unknown adults in the context of abuse or prostitution and not from consensual relations with friends. Furthermore, the principal character who contracts HIV appears to get sick and die within a matter of weeks. Far from preaching an alien Christian morality or even the humanist parallel of functional normalcy, however, the video aims instead to work within the frame of reference of the intended audience, establishing legitimacy through the challenge of authority figures and the sympathetic portrayal of petty theft. Awareness of the necessity of 'cultural sensitivity' is nothing new to the development industry, only the justification for such an effort usually lies in increasing efficacy for ultimately homogenizing social marketing campaigns. Furthermore, the cultural elements developmentalists tend to be most sensitive to are often in and of themselves instruments of domination and oppression.

If the several narrative shortcomings of *Survivors* are overcome before its final release, however, the video actually appears to have the potential to be profoundly empowering for marginal street youth. Despite the problems with any product designed to reach across many cultures, the potential of *Survivors* lies in its intent to affirm street life in much the same way that locally produced AIDS educational material in Canada often affirms gayness. 'Health,' 'development,' and the fight against AIDS itself are obviously laudable goals when they are not fronting for intervention and control; it appears that Street Kids International is at least making an effort to develop educational material that addresses HIV transmission without promoting normalcy or moralism.

The Views from the South

Most Third World governments have gone the route of the development industry, either medicalizing or moralizing the epidemic. Two posters – one from an official Jamaican campaign and one drawn by a high-school boy in Zambia – reflect these problematic tendencies (see plates 47, 48). While the Jamaican example uses the magnifying glass as an icon of science and the Zambian poster sticks with the more traditional colonial icon of the cross, both serve to chastise the viewer who has not adequately bought into the de rigueur medically and morally clean lifestyle.

But just as affected communities in the North have asserted broader political rights in their struggle for a liberating representation of AIDS-prevention information, the most profound resistance to the pandemic in the South lies of course in the counterdiscourses launched by marginal groups.

Beijo da rua means 'street kisses' in Portuguese, and it is the title of a bimonthly tabloid newspaper started up by a retired prostitute in Brazil (see plate 49). Rather than using AIDS as an excuse to scapegoat sex-industry workers and leave them vulnerable to further exploitation, the paper serves as a forum not only for health information, but for legal updates, documentation of street actions at Carnival, art, affirming interviews, and the regular 'Queridos clientes' (Dear Customers) column. AIDS information affirms the expertise and self-worth of the reader, passing on information updates and reminders rather than condemnations. Given Brazil's fairly high levels of illiteracy, the paper is probably more useful as a public-relations and lobbying tool than as an educational device, and a number of the articles (such as the 'Dear Customers' column) seem oriented to an audience of politicians. Nevertheless, the paper is a strong example of how the fight against AIDS can be complementary to a broader progressive political discourse.

TASO, 'The AIDS Support Organization,' in Kampala, Uganda, is another good example of a community-based group that opposes the scare-and-shame tactics of official AIDS prevention campaigns by proposing and promoting counterdiscourses to medicalization and moralization. TASO was founded by a group of HIV-positive women whose husbands had died of AIDS.

Like persons-with-AIDS groups in Canada, TASO counters medical and moral horror stories by giving a forum for people with AIDS to speak out and assert their humanity and their ability to live with dignity. Organizational philosophy and priorities are reflected both in its audience, which ranges from PLWAs to family members to health professionals, and in its programs, which refuse to stick to the accepted PLWA terrain of counselling and support by including education, care, and health-professional training. By giving a voice to people with AIDS, TASO serves as an example to all of us by asserting our collective expertise while challenging the 'experts' who seek to disempower.

Conclusions

The mainstreams of development discourse reinforce the oppression, domination, and subjection of women, men, and children in the Third World. On the scale of social formations as well, Third World peoples are, if not erased, at least threatened with being overwhelmed by an as yet unsuccessful assertion of 'global culture.' As AIDS and sexual health are incorporated into the modernist project, the efficacy of this process increases dramatically.

Is the answer to refuse to acknowledge AIDS and its consequences? To accept or reinforce traditional modes of power as resistance to new ones? Or to retreat into cynical despair? All such strategies are clearly unacceptable. There is already a rich history of counterdiscourses to developmentalism, though those who formulate and promote them recoil at the increasing skill with which the dominant discourse absorbs, co-opts, and destroys notions such as basic human needs, gender politics, and social and economic rights. But rather than denial or despair, we need a recognition that struggle and progress necessarily follow from co-optation. A multiplicity of resistances needs to be strategically developed to be able to shift the terms of reference of power as they are co-opted.

Above all, difference must be asserted and normalcy must be denied. The challenge of AIDS is to resist the easy temptation to define necessary or fundamental values and instead to proclaim joy and life in diverse ethics and diverse practices of sexuality, healing, and community evolution. In the incomplete triumph of modernism, many Third World social formations have an advantage in this over the industrialized world; tensions between regimes of power present particular opportunities for effective struggle. The role of the progressive cooperant or development activist is to support these moments, and in doing so learn how better to codify our own resistances.

PORTFOLIO ONE

Posters from the Visual AIDS Exhibition, London Regional Art and Historical Museums

11–20 OCTOBER 1988

The Visual AIDS Exhibition originated as a class project of the 1988 Frontiers of the Humanities Seminar on AIDS and the Arts at the University of Western Ontario. It had its North American première on 11 October 1988 in the Community Gallery of the London Regional Art Gallery (as it was then known) and its first European showing the following March at the Splendid Palace bookstore in Bern, Switzerland, under the auspices of the AIDS Info-Docu Schweiz. By the spring of 1991, after two years of touring, Visual AIDS had expanded to include an archival collection of approximately 1000 AIDS Awareness posters from over fifty countries; three curated exhibitions that have travelled to seven countries; an extensive series of critical commentaries on the contents of these exhibitions; and a slide library documenting every image in the collection.

The main objective of the project has not altered during this period of expansion. It is to heighten public awareness of the AIDS crisis as a global problem, and to foster socially constructive attitudes towards people with AIDS and their caregivers by illustrating how people all over the world are coping with the enormous challenges of AIDS education. Visual AIDS is also intended to alert viewers to the various ways AIDS has been used by its advertisers to articulate deep-seated prejudices against sexual minorities, people of colour, immigrants, and women.

The posters in Visual AIDS are divided into four iconographic groups reflecting four competing conceptions of 'AIDS awareness': Images of

Death; Images of Defiance; Images of Defence; and Images of Desire. The Death group reflects an AIDS awareness based on a deep fear of mortality and a morbid hostility to sex. The Defiance group promotes collective anger at oppression as the driving force behind AIDS activism. A liberal faith in human progress, particularly through the intervention of the arts and sciences in the 'management' of the crisis, underlies the awareness advertised in the Defence group. Countering the morbidity-and-mortality campaigns, the Desire group encourages a resolutely sex-positive, at times humorously erotic, attitude towards life in the Age of AIDS.

All four groups are illustrated, with three posters apiece, in the selection from Visual AIDS reproduced in this portfolio (after p 184). The contents of the portfolio were all produced by public-health agencies in developing countries or by socially marginalized groups within developed countries. The only exception is the twelfth poster (from a clinic in Poland), which presents an appropriately metallic image of desire from the now fairly rusty world of the Iron Curtain.

The exhibition would have had few samples of AIDS publicity from the Third World if Ruth Wilson, a health-education officer with Canadian University Students Overseas, had not donated a large number of African posters to the show and encouraged fellow CUSO workers around the globe to do the same. In her moving address to the 'Representing AIDS' conference, she discussed the discriminatory representation of women in the Zambian poster campaign of 1988:

> There is general agreement among everyone that I spoke to that these are bad posters. As one Zambian health officer pointed out to me, 'even the fat woman looks unhealthy' [see figure 1 in the portfolio]. Yet it is difficult for me to be critical of these posters. I know that they are the efforts of one or two people. I know that they had a difficult time finding someone to draw the pictures. The printing had to be done by a private company and then thousands of them were destroyed when rain came in through the windows of the decrepit building where they were stored. Distribution is a problem, and these posters and other materials sit in piles in a home in Lusaka waiting for people to come and get them. Their message is not clear enough, and their producers realized quickly that they would have to change it. But of course there was no consulting firm to help get the image right, no media testing to get the message right, no fancy paper, and no agency to market the final product.

Then, considering the cultural impact of such publicity when it does get distributed, she concluded ruefully: 'The problem is that at the moment this is all there is. In these critical initial months of the education campaign, women have been portrayed as the spreaders of this disease. So many people, women especially, can't read, and these posters are what they see and therefore learn about AIDS.'

The exhibition committee wishes to thank Ruth Wilson for clarifying the social context of these posters; Tom Lennon, dean of the Faculty of Arts at the University of Western Ontario for his encouragement of the project; and John Tamblyn for his technical expertise and unfailing patience as photographer of the collection. Funding for Visual AIDS has been generously supplied since 1988 by London Life.

James Miller

Images of Death

1 ZAMBIA: Ministry of Health, Lusaka (1987–8)

This before-and-after image locates the AIDS crisis in two endangered sites: the bodies of sexually active black women (specifically their vulnerable genital area); and the purses and pockets of Westernized Zambians (symbolizing their vulnerable economy). Physical plenitude and sexual potency are equated here with economic development and political vitality. The top caption was taken from a poster published in 1986–7 in Britain, where 'go' in a sexual sense is more or less equivalent to the North American 'cum.' Getting yourself 'totally wasted' by just one 'go' in this African context, however, signifies not only physical debilitation for the well-developed individual but also economic ruin for the developing country. Underlying this allegorical schema is the horror of the Fall. Like prelapsarian Eve, the Before Woman is innocently confident of her flourishing sexuality (symbolized by the flower on her breast) while her After self is a grim icon of the fruits of unsafe sex and the wages of unproductive sin. Ironically, this design reverses North American stereotypes of the Beautiful Thin Woman and the Loathely Fat Lady.

2 SENEGAL: Comité National de Prévention du Sida (late 1980s)

'AIDS – A Threat to Our Health' is the message proclaimed by this macabre trio, who recall the Memento Mori figures in the plague art of the later Middle Ages. Judging from the 'healthy' figure on the left, one would have to say that health is an unenviable condition among Senegalese males: they appear to have bluish-white skin and no external genitals. When they contract AIDS, which obviously cannot be by the usual routes of sexual transmission, their skin not only sags and shrinks appallingly. It turns brown. They become 'niggers' in the old nineteenth-century colonial sense: abject, powerless, doomed creatures enslaved by history and castrated by fate. This dramatic dermatological symptom speaks volumes about the perpetuation of the old racist equations White = Power = Health, and Black = Weakness = Disease in post-colonial Africa.

3 JORDAN: Ministry of Health, Amman (1988)

Swooping down out of a black sky, two yellow genie-like hands have scared the hair off a whole crowd of perplexed Jordanians. Well may we wonder (like the man with the question mark tattooed on his pate) what is going on here in this apparent parody of a *Time* magazine cover. The Arab version of the AIDS Apocalypse is literally upon us. Besides a xenophobic horror of the Virus that Came from Beyond, this poster seems to reflect the rigid conformist ethos of the conservative élite in Jordanian society. In their pale faceless ranks the scared citizenry looks like the army of cadavers that once marched through medieval nightmares of the Triumph of Death. Though the menacing hands are explicitly glossed as 'El AIDS,' there is an implicit political reference in the image that may not be apparent to Western eyes. On murals and posters throughout the Middle East, America is commonly represented as an eagle swooping down from the clouds and snatching up all it can get from the Arab nations with its yellow taloned feet. AIDS, which is often constructed in the Third World as the 'American disease,' here serves as a conveniently frightening metaphor for American imperialism.

Images of Defiance

4–6 CANADA: The Association of Iroquois and Allied Indians, Health and Welfare Canada (1989)

This intensely allegorical triptych (figures 4–6) says far more about the cultural fears and defiant political agendas of its native Canadian producers than it does about AIDS. Though the headlined captions proclaim the international need for effective AIDS education – AIDS being constructed pedagogically as 'a worldwide problem that everyone has to know about' – the specific lessons conveyed by native artist Norman Knott's images are really about tribal values under siege by the White Man's corrupt and corrupting society. The epidemic serves as a vehicle for a complex extended metaphor about the woeful Indian past, the perilous Indian present, and the ideal Indian future. In all three posters HIV is represented as a verminous mutant sperm complete with demonic tail and sickly green body containing the fatal acronym AIDS. Besides confusing the virus (and HIV infection) with the syndrome it may precipitate, this embryonic fantasy identifies AIDS with sex in general, and with male sexuality in particular, in a way that suggests the deep impact of erotophobic missionary discourse upon the collective consciousness of the First Nations' peoples. In the first poster, which grimly evokes their past, the demon seed has penetrated the ovum-like circle of tribal unity and can be glimpsed amid the flames of Hell that double as the flames of Sex. With this first rupture – a parodic conception resulting in the death of the Old Order through intermarriage outside the tribe – all hell breaks loose within the sacred circle. Booze floods in. Reefers fall into the flames. Syringes squirt their fatal brew of heroin and HIV.

What will it take to make the mystic circle of cosmos and culture strong again? With its intergenerational image of tribal unity, the second poster in the series provides a boldly simple native answer: solidarity and communion with ancestral spirits. The present (symbolized by the child) can only be healed by the wisdom of the uncorrupted past (embodied by the old man but derived from the ectoplasmic figures beyond the circle).

With its utopian look to the future, third poster in the series is the ecological mandala of a revived ancestral universe where nothing ever changes for the worse because Man and Nature are in harmony. Against a glowing technicolor sky an ideal native family walks off hand in hand into the sunset, looking (but for their Hollywood costumes) like a fifties-style suburban nuclear family out on a camping trip. Since their purified universe roughly parallels that of the Tory government in Ottawa, it's not surprising that the triptych, funded by Health and Welfare Canada, covertly celebrates an ironic yet happy coincidence of conservative tribal values and Conservative family values in the 1980s.

Images of Defence

7 UGANDA: Ministry of Education, Ministry of Health, Kampala (1990)

Education, specifically medical education, is often advertised as the surest line of defence against the epidemic, and in this poster produced with UNESCO funding for a high school 'health kit,' the beleaguered medical community in Kampala seems to be arming students with all they need to know to combat AIDS anxiety. The popular notion of AIDS as a discrete disease literally deconstructs itself before their eyes: AIDS is represented as an insidiously protean illness that tricks the uneducated eye by disguising itself as many other debilitating conditions visible on the streets of the Third World. The illustrations place the students in the nervous position of a health-care worker surveying a wide range of ambiguous symptoms. Is the woman on the lower right 'presenting' AIDS, or are her lesions wholly unrelated to HIV infection? Is the skinny child suffering from 'Slim' (as AIDS is commonly called in central Africa) or simply from a poor diet? Ironically, the effect of this seemingly helpful display of symptoms is not to teach but to confuse the students supplied with the kit, so that they will not 'play doctor' and 'spread rumours.' Medical information is thus used to increase AIDS anxiety in order to promote the authority of the medical community.

8 AUSTRALIA: Commonwealth Department of Community Services. Aboriginal Health Workers of Australia (1987–8)

Written in a form of 'nation language' (cultural dialect), this poster attempts to overcome male reticence toward condom use by suggesting not only that latex is Man's best defence against AIDS but that safer sex is for superheroes. The aboriginal health workers who produced this much-imitated ad clearly also intended it to be a manifesto of ethnic pride and cultural independence expressed in the popular idiom of the comic book. Its political subtext asserts that as a separate underclass aborigines must protect themselves. They cannot depend on white supermen with bibles and antibiotics anymore. Dominating the landscape on his sexual walkabout, Condoman sheathes his head (and presumably also his penis) in indestructible material. With one first clenched, and the other carrying his talismanic box of condoms, he assures his admirers that their ethnic identity and erotic potency will not be compromised by the use of this particular product of Western capitalist culture.

9 MEXICO: CONA SIDA, Centros de Información sobre el SIDA (1988–9)

This surreal version of the Condom-as-Defence motif stresses the collective power of 'El Preservativo' while pointing out the limits to that power. Here we discover that old condoms never die: they either enlist in the safer-sex army to conquer the world or join ACT UP (The Alliance of Condoms To Unleash Power) to march in demonstrations of solidarity through Mexico City. 'Our best weapon against AIDS is prevention,' the main caption proclaims, while the proclamations on the banners held by the activist condoms echo the militant rhetoric: 'We'll beat the virus'; 'The virus will not break our ranks'; 'Join the fight.' To the CONA SIDA slogan 'the Condom is a means of prevention' is appended an encouraging message from Command Central: 'Happily there is an effective way to prevent the infection of AIDS. Which way? By using condoms correctly each time you have sex. Besides preventing the transmission of the AIDS virus, the condom also prevents other sorts of sexually transmitted diseases – syphilis, gonorrhoea, various kinds of herpes, and hepatitis B. Take care!' Though some of the enlisted condoms in the front ranks look a little tired – even bombed out – their determined expressions and furrowed brows would daunt even the most aggressive virus.

Images of Desire

10 PAPUA NEW GUINEA: Department of Health (1988)

Written in Melanesian pidgin, a lingua franca incorporating many English words (eg, 'slip' = 'sleep, go to bed with, have sex with'), the text of this government poster may be translated: 'Think before you have sex with another person ... with either a man or a woman! AIDS. This disease kills people and there is no cure for it. The disease is acquired when a person has sex with a person who is sick with AIDS. Stick to one partner only, either a man or a woman.' In sharp contrast to this cold shower of warnings is the hot romance going on inside the valentine: this heterosexual couple evidently has not seen the 'poisoned valentine' posters emanating from Britain, via Africa, with the cheery message that 'your next sexual partner could be that very special person – the one that gives you AIDS.' Of course, if the one partner you stick to happens to be infected with HIV, you're probably in big trouble. The fidelity 'rule,' in this case, is hardly proved by its exceptions.

11 SRI LANKA: Ministry of Health, Planned Parenthood, Colombo (late 1980s)

You would never know from the Singalese text on this poster, a prosaic warning about preventing AIDS (and unwanted pregnancy) through the use of 'Durex' condoms, that the world had been set on fire by lust. For that information you have to consult the accompanying image – red flames engulfing the red silhouette of two lovers embracing against a blazing yellow sky – which looks like a movie poster for an Asian remake of *Gone with the Wind*. Is this a sex-positive poster? Or is it an image of desire doubling as an apocalyptic warning about the viral damnation in store for the lustful?

12 POLAND: Nakladem Venereology Institute, Warsaw (1988)

If you're having difficulty screwing because your bolt's rusty and corroded, this Freudian poster from a venereology and dermatology clinic (where most AIDS cases are treated in Poland) reminds you that 'you are getting treatment.' Perhaps you're meant to repeat this reassuring fact several times a day in case you forget what's happened to your bolt and take it by accident to a mechanic. Knowing how hard it is to get spare parts behind the Iron Curtain, the poster designer Zametski also urges you to 'remember your partner's health' – though Catholic modesty (perhaps) prevents him from recommending a stainless steel condom for safer sex. If you're being treated at the clinic for AIDS-related lesions, the final message on the poster may strike you as somewhat ironic: 'Treatment at a dermatological clinic – discreet and efficacious.'

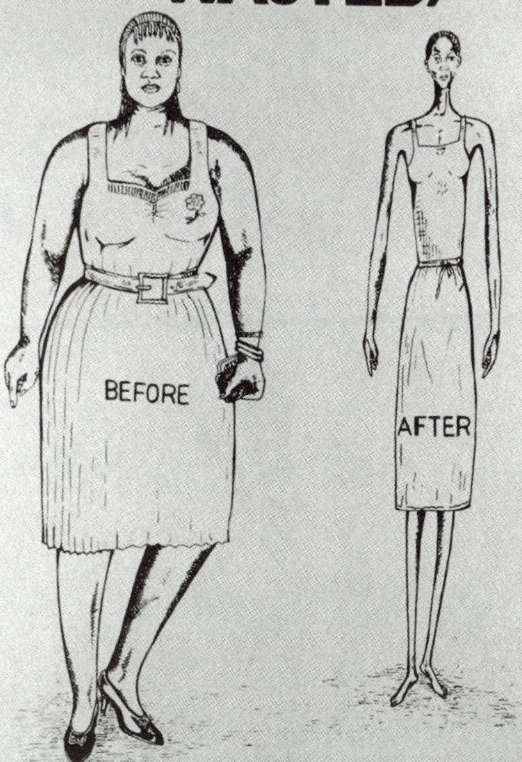
JUST ONE GO CAN
GET YOU TOTALLY
WASTED!
BEFORE
AFTER
"BEWARE OF AIDS!"
PRODUCED BY THE HEALTH EDUCATION UNIT, MINISTRY OF HEALTH, LUSAKA 1988
EASTERN SUN PRINTERS

1

2

SIDA

UNE MENACE POUR NOTRE SANTE

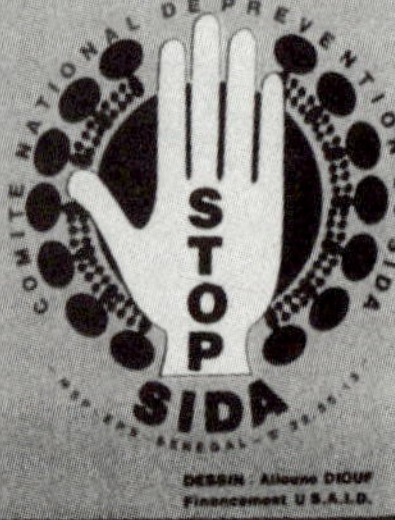

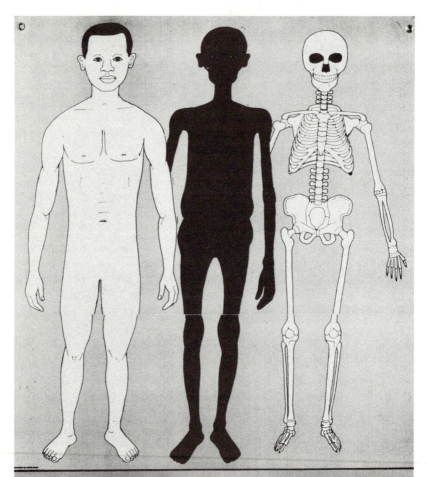

DESSIN : Alioune DIOUF
Financement U.S.A.I.D.

SERVICE DE L'EDUCATION POUR LA SANTE - M.S.P. - C.N.P.S. - SENEGAL

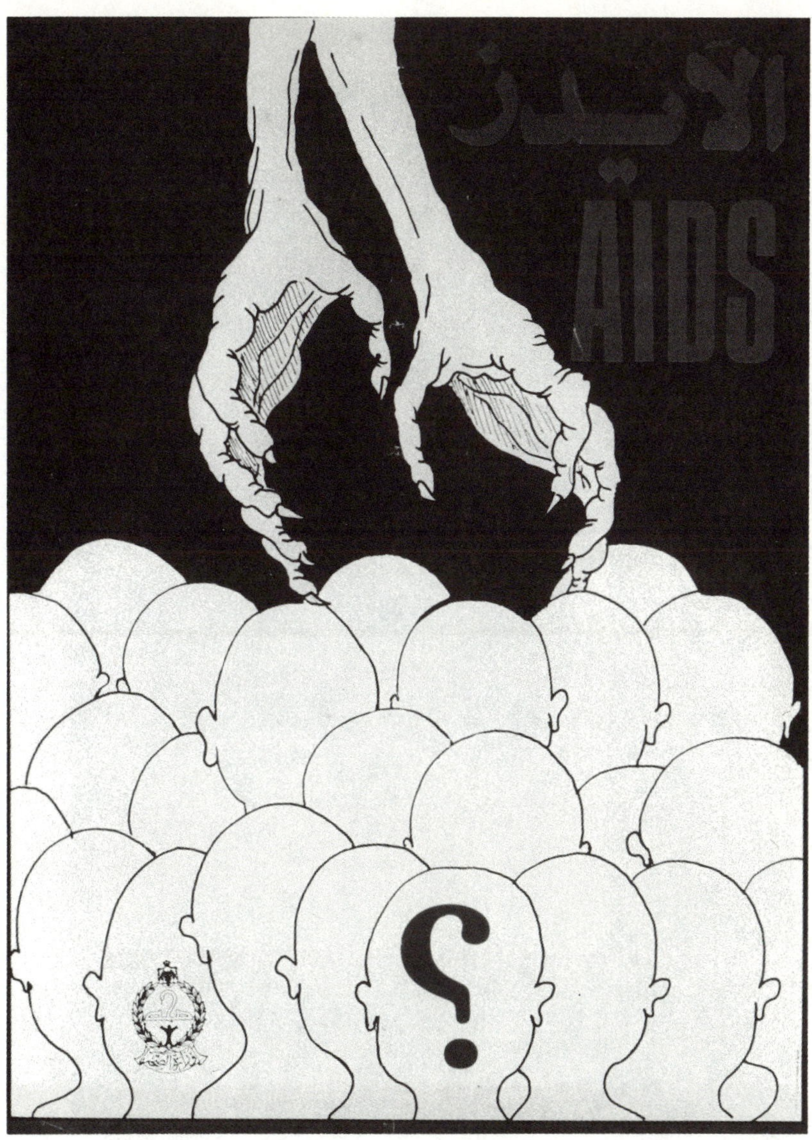

3

AIDS

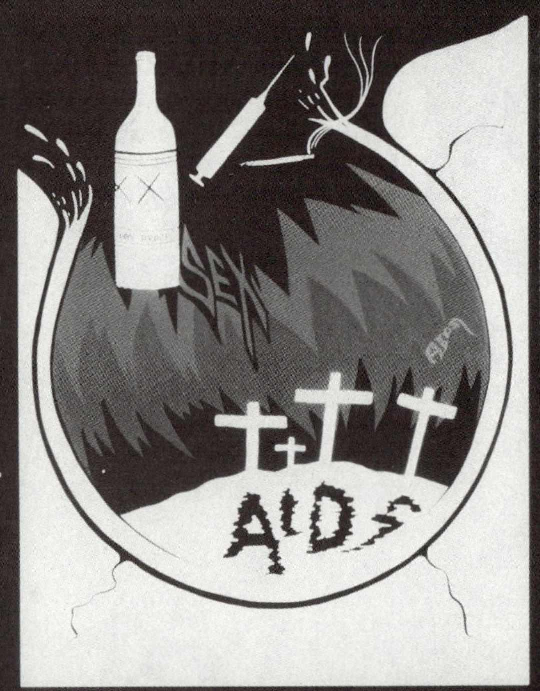

FIRST NATIONS
PEOPLES
ARE NOT IMMUNE
TO AIDS.

LEARN
HOW TO PROTECT
YOURSELF.

A DISEASE
THAT WILL KILL YOU
IF YOU GET IT

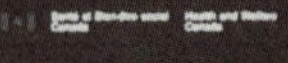

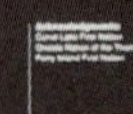

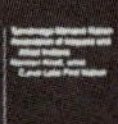

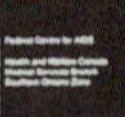

Canada

AIDS

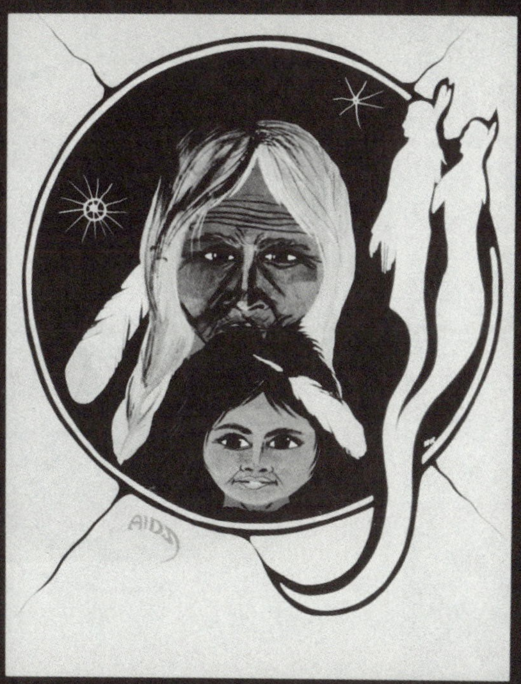

LEARN

TO MAKE HEALTHY

CHOICES.

KEEP THE CIRCLE STRONG

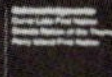

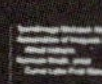

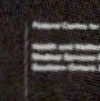

Canada

5

AIDS

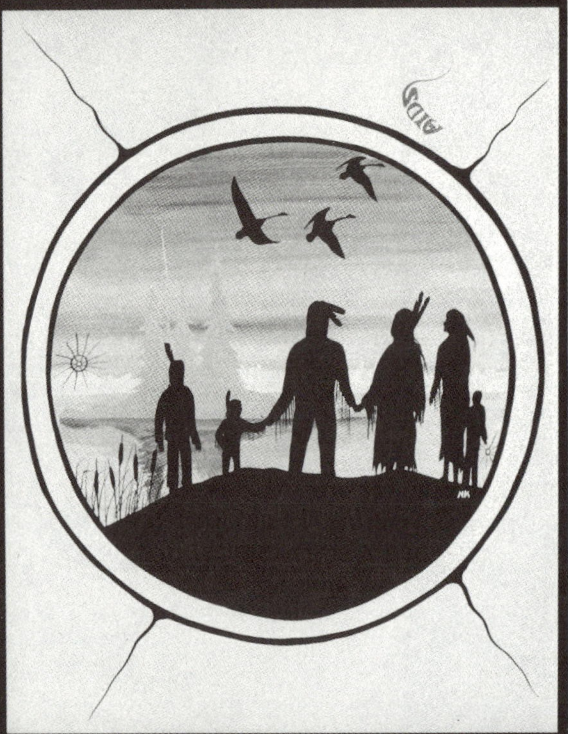

FIRST NATIONS
PEOPLES
NEED TO KNOW ALSO.

LEARN ABOUT AIDS
AND LEARN HOW TO
MAKE HEALTHY
DECISIONS.

A WORLDWIDE PROBLEM THAT EVERYONE HAS TO KNOW ABOUT

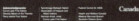

Canada

What Does A Person with AIDS Look Like?

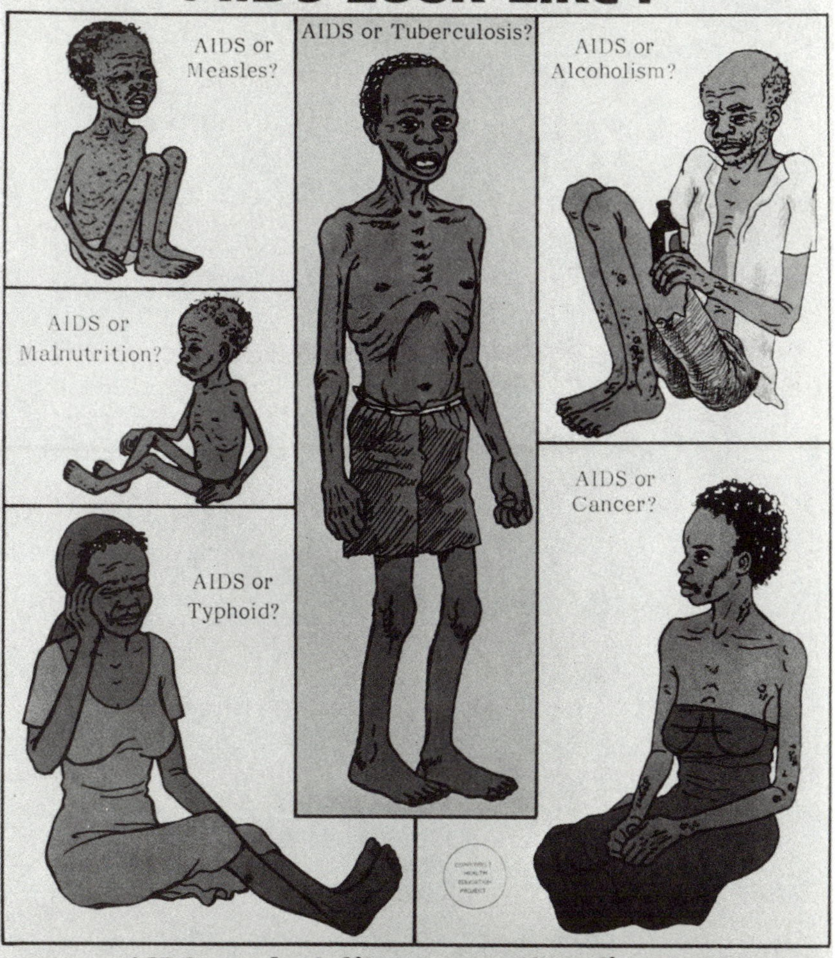

AIDS can look like many other diseases.
Don't be confused. Don't spread rumours.

See a qualified medical person for tests if you think you or someone you know may have AIDS.

Uganda School Health Kit on AIDS Control (Item 6)
Ministry of Education, Ministry of Health (AIDS Control Programme), UNICEF Kampala

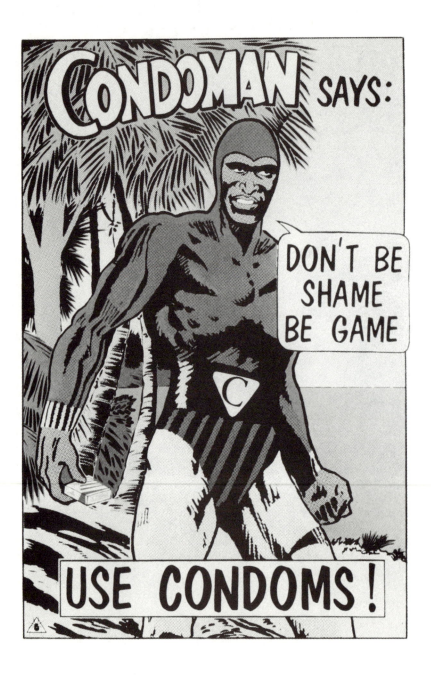
CONDOMAN SAYS:
DON'T BE SHAME BE GAME
USE CONDOMS!

Nuestra mejor arma contra el SIDA es la prevención

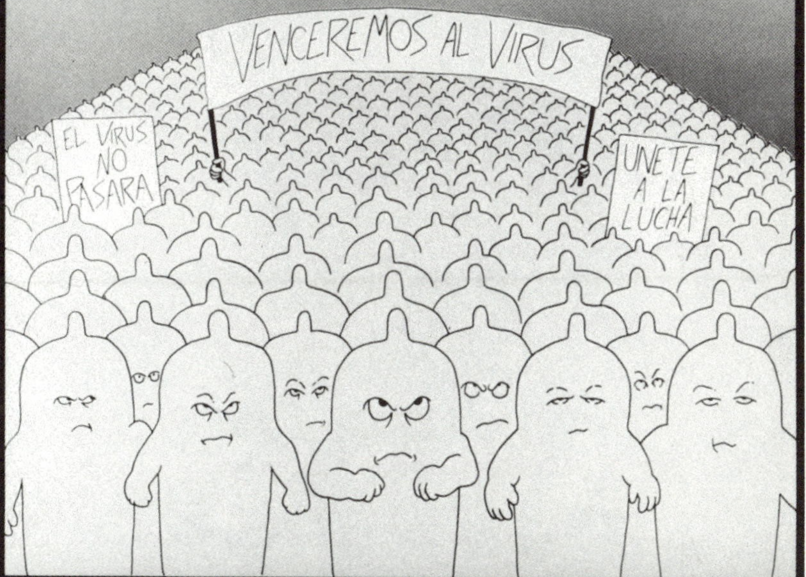
VENCEREMOS AL VIRUS
EL VIRUS NO PASARA
UNETE A LA LUCHA

El condón hace la prevención

Por fortuna, existe una forma efectiva de prevenir la infección por el virus causante del SIDA. ¿Cuál? Usando correctamente el condón cada vez que tengas relaciones sexuales. El condón, además de evitar el paso del virus causante del SIDA, previene otras enfermedades de transmisión sexual, como la sífilis, gonorrea, herpes en sus distintas variedades y la hepatitis B. ¡Cuídate! Y recuerda que: ¡El condón hace la prevención!

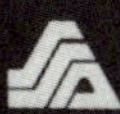

CONA
SIDA

TINGTING PASTAIM BIFO YU LAIK SLIP
...WANTAIM NARAPELA MAN OR MERI !

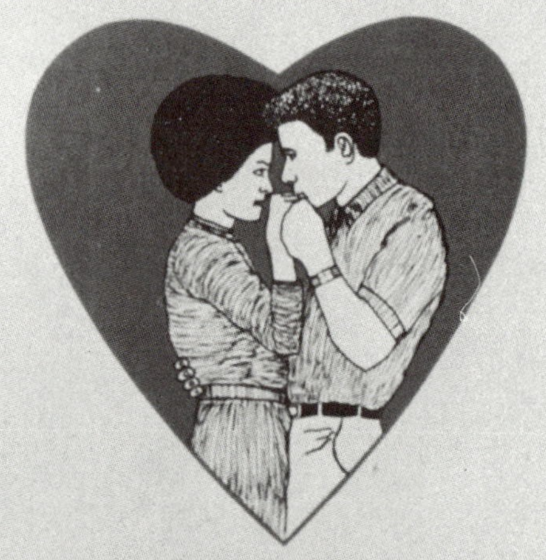

AIDS

EM DISPELA SIK I SAVI KILIM MAN NA I NOGAT MARASIN BILONG RAUSIM. SIK KAMAP LONG TAIM WANPELA I SLIP WAN-TAIM NARAPELA I GAT DISPELA SIK AIDS.

MAS ISTAP PAS WANTAIM WANPELA MAN NA MERI TASOL.

PUBLISHED BY THE DEPARTMENT OF HEALTH 1987

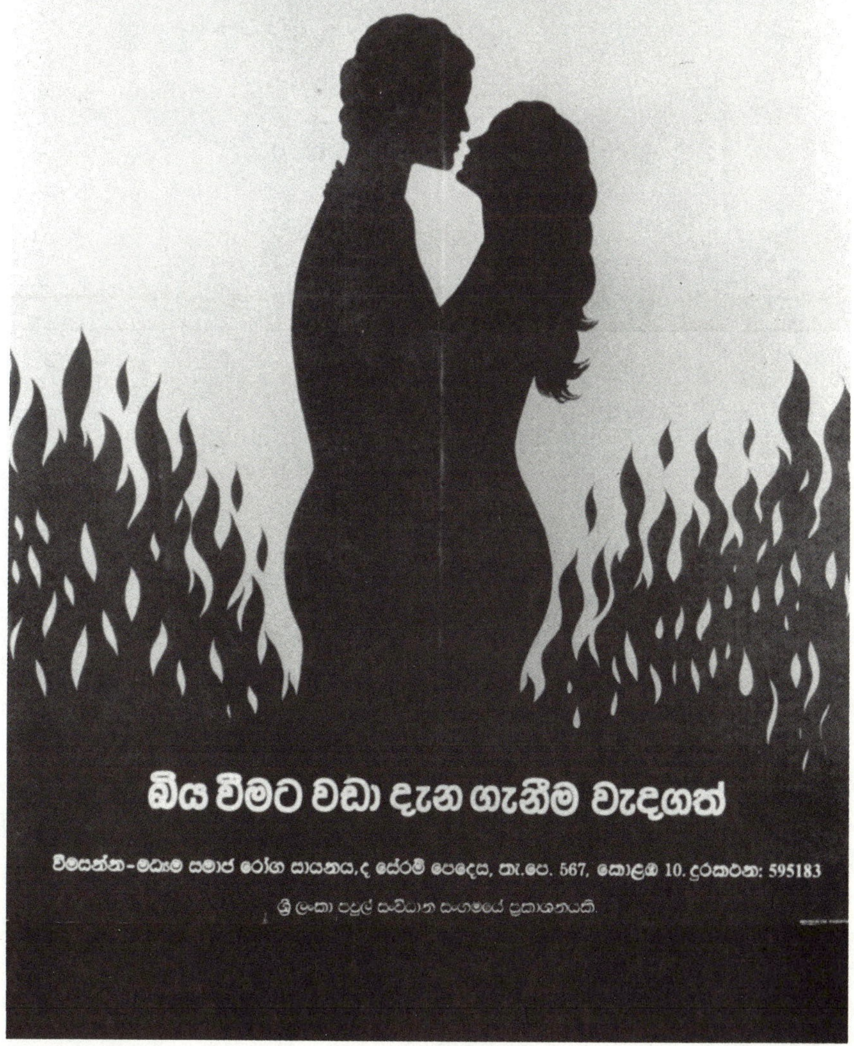
ඒඩ්ස්
දැන් ලොව පැතිරෙන භයානක රෝගයකි
බිය වීමට වඩා දැන ගැනීම වැදගත්
විමසන්න-මධ්‍යම සමාජ රෝග සායනය, ද සේරම් පෙදෙස, තැ.පෙ. 567, කොළඹ 10. දුරකථන: 595183
ශ්‍රී ලංකා පවුල් සංවිධාන සංගමයේ ප්‍රකාශනයකි.

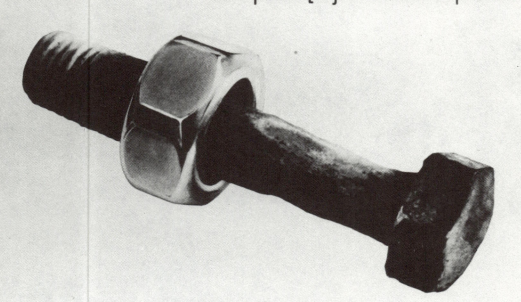

12

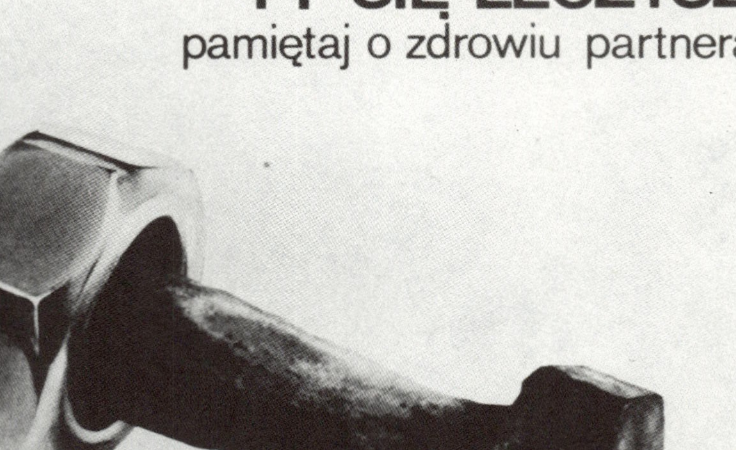

TY SIĘ LECZYSZ
pamiętaj o zdrowiu partnera
LECZENIE W PORADNI DERMATOLOGICZNEJ DYSKRETNE I SKUTECZNE

Criticism as Activism

JAMES MILLER

'The World Is Sick ...'

At the opening ceremonies of the Fifth International Conference on AIDS, which took place in the vast assembly hall of Montreal's Palais des Congrès on 4 June 1989, I found myself sitting beside a middle-aged doctor from the Atlanta Centers for Disease Control. We were both waiting for the conference to begin on its scheduled Apollonian note, with a string orchestra playing music from the Age of Reason. But the orchestra was late, the throngs of delegates and reporters were growing restless, and something oddly discordant was happening in the corridors outside the hall. It sounded like Dionysian drumming.

I blocked out the unscheduled noise and focused my attention on the conference catalogue, which lay open like a telephone book on my lap. Noticing my search for a hopeful paper in the clinical sections of the catalogue, the doctor from the CDC warned me not to attend the Monday morning sessions on dermatology if I wished to keep my breakfast. 'You have to have a strong stomach to take what the dermatologists dish out in their slide presentations,' he warned. 'Skin-flicks we used to call'em in med school.'

I laughed uneasily. I had no wish to be an AIDS voyeur, but there I was, with my catalogue before me, looking as if I was looking for a good show. The doctor assured me that the skin-flicks on AIDS would be 'pretty horrendous' because they showed 'the real world of the epidemic' by which he seemed to mean not only the erupting field of lesions and rashes and ulcers on the surface of the skin but also what lay beneath it, the microscopic combat zone of viruses and killer T-cells. Viewer discretion was advised.

While the epidemic (as represented by the conference organizers) seemed strangely unreal to me at that moment – as if it were no more than a spectacle of symbolic confrontations far from the field of action – to the doctor on the front lines it was World War Three. 'The War on AIDS,' he declared, echoing Reagan's old script for the War on Drugs, 'must be won if we're to survive as a nation.' I'm sure it was just a slip. He didn't mean to imply that we were all in the fight for America's sake, though as a Canadian I felt duty-bound to point out that other nations besides his were fighting for survival during the crisis. Kenya sprang to mind. Kenneth Kaunda, the Kenyan president, was scheduled to address the assembly at the end of the opening ceremonies. 'Words, word, words,' the doctor complained. He seemed to have a point, and I conceded it in silence.

The silence was broken with more drumming sounds from the corridors: the percussion of dissent. 'One thing I'll tell you,' he confided, frowning at the disturbance, 'the War on AIDS will not be won by waving placards at doctors and politicians.'

He was referring to a demonstration that had just broken out at the back of the assembly. A coalition of three protest groups – New York's ACT UP, Montreal's SIDACTION, and Toronto's AIDS ACTION NOW! – were bursting into the hall waving tall thin placards with bilingual variations on the same complaint. 'The world is sick ...' was printed in black block capitals on the upper half of each English version of the placard, while in crudely hand-painted lettering on the lower half appeared various phrases to complete the message (see plate 50, following p 214). 'The world is sick of your protocols,' declared one impatient sign. 'Le monde est tanné de ta lenteur,' read its French equivalent, referring to the slowness of drug trials and other politically regulated research procedures. Other signs expressed the world's frustration with quarantines, medical negligence, AIDS hysteria, and 'génocide gouvernemental.'

As more and more of these signs bobbed into view, I was struck by their collective defiance of the conference's carefully promoted image of a world united against AIDS. There seemed to be two AIDS worlds colliding here (quite apart from the 'real world' observed by the CDC doctor). One of them was the privileged corporate world of the conference, its logo a globe harmoniously wedded to a cross-section of the human immunodeficiency virus. The other was the raggedy world of radical activism with its mohawked guerrillas, militant gays with 'Read My Lips' T-shirts, and the red-sequined Scarlet Harlot (an advocate for prostitutes' rights) twirling through the flashing ranks of the media. The radicals had their own logo to brandish at the corporate world-virus: a pink triangle borrowed from the Nazi concentration camp insignia by way of the American Gay Liberation Movement. It appeared in the centre of black placards bearing the popular ACT UP slogan 'Silence = Death.'

As the protesters forced their way past the security guards and headed down the central aisle towards the podium, they were evidently determined to make Noise and Action equal Life. They clapped their hands, beat their placards like drums, and chanted 'Not Patients! Not Victims! But People Living with AIDS!'

Their lively procession, which resembled the street-theatre protests of the late sixties, did not amuse the CDC doctor. 'AIDS patients *are* victims,' he muttered. 'Just ask Kaunda. His son died of it.' When I ventured to question his implicit identification of AIDS patients with passive casualties of war, he responded with a world-weary frown. It was his turn to keep silent, but not as a sign of concession.

Since I did not bear a green name-tag identifying me as a scientific delegate, communication between us was bound to be limited. He had evidently sized me up from my black name-tag (which placed me on the 'Audio-Visual Program Committee') as an art-world infiltrator of the conference. His suspicion that I sympathized with the activists was confirmed when I rose from my seat to cheer them on.

They were not all strangers to me. In their midst I spotted my graduate student David White next to British AIDS activist Simon Watney before the current of protest swept them away to the distant podium where their leaders were preparing to read 'Le Manifeste de Montréal' (see appendix to this article). It was not the political goal of the radicals to stop the conference before it had started, but to open it on a corrective note with the self-enfranchising voice of a person living with AIDS.

They were there to form, or at least to propose, a coalition with the delegates in the 'official' AIDS world. Were the researchers not facing the same enemies as the radicals? Besides the intransigence of the virus, were they not all outraged and frustrated by the financial unresponsiveness of conservative governments? If the researchers should need more funds for their drug trials and prevention projects, as they surely do, then let the radicals with their impassioned will and media savvy lobby for them against the indifference of the politicians and the greed of the pharmaceutical companies.

Communication between the two AIDS worlds was essential for this coalition to form. As the resounding cheers of the delegates merged with the riotous chanting of the protesters, I there and then resolved to infiltrate the scientific sessions, come what may, in order to give the lie to anyone who unquestioningly assumed that communication between medical experts and cultural critics was impossible or virtually useless in the AIDS crisis. I was prepared to face with an unflinching eye – and a full stomach – all the skin-flicks the doctors had to offer in their private screening rooms.

Oral Manifestations

What I was not prepared for, however, was the 'whole panic scene' of colliding and disintegrating discourse (as Arthur Kroker would put it) played out the next day in Room 401 before a full house of dermatologists, dentists, and other specialists who had gathered for a session on 'Oral Manifestations of AIDS.' By the time I found the room, which took some doing in the multilevel labyrinth of the Palais des Congrès, it was already darkened like Plato's cave for the presentation of fascinating (though transient) images of the 'real world of the epidemic.'

A paper was in progress. For a tense moment I thought I had actually stumbled into a skin-flick in the usual sense: a pair of swollen lips, half-opened, flashed over the screen, while out of the darkness came a husky West Coast voice inviting us all to consider the possibilities of 'oral-anal sex.' In the gloom, I consulted my conference catalogue to find out who was speaking. He turned out to be a dentist from the Schools of Medicine and Dentistry, University of California, San Francisco, and his paper, co-authored with five other San Franciscan researchers, was entitled 'Sexual Practices as Risk Factors in Candidiasis and Hairy Leukoplakia: The Oral AIDS Epidemiology Project.'

Despite my defiant sense of mission, I was beginning to feel like a child accidently initiated into the mysteries of the primal scene. I felt distinctly odd. Not nauseous, mind you, just incongruous. For what had a spy from the Unreal World of the Arts to do with candidiasis and other afflictions of the tongue?

I had to stay and see. I had to break through the force field of scientific expertise and find some connection with the dentist's 'cohorts' (as he called his gay male subjects) in the War on AIDS. While phrases like 'odds ratios for CD and HL' and 'immunologic measures' went over my head, I wondered how this speaker could detach himself so cooly from the mouths and throats he peered down with his instruments.

Letting down my cynical deflector shields, and sharpening my resolve to listen closely to what medical experts were telling each other behind the scenes, I managed to overcome my impulse to flee the room before the slide show slid me further down some nameless PWA's 'oral cavity.' I had to cut through the interference from my own discursive field. That meant tuning out all literary allusions from my brainwaves, I realized, for if I was to mind-link with the dentist and his world – even momentarily – I had to acknowledge the world of difference between our mentalities. Where a literary type would bleakly philosophize about sex and death in the Age of AIDS as foreshadowed, say, in Thomas Nashe's 'Litany in Time of Plague' (1592) –

> Fond are lifes lustfull joyes,
> Death proves them all but toyes ...
> Phisick himselfe must fade.
> All things to end are made ...[1]

– a modern proponent of physic would rather cast a purely clinical gaze at sex and thrush in the mouths of seropositive gays as statistically investigated by epidemiological examiners 'blind to serostatus.' I could not help wondering, with Nashe, 'what vaine art can reply' when challenged by 51 mouths blanched with candidiasis and another 110 coated with the furry scum of leukoplakia.

The dentist's reply was statistical: the correlation between subjects who engaged in genital-oral sex and those who manifested leukoplakia was 3.87, while the odds were considerably lower (0.94) for anal-oral subjects turning up with hairy white tongues. A similar difference in odds, depending on sexual practices, was detected in seropositives manifesting common candidiasis. 'The increased risk of both infections with oral-genital sex,' he concluded, 'implies that both may be contributed to by sexual activity.'[2]

Life's lustful joys were being bad-mouthed, I suspected, as the Babel decoder in my brain strove to translate the moral of the dentist's paper into street talk: don't suck cock or kiss ass or your tongue (parts of it at least) will be cut off and subjected to microscopic examination at the Oral AIDS Centre. I did learn a few other things from the paper, such as this medical tidbit: you can scrape candidiasis patches off the tongue easily enough, but when you try to do the same with hairy leukoplakia you scrape off the tongue. Cold comfort, indeed, for the high-risk 'cohorts' left behind in San Francisco.

'Wit with his wantonnesse,' Nashe cried, 'tasteth deaths bitternesse.' That was the taste left in my mouth after the dentist's presentation all right, but it was not his fault as an oral AIDS specialist or the fault of his medical language but the sad result of my own defensive irony, my own wanton wit. I could not look AIDS in the mouth, literally, until I had purged the last poetic allusion from my mind (it was St Peter's satiric apostrophe 'Blind mouths!' from Milton's *Lycidas*) so that some kind of critical illumination might follow directly from my espionage. The whole experiment in discursive infiltration would be reduced to the absurdity of a memento mori meditation if I were to leave Room 401 without some insight into the contemporary cultural significance of the conference and its conflicting signs.

It came to me in a flash during the question period when a Zairean researcher, who had previously spoken on oral symptoms of HIV infection among patients in Kinshasa's Mama Yemo Hospital, pushed his way through the darkness to the floor microphone and in heavily accented English anxiously asked the dentist for a diagnostic definition: what did he mean by the term 'hairy leukoplakia'? When the San Francisco definition was provided, the questioner, in perplexity, remarked that 'hairy leukoplakia' meant something a bit different in Kinshasa and so all the African data about its manifestations were bound to seemed 'cooked' from an American viewpoint. The San Francisco definition was immediately defended as the true one by a dentist who worked with the presenter on the Oral AIDS Project. 'But that's not quite what we mean by HL either,' complained a British doctor, who spelled out a number of subtle diagnostic differences between the rival definitions. He thought the African researchers were confusing it with various kinds of candidiasis, though just which white patches were hairy and which ones were not, he confessed, was sometimes difficult to say. Mouths did not come with neat white labels.

In my naïveté I thought that something as impressively technical (or technical-sounding) as hairy leukoplakia would be wholly unambiguous in its diagnosis and definition, but apparently not. Diagnostic labelling, like safer sex, was not practised with rational consistency in all parts of the world.

As a result, heated confusion was erupting on the normally cool ground of medical expertise. The international façade of scientific authority seemed to be cracking (microscopically) under the impetuous efforts of the San Francisco dentist, the Zairean epidemiologist, and the British clinician to defend their local definitions of leukoplakia. It reminded me of the confusion of tongues on the Tower of Babel. The looming presence of a simultaneous translation booth in Room 401 did little to cool tempers at the podium, or to dispel the growing anxiety in the aisles.

Something unexpected had been revealed to the witnesses of this backstage debate, something scary, and their unexpressed panic was quite unlike the officially orchestrated scene of clashing discourses and full-blown AIDS pandemonium the day before when the passionate PWAs of the activist groups opened the conference in their own terms, with their own words, breaking the silence that equals death. Now it was speech that seemed deadly, not silence.

If leukoplakia meant this here, and that there, and this or that over yonder, did it have any global significance at all? Were all the terms in the medical arsenal susceptible to international meltdown at a moment's notice? I wondered how all these champions on the front lines of the Thrush Campaign could ever be expected to halt the Viral Huns when they were not even able to settle minor terminological disputes back at Command Central. Was it possible that medical experts could not get their acts together on diagnostic definitions *eight* years into the epidemic? Word was out: the doctors might not know what they're talking about after all – even among themselves.

I felt the Deconstructive Labyrinth opening up in Room 401 and the Void of Indeterminacy yawning just outside the door. Nashe threw me some more life-lines as my spirits sank:

> Brightnesse falls from the ayre,
> Queenes have died yong and faire ...

But I found myself shuddering at the ironic significance of these lines in the context of the 'gay plague': AIDS had randomly generated a new lyric out of the old litany. Even as the epidemic has no fixed meaning, neither does its poetry – or the prose of the experts.

Appalled by this thought, I looked to the conference-room screen for illumination during the diagnostic crisis. There, looming large over the debate, a silent emblem of it all, deathly white, obscene, hung the image of a diseased tongue.

I left the room muttering activist slogans under my breath. Not patients, not victims, but tongues living with thrush. Tasting death's bitterness again, I had a sudden attack of sympathy with what philosopher Richard Mohr, comparing the Plague of Athens to the AIDS crisis, calls 'the common mind searching for meaning in things.'[3] That search underlies all activist initiatives aimed at ending the crisis, I suspect, as it does the multitude of medical projects represented at the conference. The conference itself, by bringing the experts and the activists face to face, could be seen as a collective defiance of all easy allegories and meaningless voids that may invite us, when our guard is down, to lower our voices against this outrage, to give in to the silence, to close the lines of communication between Physic and Art merely because hell's executioner (as Nashe called Death) 'hath no eares for to heare.'

A Crisis of Representation

Listening with a critical ear to what other people have to say about the epidemic – repulsive as their narratives and commentaries may be to those who have ears to hear – requires a willingness to stop listening to oneself on the subject for a while. As with listening, so with looking: in order to look with a critical eye at art's myriad responses to AIDS (not all of them vanities, pace Nashe) one must set all personal views of the crisis against the backdrop of conflicting signs held up by diverse people from the various 'AIDS worlds' that collided at the Palais des Congrès.

For those who have eyes to see, the AIDS worlds turn out an enormous variety of images. Examining what other people have glimpsed, imagined, painted, photographed, or diagnosed from their angle on the 'whole panic scene' takes a reckless sort of courage that not everyone is willing to muster for the grim reward of staring at slides of diseased mouths, or confronting what television reporters like to call 'the human face of AIDS.' There is of course no Human Face of AIDS, just billions of human faces with eyes to see for themselves what the epidemic is doing to some people here, other people there, and what it means in an intimate physical and social sense to be living with AIDS.

Contemplating this multitude of visions is a 'high-risk activity' for even the most courageous of spectators because it leads to a sceptical and then increasingly polemical engagement with the cultural dialectics of what Simon Watney has perceived as a crisis of representation, 'a crisis over the entire framing of knowledge about the human body and its capacities for sexual pleasure.' His trenchant Foucauldian objections to mainstream AIDS commentary should be heeded by everyone concerned with the impact of the syndrome on human relationships and humane values. He is surely right, even in his ironic choice of Grand Guignol rhetoric, when he claims that 'AIDS has been used to articulate profound social fears and anxieties, in a dense web of racism, patriotism and homophobia. It is this web, spun out of words sticky with blood lust, contempt, hatred, and hysteria, which hangs across the entire media industry of the Western world.'[4] The point of his world-indicting polemics was brought home to me, quite literally, by an AIDS poster I found in the winter of 1988 on a bulletin board at the University of Western Ontario where I teach English and philosophy. Stark white capitals on a black background spelled out the warning of the decade: DON'T DIE OF IGNORANCE.

Though the poster itself (plate 51) was an official product of Western's Student Health Services, the fearful slogan did not originate with the excellent staff of this agency. When I traced it to its source, I was more than a little perturbed to find out that the slogan and much of the text had been taken from the Thatcher Health Ministry's 1985 billboard campaign against the spread of AIDS to the mythical General Public. The conservative tenor of the original British poster, which Watney exposed in 1987 as an example of the crisis of representation, lost little in its translation across the Atlantic to my university – though the key term 'ignorance' did acquire new implications when it was transferred from a general (that is, normative white heterosexist) context to a specifically intellectual environment.

However well-intentioned, Western's version of the poster implied that people who died of AIDS (over forty in London, Ontario, by 1988) were ignoramuses not worthy of serious academic concern; that they died because of their own native ignorance instead of governmental failure to fund any effective safer-sex education campaigns; that they were therefore responsible in some intellectual sense for their own deaths just as students who do not study hard enough are responsible for their low marks; and that AIDS is really a *simple* epistemological problem for which easy solutions have been worked out by the Authorities.

I felt that if these were the kinds of messages that universities were unwittingly or (worse) wittingly communicating to students – let alone what governments were broadcasting to the proverbially uncritical General Public – then the time had come for a critical examination of the cultural framework (the Watneyian 'web') in which such representations were being spun. Finding myself suddenly caught up in the politics of AIDS representation, I decided to offer a graduate course on AIDS and the Arts that would challenge the normative thinking behind all AIDS education campaigns aimed at the General Public.

The course was taught at Western in the fall term of 1988. A year later, an undergraduate version of 'AIDS and the Arts' was taught by my graduate student David White in the wake of his experience as an activist at the Montreal conference. The students in his class designed a pair of safer-sex posters for their straight and gay peers (see plates 52, 53) to counter the 'Ignorance' sign, which was still on display in the University Community Centre. Their 'Get It On' posters proved such a success with the majority of students at Western that the Student Health Services placed copies of both versions prominently in their glassed-in bulletin boards and defended the new campaign from the moral rage of a small but vocal group of Christian students who championed the sovereign joys of chastity. Threatened by the posters' radically sex-positive message, an advocate for abstinence wrote a letter to the student newspaper condemning the 'Get It On' campaign as 'beautiful but pornographic.' Ten courageous letters defending the design were published in subsequent issues.

Polemical engagement with – or against – the radical-activist vision of the AIDS crisis is bound to threaten the stability of personally cherished views of the medical crisis, which in turn provokes a painful review of society's fundamental attitudes towards sex, death, nature, beauty, money, physic, art, the law, the state, the world, the flesh, and the devil – Nashe's whole litany of obsessions, and then some. Courage is always needed when there's a risk of radicalization on so many fronts, and the risk of turning over a new political leaf in the AIDS crisis is higher than you might think, even if you're not immediately inclined to equate Silence with Death.

Crisis and Criticism

As everyone involved in the AIDS and the Arts course soon discovered, the very notion of 'crisis' in the context of AIDS raises critical questions about the politics of representation. Apart from headlining the epidemic, making it horrific news on a par with wars and stock-market crashes, what has the term 'crisis' done to organize our perceptions of the syndrome and its cultural impact? How has it constructed AIDS for us without our having to think about it, plotting the rush of biological events, individual life histories, scattered community responses, tardy government campaigns, and brief international get-togethers into a comprehensible story?

Still latent in 'crisis' is its ancient Greek sense of 'choosing' or 'picking out,' hence a 'decision' or 'judgment,' particularly in a legal context where a judge resolves a dispute by identifying a victim, picking out a winner, deciding against this or that side, handing down a sentence. Since a crisis served as the decisive turning-point in a wrangle, it inevitably implied authoritative intervention, hierarchical control, and effective resolution. To reach a crisis, then, meant to impose a set of clearly defined social roles on a quarrelsome crowd of people and to unravel their tangled conflicts into a straight course of events with a beginning, a middle, and an end. The events provoking the dispute made up its beginning; the dispute itself was the middle; and with the crisis, which could be considered the end of the middle or the beginning of the end, a resolution to the plot was legally created, secured, worked out. The imperative of irreversible closure, the full stop, charged the word with deus-ex-machina efficacy.

In the mid-sixteenth century, when 'crisis' entered English as a learned borrowing, it had shifted from a legal to a strictly medical context, but its decisive sense of resolution through intervention was retained. It signified the turning-point in the 'progress' of a disease when something happens – a fever breaks, a pustule erupts – to mark the imminence of either death or recovery. The intervening force was often conceived astrologically as a favourable or unfavourable conjunction of the stars, but angels, devils, daimones, saints, witches, alchemists, mages, barbers, and chirurgeons also figured as the agents of resolution. Since Renaissance medicine habitually constructed the human body in legal and political terms, diseases being discordant disputes among the members of our 'little state,' we should not be surprised by the appropriation of quasi-juridical power by ambitious practitioners of physic: if physicians could read the signs of crisis in the body as astrologers read them in the stars, might they not also be able to plot the events of the disease and impose critical resolutions on organic disputes, ending the unnatural suspense of illness, restoring the natural concord of health? Of course they could, and did, with a ghastly array of arbitrary 'treatments' from blood-letting to mercuric baths. A medical crisis increasingly demanded purely medical intervention. The doctor-ex-machina hit the boards.

In the seventeenth century, during the disputatious prelude to the English Civil War, crises began to appear in the discursive fields of politics and history. The old medical model of a 'critical illness' clearly underlay these new social visions of the suspenseful but negotiable turning-point (for instance, Rudyard's complaint in 1627: 'This is the Chrysis of Parliaments: we shall know by this if Parliaments live or die.'[5]). Puritan crises, which included the spiritual kind, were useful points or phases to see coming or to look back on – however difficult they were to get through – because they assured the vigilant soul that every frightening course of events had a determinable structure with a morally fitting resolution. Though the eighteenth century tended to emphasize the insecurity, suspense, and difficulty experienced by heroic souls during the 'great crises in Church and State,' such times, dark as they seemed, were brilliantly reconceived as social and spiritual challenges to mankind's ultimately invincible powers of reason by that decisive new arbiter of social value and cultural excellence, the Enlightenment 'Critick.'

It was an offspring of the German Enlightenment, neoclassical critic Gustav Freytag, who turned 'crisis' into a popular literary term by lending its already fateful ring a tragic cadence, a dying fall, that it had never had before the nineteenth century. In his monumental *Technique of the Drama* (1857) – which was to fix the ideal 'pyramidal' form of tragedy as a rising action, climax, and falling action in the minds of generations of literature students as if it were a divine truth handed down to the Victorians from the ancient Egyptians by way of the Greeks – Freytag defined 'Krise' as the turning-point in the tragic plot after which the protagonist is unable to control the action or prevent his own destruction.[6] From this gravitational kind of crisis, which precipitates a collapse rather than resolves a conflict, it's downhill all the way to the catastrophe. Forget about free will at the end. Abandon vain hopes of divine intervention. Don't even bother with first aid. The hero's thread is cut at the critical moment he ceases to be a hero and becomes a victim, a sacrifice to the schoolroom gods of pure aesthetic form.

What sort of crisis, then, is the 'the AIDS crisis'? That would seem to depend not wholly on the biological peculiarities of the syndrome itself or on the relentless spread of HIV from this population to that, as one might at first suppose. Rather, given the long evolution of 'crisis mentality' in the West as a perceptual habit designed to organize events into a decisive plot, one can only conclude that it largely depends on certain cultural (that is, political, economic, religious, and even aesthetic) factors that have little to do with the 'real world' of infected cells and hairy tongues and a great deal to do with the fantasy world of social agendas and conflicting discourses. What sort of AIDS crisis you find yourself in depends, then, on who constructs the narrative around the imagined turning-point, what sort of narrative is constructed, and why such a construction is formed at such a time in such a place.

For instance, if Michael Callen (a founding member of the American PWA Coalition) is telling the story of AIDS as he did to a bewildered reporter on Canadian television during the Montreal conference, insisting in his provocative way that 'politics is the only cure for AIDS,' then the narrative is plotted like an unfolding political battle punctuated with government showdowns, courtroom conflicts, radical resistance strategies, collective and personal victories. The AIDS crisis in Callen's vitally optimistic, bravely democratic world resolves into a series of social decision-points, crises in the ancient Greek sense, with principled PWAs successfully defending themselves in the arenas of social arbitration and resolving in time all the racist, sexist, rightist, and leftist conflicts stirred up by the epidemic.

By contrast, if you turn to Peter Jaret's microcosmic account of our embattled immune system in *National Geographic*, the AIDS crisis is constructed along quaintly medical lines reminiscent of the disease-as-discord theory prevalent in the sixteenth century. Like a stoical Elizabethan doctor, Jaret delivers a serene panegyric on the civilized political order of the healthy human body – he even hails the 'biologic democracy' of lymphocytes and macrophages! – as a Galenesque prelude to his main theological fantasy: an allegorization of AIDS as demonic scourge.[7]

The mythical 'AIDS virus' here assumes the supernatural role of an incubus, a nocturnal spirit capable of stealing through the secret portals of the body and robbing our normally carefree souls of sleep. 'Then suddenly there was AIDS – a new, virulent scourge that relentlessly disarms the immune system,' he shudders to relate. 'Into our peaceful sleep has crept a nightmare, putting the quest to understand the body's defenses on a crisis footing.'[8] Lady Macbeth's doctor could not have diagnosed the crisis more ominously: a sudden mysterious disruption of our collective psyche, causing a fantastic acceleration of the once calmly scientific 'quest to understand,' serves as the critical sign that humanity is heading either for extinction or salvation. We are all, it appears, suffering from AIDS-induced delirium, a critical condition that causes us to walk about like seropositive zombies thinking on death and trying to wash our hands of the whole scary business. But this absurd condition will prove fatal for the body politic, if the American medical and technological establishments (whose leading representatives strike attitudes of resolute sagacity in photographs of the Quest-in-Progress throughout the article) are not paid to intervene as epidemiological exorcists at the critical moment of HIV possession.

Whenever the AIDS story is plotted as a moralized chronicle of hideous suffering on a grand scale, violent clashes between natural and cultural forces, and epic battles between virtuous and villainous 'personalities,' the turning-point in the narrative is a moment of public enlightenment when reason (in the morally fortified eighteenth-century sense) glimpses the glorious or ghastly truth about the state of things and exerts itself, through its heroic human agents, to take arms against a sea of troubles and by opposing end them. This kind of crisis mentality is endemic among journalists and broadcasters who pride themselves on presenting both the Big Picture and the Human Face of AIDS. Chronicler Randy Shilts is the best-selling doyen of their school, and from his celebrity viewpoint the moment of enlightenment for America (and hence the world) was the death of Rock Hudson – a tabloid event that brought the nation to its senses about the Threat to Us All. The tide of public opinion turned at this point away from its cosy Reaganite fantasies of small-town prosperity towards the awful Truth that homosexuals, those creatures of perverse irrationality, were polluting the bodily fluids in the American mainstream.[9] Reason's valiant negotiators in this 'crisis situation,' a massive complication in the Patient Zero plot formally invented by Shilts, are his own glowing culture-heroes: gay prophet Larry Kramer, CDC investigator Don Francis, and himself.

Also written as an enlightenment critique of history, though not in chronicle form, is Masters and Johnson's epidemiological thriller *Crisis: Heterosexual Behavior in the Age of AIDS* (1988). The title says it all. Until HIV leaked out of the polluted gay underworld into the mainstream there was no AIDS crisis: the punctuating 'event' between the safe Before and the perilous After, the critical tide in the affairs of men, was 'the outbreak of AIDS in the heterosexual community in the United States,' as bravely documented by our two celebrity sexologists acting in the public interest. They alone (through their disciple Robert C. Kolodny) now speak with the voice of Reason against even the voices of other widely respected authorities, including Washington health officials, who 'are greatly underestimating the number of people infected with the AIDS virus in the population today.'[10] The prestigious names of Masters and Johnson, no small commodity in their upscale world, were put on the line for what Reason had revealed unto them through the moralized lens of promiscuity surveys. Their formal invention of a new cultural period, the devastating 'Age of AIDS,' implicitly structures their Ladies' Home Journal of the plague years along apocalyptic lines.

Truths stranger than fiction, such as the scientifically conceivable risk that you can 'catch AIDS from a toilet seat,' vie in their pages with fictions stranger than truth, most notably the existence of a single monolithic 'heterosexual community' poised on the brink of viral extinction.[11] When did this ideologically uniform group of straights emerge in the U.S. population? How can Reason save them from their promiscuous passions? What Castro can contain them?

'Does this terrible tale have a moral?' asked Dr Robert C. Gallo of the National Institutes of Health, striking, for a moment, the judicious pose of an Enlightenment Critick in his 1987 *Scientific American* article on the proteinaceous grenade he dubbed (how injudiciously!) the AIDS virus. His answer, of course, was

> Yes. In the past two decades one of the fondest boasts of medical science has been the conquest of infectious disease, at least in the wealthy countries of the industrialized world. The advent of retroviruses with the capacity to cause extraordinarily complex and devastating disease has exposed that claim for what it was: hubris. Nature is never truly conquered. The human retroviruses and their intricate interrelation with the human cell are but one example of that fact. Indeed, perhaps conquest is the wrong metaphor to describe our relation to nature, which not only surrounds but in the deepest sense constitutes our being.[12]

At first this sounds like moralized history welling up from the depths of Stoic melancholy: but at the mention of 'hubris,' followed by a gloomy soliloquy on failed 'conquest' and invincible 'Nature,' the terrible tale betrays its true literary colours. The co-discoverer of HIV, a giant among virologists, has constructed the story of AIDS as a neoclassical tragedy with an elemental conflict between Man and Nature at its raging heart. Gallo himself is the tragic hero, the promethean mediator between conservative Nature and progressive Culture. In the past two decades, like the medical science whose proud spirit lives in him, he has had everything going for him – oracular agar plates, miraculous scientific breakthroughs, and the favour of the project-funding gods.

Enter his relentless antagonist, the AIDS Virus, an invisible foe who cannot just pop up out of a trap door in the style of a stage villain. HTLV-III (as Gallo first called HIV) must have a mythical origin like the Hydra, springing many-headed from the poisonous blood of a Green Monkey, and an apocalyptic 'advent' like the Antichrist, heralding the ghastly end of the industrial world. Howl we must, therefore, like the hapless chorus during the Theban plague, when the Virus marches its legions of mutant RNA clones out of Africa into America where AIDS is first recognized as Nature's ultimate threat to medical science and the civilization dependent on its victories. The rising action reaches its climax when Gallo, the Scientific American par excellence, heroically captures the attention of the world media by 'discovering' his secret foe, and this he manages to do against all odds, despite every complication in the plot, including the message just in from Paris that Dr Luc Montagnier of the Pasteur Institute may have discovered the damn thing first.

Thus are we brought to the tragic crisis: Gallo's other discovery, this paralysing anagnorisis concerning ... himself. Like poor tormented Hamlet unable to act after discovering Claudius at prayer, Gallo, for all his intimate knowledge of the foe, is unable to kill it where it lies and purge the rotten state of its infernal presence. Science does not grant him power over it, or over its dark mother, Nature, who having constituted 'our being' too turns out to be (O Oedipal horror!) his own mother. No one can conquer her. Not even him, the conquering hero. And why not? Because the gods of healing, who refuse to come down to earth in their old machines, have evidently decided to punish him for his hubristic attitude towards Nature.

A perfect Freytagian pyramid is thus implicit in Gallo's soliloquy on conquest. All the great doctor can do, looking ahead to Nature's inevitable victory over him at death, is to meditate on the falling action of the plague and on the pervasiveness of his greater enemy, who like a Fury not only hounds him but possesses him 'in the deepest sense.' And what that mysterious sense might be only a tragic hero has the depth of soul to know.

Does this terrible moral have a tale? No – many tales. Or if one only, then it is the continuing story of how Gallo, and Masters, and Johnson, and Jaret, and Callen, and all the rest of us are constructing our own versions of the AIDS crisis to realize individual and collective fantasies of cultural intervention.

In so far as we have discovered 'crisis' itself to be a formal invention designed to give shape and significance and the promise of resolution to an otherwise frightening course of conflicted events, the AIDS crisis should be confronted and combatted not only by virologists and sexologists and other researchers mantled in scientific authority but also – perhaps principally at this time – by cultural critics working out of the arts in close cooperation with activist artists critically attuned to their work. I would even go so far as to argue, against Gallo, who in Montreal flaunted his hubris by arguing for the expulsion of all pesky non-scientists from future international AIDS conferences, that the AIDS crisis is properly our domain of study, not his, however rudimentary our knowledge of hairy leukoplakia and the glycoproteins studding the membrane of HIV. The arts world has its frontiers of enlightenment too, and its fronts in the field, and we must not allow ourselves to be expelled from this battle.

The Rising Action

If the only function of activist criticism was to produce sceptical spectators of the crises in the 'AIDS tragedy,' necessary as that function is at the outset to encourage transdiscursive infiltration and counter-discursive questioning, the effort would not amount to much in the end. Marshalled at the Arts Front would be a cadre of disgruntled dialecticians slowly sinking into the Slough of Despond. The AIDS crisis is an absurd fantasy not worth fighting for or against, they would grumble, because there is no plot or moral in the whole mess, no single live-or-die turning-point, no possibility of a morally fitting resolution to the myriad conflicts, no hope of effective cultural arbitration, no protagonist to die at the hands of an implacably vengeful Nature, in fact no Nature, nothing with shape or significance, nothing, nothing, nothing. Nothing but words tripping off a diseased tongue.

It does not take much to push a sceptical spectator of the AIDS scene over the edge. A lecture on hairy leukoplakia almost did it to me. You might be driven to the howling brink by almost any network broadcast on the epidemic, any government-sponsored poster on abstinence as a form of safer sex, or any pious statement by Jesse Helms on the gay threat to family values. However sane it may seem to suspend judgments for a while, to listen to other discourses before defending or revising your own agenda in the midst of the plotless turmoil, the time must come to pull back and not give in to the 'falling action' if you truly question and reject the various crisis mentalities constructing the Age of AIDS around (or within) you.

Unless you take action at the brink, a resolutely rising action, you risk sliding off the beaten path of dialectical scepticism into the quick sand of cynicism – where apathy (in the old Stoic sense of 'unfeelingness') is the only breathing straw left for the philosophical soul struggling to keep reason alive. From there you may be drawn into the pit of nihilism where all thought is crushed out of existence by the romantic pressures of irresolvable paradox, which may indeed suit you if you're half in love with easeful death. Or you may opt for intellectual suicide by another route – conversion to right-wing fundamentalism – where beliefs are apocalyptically 'saved' along with your soul by the eternal lifeline of organized paranoia.

That way madness lies. And sometimes money. But what reasonable way leads back from the paralysis of terminal irony and the palliative care of apathy to a valid and vigorous recovery for the critical spirit in the Age of AIDS?

The rising action of criticism-at-the-edge takes off from a decisive belief in the possibility (even the merest possibility) that cultural critics, in close cooperation with activist artists, can actually save lives while 'the plague full swift goes bye.' This we can do, we must tell ourselves. This we can do by fiercely resisting the fatally twinned discourses of sexual repression and social oppression working at large in the world to construct the AIDS crisis in ways that blatantly victimize PWAs and their caregivers while blindly hindering their constructive efforts to halt the spread of HIV through effective safer-sex education and clean-needle programs. This we can do by applying what arts faculties banally call 'theory' – the radically sceptical methodologies developed in the last two decades by formidable opponents of the modern surveillance state – to the crush of cultural problems caused or exacerbated by the epidemic at every social level, across every discipline, in every afflicted and conflicted realm of Nashe's 'uncertain world' lying just outside the university gates. This we can do by empowering ourselves with the realization that even as the crisis can come under criticism, so criticism can take on the crisis.

If AIDS criticism is to be more than just another exercise of wanton wit, another symbolic show of 'AIDS awareness,' we must construct an agenda for it to translate its subversive sceptical theories into life-saving activist practices. What we should do must be doable, of course, but it must also be done – right away – in stride with those people with AIDS (like Michael Callen and John Gordon) who have been struggling at various counterdiscursive fronts since the epidemic was first madly perceived as a crisis for the microscopic 'immune system' and then for the monolithic 'general public.' It is, we must continue to tell ourselves, a crisis for us.

Resisting my own inclination to flee from the Diseased Tongue into the contemplative quietude of the Academy, I propose that the following six collective aims (at least) be on the main agenda of an activist criticism for the Age of AIDS:

1 To select, from the variety of contemporary critical theories, those lines of cultural analysis that will lead to a singularly clear but multi-angled understanding of the 'Crisis of Representation' as it affects the political process of constructing the syndrome at a micro-level, the epidemic at a macro-level, and the human body caught between them;
2 To extend those lines of cultural analysis from the Holy Mountain of the Arts (our traditional grounding in the aesthetic practices and products of High Culture) into the fairly unholy but lively Cities of the Plain, the suburbs and ghettos and business districts of popular culture, monitoring in particular the media's obsessive mythologization of the epidemic and the experts' incessant reinvention of the crisis;
3 To judge, fearlessly, with the courageous reasonableness of Enlightenment Criticks but without their moralistic twaddle or aesthetic perfectionism, the socially constructive representations of AIDS from the harmful ones, on the politically and aesthetically radical basis of whether they further the critical cause of saving and sustaining lives;
4 To introduce into university curriculums interdisciplinary arts courses on the representation of AIDS in both academic and popular cultural contexts, transforming normally complacent classes into radical cells of resistance to homophobia, erotophobia, and the mainstream discourses constructing the epidemic;
5 To spark debate on AIDS issues at a local level among principled representatives of the critical circle, the PWA support groups, the university community, the medical establishment, the municipal administration, the school systems, the art galleries, the churches, and any other concerned institutions, leading to local changes in policy and practice vis-à-vis safer-sex education and anti-drug programs; and
6 To devise, in close cooperation with community-based AIDS groups and activist artists, some kind of accessible vehicle to

> carry the analytical conclusions and critical judgments of the activist collective out from the university into the community surrounding it, and further afield, if possible, into the national and international scene.

The temptation to substitute rash social action for rigorous critical thinking may be hard to resist at this point, when there is so much to be done in the world of ACT UP and AIDS ACTION NOW!, but resist it we must within the world of the arts – for the short time it takes to collect our thoughts – before venturing to take such an agenda into the mean streets and meaner strata of society. Socially constructive action on the part of the arts to end the AIDS crisis (rather than 'to transcend it,' as Douglas Crimp has pointed out[13]) should grow out of, be spurred on by, hard thinking about who's getting what out of the calamity. Little good would be done for the sick or the well by promoting a nostalgic return to medieval 'contemptus mundi.'

The Middle Ages got a few things right, however, and one of them was the championship of rigorously disciplined contemplation that extended itself unflinchingly into the mucky realm of life's lustful joys, mortal dreads, and dire uncertainties. If we were to spurn the 'contemplatif lyf' entirely in our advocacy of activism, the 'actif lyf' would become no more than a directionless scramble for temporary personal gains and political handouts lacking even the levelling impetus of the danse macabre. Activist criticism must unite the contemplative with the active life if it is to help save lives by sustaining the critical belief that lives can be saved from the plague, and are worth saving, through cultural intervention.

Arts Action Now

If the hard thinking at the core of what might be called the 'Arts Action Now' agenda takes any one modern source as its starting-point, it is the social philosophy of Michel Foucault. In so far as Foucauldian theory levels all cultural productions to the dynamic political status of institutional signs, its sceptical thrust tends to undermine the old static hierarchy of 'high culture' and 'low culture.'

Things neither commonly presented nor commonly perceived as works of art can suddenly assume aesthetic power beyond the éclat of masterpieces, and instructive control beyond the élan of propaganda, when seen from the marginal angle of the disenfranchised. The slide of hairy leukoplakia was certainly no *Guernica*, yet it struck me for a moment as a more powerful icon of powerlessness than any that High Culture could show me – because the Diseased Tongue was so still and silent, so paralysed by the potent medical gaze, so insulting to the unheard patient whose hair-raising scream was thus suspended by audiovisual technology at the push-button command of a specialist.

In applying Foucauldian theory to the fulminant yet sill largely unanalysed domain of AIDS representations, those who follow the 'Arts Action Now' agenda should routinely extend their critical gaze from the old high grounds of academic culture to the new flickering cave of media-based popular culture, and back again, breaking down the perceptual barriers between these two worlds (both fantasy worlds in their own right, one no realer than the other). Thus will they reveal the interdependence of élitist and populist agendas, transcendental and confrontational impulses, mainstream and underground discourses that are still at work in constructing the highly unstable narratives of the Crisis.

The authors in this volume offer numerous examples of this crossover strategy in operation. Monique Brunet-Weinmann, for one, has analysed an Australian AIDS poster (the producers of which probably never even viewed it as bad art) as if it were a detail from some weird postmodern extension of the danse macabre frescos in the Cemetery of the Holy Innocents. Little did the public-health officials down under realize (or did they?) that their Grim Reaper ads promoted a highly conservative, intensely moralistic theology of AIDS that had its roots in the era of the Black Death (see p 149 in this volume).

The subversive critical practice of confounding high and low also works in the other direction, as in Andy Fabo's Foucauldian art books. These highly academic works, filled with learned allusions to Renaissance painting and sculpture, test Foucault's theory of power-knowledge against lived experience – the constant physical suspense of a PWA, the policed yet empowering desires of a gay man, the militantly regenerative instincts of a figural artist. Yet, as David White shows in his probing essay on Fabo's activist art, its basis, literally, is not hoity-toity theory or high-brow painterly convention but a series of grass-roots shop manuals upon which the artist has constructed his often fantastic imagery as if grounding it in the practical world of drill-bits and screwdrivers. Similarly, André Durand's Neo-Renaissance altarpiece *Votive Offering*, a monarchist fantasia on the theme of mystical healing, turns out to be based on common media images of Princess Diana and a sensationalist photo 'spread' of an American PWA in *Life* magazine. In the fine Foucauldian confusion of aesthetics and politics, AIDS images like these lose their romantic mystique as artistic 'objects' existing on their own for art's sake but gain in cultural resonance as social 'constructions' promoting the value systems of their producers.

Since activist critics rarely recoil from defending or attacking what they study – they are not polite 'New Historicists' wary of expressing allegiance or opposition to ideological values – their pages fairly bristle with sharp judgments and brusque rebukes. In many cases their political and aesthetic judgments were roughed out in the dialectical excitement of pioneering classes such as Simon Watney's 1985 'AIDS and the Media' course at the London Polytechnical Institute, Jan Grover's 1986 'Media(ted) AIDS' course at the California Institute of the Arts, and Douglas Crimp's 1987 AIDS activism seminar at Rutgers.

In their wake I taught my interdisciplinary graduate course 'AIDS and the Arts' at the University of Western Ontario in the fall of 1988. During the ninth week of my course, from 9 to 11 November, a weekend conference on the cultural representations of AIDS was held at the UWO's University Hospital – a fittingly Foucauldian venue – with Watney, Grover, and Crimp in attendance. Since 1988 there have been at least two further activist 'cells' started up in institutions of advanced learning: an undergraduate version of my course taught by David White at the UWO in 1989; and concurrent with it, Professor William Hardy's seminar on the AIDS crisis and the media in the Department of Radio, Television, and Motion Pictures at the University of North Carolina at Chapel Hill.

These classes, I must point out, were not isolated from each other. Like a foreign correspondent, Grover sent weekly letters from San Francisco to my graduates while we were struggling over the discursive ground she had broken two years earlier. Watney and Crimp both delivered papers at the UWO conference, and discussed their activist agenda in person with White, then an auditor in my seminar. I, in turn, delivered the opening lecture at Hardy's UNC seminar to a new group of students who were about to read Watney, Grover, and Crimp in the now legendary AIDS issue of *October* magazine. Clearly, momentum is growing at the fourth stage of the 'Arts Action Now' agenda.

Visual AIDS

As for the social-outreach stages of the agenda, the expansion and transformation of activist criticism into critical activism beyond the university gates, I can only offer a local example of social cooperation in the effort to alter prevailing 'general public' constructions of the crisis: what the UWO classes in AIDS and the Arts have done in London, Ontario – a prosperous middle-sized city of largely white home-and-garden English Canadians – reflects our critical understanding of the cultural manifestation of the epidemic in our social environment. Bearing in mind Grover's crucial point that there is no single AIDS epidemic but a multitude of diversely manifested and constructed epidemics across the cultural spectrum of the globe, we realize that our version of cultural activism may not work in places only a few hours' drive away – like Detroit, where the epidemic has a very different ethnological and epidemiological character.

London is a life-insurance centre, the Hartford Connecticut of Canada (minus the racial violence). With a sizeable proportion of its population dedicated to the pursuit of financial security by the age of fifty-five, it is not a hotbed of political or cultural radicalism; nor is it, like Toronto, a media-wired theatre where confrontational politics or civil disobedience in the New York ACT UP style would be likely to get effective coverage. AIDS ACTION NOW!, I recall, valiantly staged a 'die-in' outside a drug-protocol conference held in a downtown London hotel during the fall of 1988 while my course was in progress. About twenty-five people showed up to lie with cardboard tombstones on the frosty sidewalk outside the hotel in front of the media – which consisted of a single shivering radio reporter unhappily recording the silence of the grave.

My students and I decided that other strategies had to be adopted in this environment to engage the public in useful debates over AIDS-related issues. Calling on the well-established arts communities in the city, we found ready allies for our program in two gallery directors: Nancy Poole at the publicly funded London Regional Art and Historical Museums; and Jamelie Hassan at the Embassy Cultural House, a small artist-run space for contemporary art located in an East London residential hotel.

After hearing what we were doing on the critical front at the university, Hassan and her board decided to complement our efforts by organizing a series of three exhibitions of contemporary art on the contextualizing theme of competitive social constructions of the body, including but not restricted to the media-constructed body of the 'AIDS victim.' These exhibitions, collectively entitled 'The Body & Society,' were London's answer to the celebrated 'Let the Record Show ...' installation at the New Museum of Contemporary Art. Works by ten Canadian artists, plus New Yorkers Leon Golub and Nancy Spero, were presented in three separate group shows (see below, pp 215ff). The third and in my view climactic show included the art books of Andy Fabo. Since the openings for these shows were strategically scheduled for Thursday evenings following my seminar, visiting artists often took the opportunity to attend the critical discussions at the university before convening at the Embassy Cultural House. Further links between the artistic and academic communities were forged by Hassan's participation on the organizing committee of the 'Representing AIDS' conference, and by Fabo's delivery of the keynote address at its opening session, which concluded with a showing of his video self-portrait *Survival of the Delirious*.

When I approached Nancy Poole at the London Regional Art Gallery (as it was then known), my expectations that space for an activist exhibition on AIDS could be found in what I thought was her conservative domain were not high. Perhaps I should not have been so surprised by her immediate approval of my plan to exhibit an extensive collection of AIDS-prevention posters from around the world that my students and I, together with Clarence Crossman and John Gordon of the AIDS Committee of London, had been putting together since the spring of 1988. Her curatorial staff were willing to take risks, she informed me in no uncertain terms, when it came to the important task of raising public awareness of the epidemic and deepening compassionate concern for people affected by it.

Thanks to her generous public-spiritedness, and the hard work of curators Marnie Fleming and Paddy O'Brien, the Visual AIDS project was launched at the Community Gallery with a première exhibition of about 150 posters from some 28 countries on 11 October 1988. In keeping with my academic-outreach conception of the show, which was to serve as an accessible vehicle to convey our critical work out into the community at large, I produced (with the help of my students David Kinahan and Brian Patton) a brief critique or 'gloss' for each poster in the show. This running commentary was designed to expose the political subtexts and cultural implications of AIDS publicity produced by community-based groups as well as government health agencies. Judgments on the prejudicial character or social effectiveness of the posters were strongly expressed in the glosses, often in provocative satiric terms, in order to engage complacent spectators in the cultural dialectics of AIDS representation.

The following excerpt from my lead-in panel essay 'Reading the Signs' sums up the sceptical objectives and cross-cultural strategies of the show:

> Visual AIDS is a poster exhibition representing the politically charged process of representing AIDS. If the international diversity of AIDS advertisements reveals anything about the new disease and the cultural turmoil it has stirred up all over the world, it is that AIDS is not a pure field of serious scientific research obscured by silly taboos and myths about sex, death, and the body. The taboos and myths are deadly serious too, and as real as HIV. They are part of the disease.
>
> AIDS posters are among the more transient representations of the epidemic, and as such, are particularly valuable in showing that the disease is anything but an immutable set of biomedical or historical 'facts' existing apart from its social constructions ... Ironically, despite the ephemeral character of the posters, their producers often claim to present us with 'the Facts about AIDS' or even 'the New Facts of Life' along with Proper Codes of Behaviour for some kind of New Age – as if they were handing us tablets of stone inscribed with grim prophecies and sacred injunctions.

Visual AIDS (which is still touring at the time of publication) invites a critical reading of these signs of cultural crisis in 'the Age of AIDS.' The organizing theme of the exhibition is the endemic tension between erotic and anti-erotic approaches to contemporary life – a life perceived as threatened by the deviously mutating (and potently mythical) 'AIDS virus.' What the exhibition represents as a whole is not any single privileged social construction of AIDS but a continuum of cultural reactions to the inward and outward consequences of the epidemic: 'At one extreme in this continuum are expressions of panic, omens of death, and militaristic threats explicitly or implicitly directed at social groups regarded as endangering the good blood or bright future of the "General Public." At the other extreme are defiantly joyous affirmations of bodily pleasure, manifestos of erotic liberation, and fantasies of safe sex springing from a frantic confidence in the prophylactic and aphrodisiac virtues of the condom, the transparent talisman of the Age of AIDS.' Between the cold sweats and the hot rubbers may be set the majority of AIDS advertisements, which are neither erogenous nor eschatological. Their designs hint at death without taking all the fun out of life. In them may be read the new age's uneasy efforts to reconcile the old claims of Eros and Thanatos, the classical gods of desire and death.

In one of those unexpected alliances of interest forged by the Crisis,

Visual AIDS found a corporate sponsor in London Life – the city's major white-collar employer and the country's largest life-insurance firm. During the first year of the show's existence, James Etherington, the vice-president for corporate affairs of London Life, generously underwrote the costs of mounting, documenting, advertising, and transporting Visual AIDS without interfering in any way with its critical activist mission. Since 1989 the project has been guided on the financial side by corporate affairs executive Catherine Finlayson. This alliance may be a first in the Canadian annals of AIDS activism: a cooperative venture linking a redoubtably cautious corporation with a radical cadre of AIDS resistance fighters.

Though Visual AIDS was originally designed for touring to small villages and towns around London, it has not been back to southwestern Ontario since its première. Before it had even closed in London, two invitations had been sent to us for distant installations: the first (January 1989) in Mary Scott's « »dl gallery in Calgary, Alberta; and the second (March 1989) in the Stauffacher Buchhandlung in Berne, Switzerland, under the auspices of the AIDS Info-Docu Schweiz. By January 1990 the exhibition had been mounted in thirteen different sites, including the Galerie John A. Schweitzer during the Fifth International AIDS Conference in Montreal (see Monique Brunet-Weinmann's article, pp 146ff); the UNC Student Union gallery in Chapel Hill (August 1989); and the Berliner AIDS-Hilfe in West Berlin (November 1989) during the exciting weeks when the Wall was falling into history. My students and I take some pride in the fact that a little over a year after its opening in little London, Visual AIDS opened in Big London on World AIDS Day (1 December 1989) at the Lighthouse, a multi-functional AIDS education and treatment centre in Notting Hill Gate.

In the winter of 1990 a second exhibition, with 350 new posters from 34 countries, was put together by the Visual AIDS committee. It opened at the DCAC Gallery in the Adams Morgan district of Washington, DC, on 23 March. A month later it was shipped to the Friends of Photography in San Francisco, where it was displayed from 3 May to 8 July in the Ansel Adams Center. I expected a receptive audience for Visual AIDS in San Francisco, and found it not only among the San Franciscans but also among the thousands of delegates who did not boycott the Sixth International AIDS Conference, which was held from 20 to 24 June in the Moscone Convention Center (just across the street from the Friends of Photography gallery). The Visual AIDS committee produced a poster (plate 54) to advertise the exhibition in the Bay area.

Copies of it were sold at the Ansel Adams Center to raise money for a San Francisco organization called 'Visual AID,' which provides art supplies to local artists with AIDS and other life-threatening illnesses.

As this volume was taking shape, I sometimes thought of it as 'Verbal AIDS': a written complement to the death-and-desire continuum of my poster exhibition, the punning title of which goes back to an article Simon Watney wrote in 1987 on public-health posters.[14] The anthology, however, turned out to be much broader in scope than Visual AIDS – which in some sense it subsumes – not only because it explores many other representational media besides graphic art but also because it involves many more authors than just myself and my students. All of us who have contributed to its dialectical structure are prepared to challenge anyone who questions our right to take on the Crisis in our critical terms. As these pages reveal, we have depended upon each other at every turn to answer the ultimate insult of the Diseased Tongue, which is to declare us all insane for countering the plague with words and images.

APPENDIX

AIDS ACTION NOW! Toronto, Canada &
ACT UP, New York, U.S.A. jointly issue:

LE MANIFESTE DE MONTRÉAL

Declaration of the Universal Rights and Needs
of People living with HIV disease

Preamble

HIV disease (infection with HIV with or without symptoms) is a worldwide epidemic affecting every country. People are infected, sick and struggling to stay alive. Their voices must be heard and their special needs met. This declaration sets forth the responsibilities of all peoples, governments, international bodies, multinational corporations, and health care providers to ensure the rights of all people living with HIV disease.

Demands

1. All governments and all international and national health organizations must treat HIV disease positively and aggressively as a chronic, manageable

condition. Ensuring access and availability of treatment must be part of the social and moral obligations of governments to their citizens.

2. Governments must recognize that HIV disease is not highly infectious. Casual contact presents no threat of infection, and irrational fears of transmission must be fought.

3. An international code of rights must acknowledge and preserve the humanity of people with HIV disease. This code must include:

a) anti-discrimination legislation protecting the jobs, housing and access to services of people with HIV disease;

b) active involvement of the affected communities of people with HIV disease in decision-making that may affect them;

c) guaranteed access to approved and experimental drugs and treatments, and quality medical care;

d) the right to anonymous and absolutely confidential HIV antibody testing. Pre- and post-test counselling must be available;

e) the right to medically appropriate housing;

f) no restriction on the international movement and/or immigration of people with HIV disease;

g) full legal recognition of lesbian and gay relationships;

h) no mandatory testing under any circumstances;

i) no quarantine under any circumstances;

j) protection of the reproductive rights of women with HIV disease, including their right to freely choose the birth and spacing of their children and have the information and means to do so;

k) special attention to the unique problems and needs of intravenous drug users, including provision of substance-abuse treatment on demand;

l) special attention to the unique problems and needs of prisoners with HIV disease and guarantees that they receive the same standard of care and treatment as the general population;

m) the right to communication and all services concerning HIV disease in the language (written, signed or spoken) of his/her choice, through an interpreter if necessary;

n) the provision of reasonable accommodation in services and facilities for disabled people;

o) catastrophic/immunity rights – the guaranteed right of people faced with a life-threatening illness to choose treatments they deem beneficial for themselves.

4. A multi-national, international data bank to make available all medical information related to HIV disease must be created. This includes all data concerning drugs and treatments, especially basic bio-medical research and the initiation of any progress of clinical trials.

5. Placebo trials must be recognized as inherently unethical when they are the only means of access to particular treatments.

6. Criteria for the approval of drugs and treatments should be standardized on an international basis so as to facilitate worldwide access to new drugs and treatments.

7. International education programs outlining comprehensive sex information supportive of all sexual orientations in culturally sensitive ways and describing safer sex and needle use practices and other means of preventing HIV transmission must be made available.

8. The unequal social position of women affecting their access to information about HIV transmission must be recognized and also their rights to programs redressing this inequality, including respect for women's rights to control their own bodies.

9. Industrialized nations must establish an international development fund to assist poor and developing countries to meet their health care responsibilities including the provision of condoms, facilities for clean blood supply and adequate supplies of sterile needles.

10. It must be recognized that in most parts of the world, poverty is a critical co-factor in HIV disease. Therefore, conversion of military spending worldwide to medical health and basic social services is essential.

Public Actions

Sunday, June 4th 4 p.m. – Palais des congrès.
Demonstration against government's AIDS track record.

Tuesday, June 6th 1 p.m. – Palais des congrès.
Rally for Anonymous Testing.

Thursday, June 8th 5 p.m. – Palais des congrès.
Demonstration for International Action to defeat AIDS.

NOTES

1 For the complete text of this song, which is from the play *Summers Last Will and Testament*, see *The Works of Thomas Nashe* vol III, ed Ronald B. McKerrow (Oxford: Basil Blackwell 1958) 282–4. Cited here are lines 3–4, 10–11, 29–33.

2 David W. Feigal, D. Greenspan, G. Overby, A. Moss, G. Rutherford, J.S. Greenspan 'Sexual Practices as Risk Factors for Candidiasis and

Hairy Leukoplakia: The Oral AIDS Epidemiology Project' (abstract) in *V International Conference on AIDS: The Scientific and Social Challenge* (Ottawa: International Development Research Centre 1989) 190

3 As philosopher Richard Mohr put it in his paper 'Text(ile): Reading the NAMES Project Quilt,' delivered in November 1988 at the 'Representing AIDS: Crisis and Criticism' conference in London, Ontario.

4 Simon Watney *Policing Desire: Pornography, AIDS, and the Media* (Minneapolis: University of Minnesota Press 1987) 8–9

5 Cited in the article on 'Crisis' in the *Oxford English Dictionary.*

6 Gustav Freytag *Technique of the Drama* trans E.J. MacEwan (New York: Benjamin Blom 1968) 114–15, 134. Freytag, in fact, distinguished three crises in the action of tragedy: the 'exciting force' between the introduction and the rising action; the 'tragic force' between the climax and the falling action; and the 'force of last suspense' between the falling action and the catastrophe. My remarks pertain to the second of these critical points – ie, the tragic moment of impasse or helplessness just following the apex of the pyramid.

7 Peter Jaret 'Our Immune System: The Wars Within' *National Geographic* 169.6 (June 1986) 709

8 Ibid 706

9 Randy Shilts *And the Band Played On: Politics, People, and the AIDS Epidemic* (New York: St Martin's Press 1987) xxi, 576–82

10 William H. Masters, Virginia E. Johnson, and Robert C. Kolodny *Crisis: Heterosexual Behavior in the Age of AIDS* (New York: Grove Press 1988) 3

11 Ibid 6, 82–94

12 Robert C. Gallo 'The AIDS Virus' *Scientific American* 256.1 (January 1987) 56

13 Douglas Crimp 'AIDS: Cultural Analysis / Cultural Activism' in *October* 43 (1987) 7

14 Simon Watney 'Visual AIDS: Advertising Ignorance' *Radical America* 20.6 (Nov–Dec 1987) 79–82. The article originally appeared in *New Socialist* (March 1987).

50

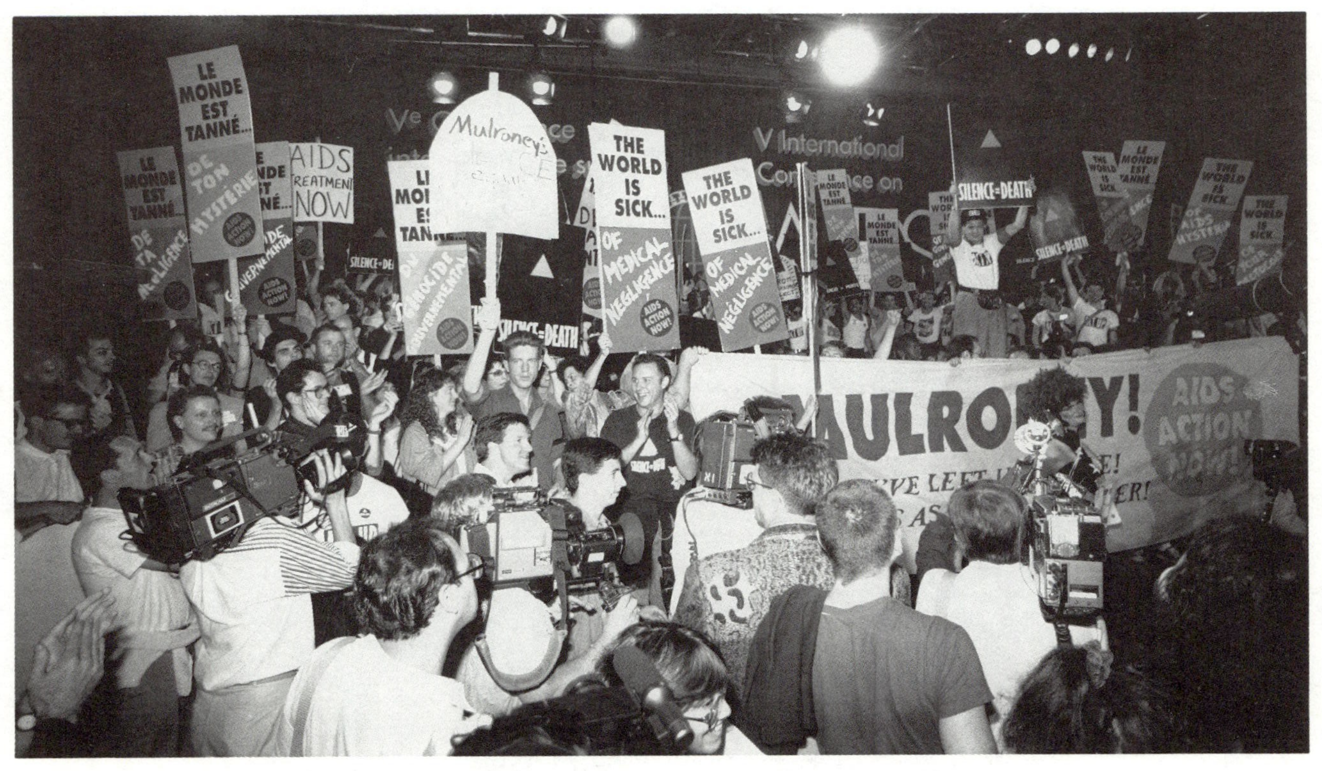
LE MONDE EST TANNÉ...
DE TON HYSTÉRIE
AIDS ACTION NOW!
THE WORLD IS SICK...
OF MEDICAL NEGLIGENCE
SILENCE=DEATH
Mulroney's
V International

50 Activists from ACT UP, SIDACTION, and AIDS ACTION NOW! open 5th International AIDS Conference with protest rally after storming podium at Palais des congrès (Montreal, 4 June 1989).

51

DON'T DIE OF IGNORANCE

1 Anyone can get AIDS. Men or women.
2 Already 30,000 people have the virus.
3 More people are infected every day.
4 Most people with the virus don't even know it.
5 AIDS is incurable and it kills.

and not even know it. In fact, most look perfectly healthy.

Think. If they can't tell, you certainly can't.

So the more sexual partners you have, the greater the risk. Either stick to the one faithful partner. Or, always use a condom. It's safer for both of you.

People who inject drugs face the added danger of infection if they share needles or equipment.

For more information, see us at Student Health Services, UCC Room 11, telephone 661-3030.

DON'T AID AIDS

Sponsored by Student Health Services

51 Student Health Services poster, University of Western Ontario (London, 1988), using slogans from Britain's Tory Health Ministry AIDS prevention campaign (1986–7)

52

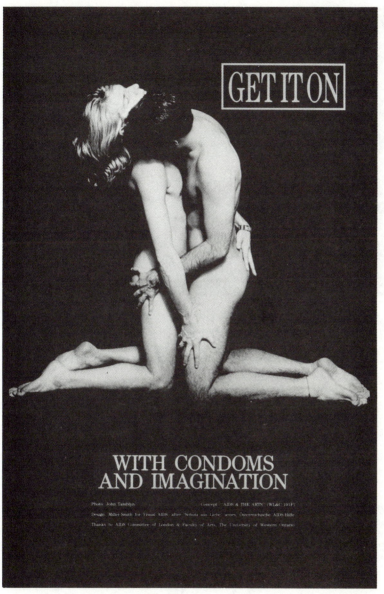

52 Gay version of 'Get It On' poster (1989) produced by 'AIDS and the Arts' seminar at University of Western Ontario. Pro-sex message counters 'Don't Die of Ignorance' (*opposite*).

53

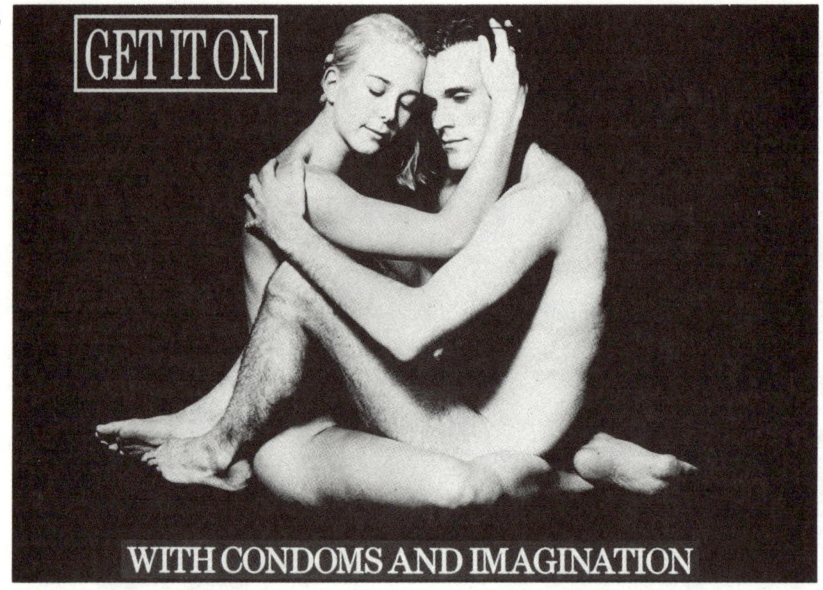

53 Straight version of 'Get It On' poster: graphic design Steve Smith, photography John Tamblyn (both versions)

54 Poster for 'Visual AIDS' exhibition (1990): concept James Miller, graphic design Steve Smith, photography John Tamblyn

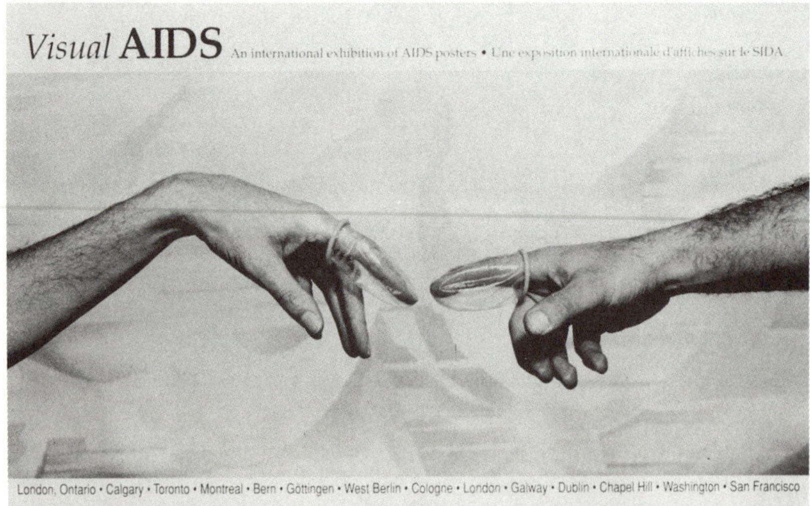

54

'The Body & Society' Exhibition: Embassy Cultural House, London, Ontario

SEPTEMBER–DECEMBER 1988

The Embassy Cultural House operated between 1983 and 1990 as an alternative artist-directed space within the Embassy Hotel in East London, hosting a varied program of exhibitions, lectures, screenings, and musical events. The unique situation of the Cultural House nurtured an interest in art not only within the Embassy Hotel itself but in the broader context of East London, which like other 'east ends' has a strong sense of its own multiracial identity on the margins of the city's predominantly white middle class. The hotel setting also played a significant role in shaping the interpretation of art within a lived experience of social mobility and marginality. Since almost two-thirds of the hotel patrons maintain full-time residency, their ongoing presence and interest in the space tended to sharpen critical attitudes towards the artists' activities in relation to the community at large. Within this context, the Body & Society exhibition was especially relevant to their concerns as well as to those of the artists.

Twelve artists were invited to participate in the three consecutive group shows that made up the Body & Society exhibition. The first show ran from 22 September to 9 October, and included works by Mary Scott (Calgary), Wendy Coad (Saskatoon and Toronto), Ed Pien (London and Toronto), and Gerard Päs (London). Exhibited in the second show, which ran from 13 October to 8 November, were works by John Brown (Toronto), Susan Day (London), Leon Golub (New York), and Nancy Spero (New York). The third show ran from 10 November to 8 December. Stephen Andrews (Toronto), Sheila Butler

(Winnipeg and London), Greg Curnoe (London), and Andy Fabo (Toronto) made up the last group of artists.

Each participant in the Body & Society exhibition addressed in his or her work the social, political, and medical issues arising from various ideological constructions of the human body. Marxists, for instance, tend to view the body as a tool for labour; fundamentalists as a vessel of corruption; and feminists as a colony for male exploitation. While the first two shows explored the broad and complex field of the sociology of the body, including its erotic 'engendering' under patriarchal control, the third focused on the social situation and political representation of the 'body under duress' in the Age of AIDS.

As a series, the Body & Society exhibition strategically coincided with a graduate seminar on AIDS and the Arts conducted by Professor James Miller at the University of Western Ontario. The whole project, in fact, was conceived as an artistic response to Miller's academic effort to examine the cultural impact of the epidemic. The Embassy Cultural House board believed that critical discussion stimulated by the images in the series would contribute in a significant way to the formation of a comprehensive framework of theoretical and practical understandings of the body, within which a critically informed awareness of AIDS could be developed locally.

The exhibition took its name from Bryan S. Turner's *The Body and Society*, an exploratory work on the sociology of the body in Western culture (Oxford: Blackwell 1984). Following Turner's lead, with additional Foucauldian prompting from the works of Douglas Crimp and Simon Watney, the organizers of the exhibition strove to further the sociological study of the body through a variety of materials and approaches. Their concerns included the analysis of disease and desire, and the interplay of power relations and sexual roles. Much of the language that has developed around the AIDS epidemic functions in tandem with the policing mechanisms of contemporary society in the West. As Foucault suggested in his phrase 'the government of the body,' our bodily existence is a zone of political activity, and our bodies a site where various acts of control (including state oppression) are inflicted on us from birth to death.

While the exhibition as a whole could be regarded in this theoretical light as complementing the AIDS and the Arts seminar, it was not primarily or exclusively an AIDS exhibition. Rather, it served to position AIDS as a cultural crisis within the broader field of inquiry opened up by the artists. As such it could be viewed as a critical response and a contextualizing extension to polemical AIDS exhibitions like 'Let the Record Show ...' (1987) at the New Museum of Contemporary Art in New York.

The coordinators of the Body & Society exhibition were Wyn Geleynse, Jamelie Hassan, and Jean Spence. The project was generously funded by the Canada Council and the Ontario Arts Council through the Special Projects Grants to Artist-Run Centres.

Jamelie Hassan, with Wyn Geleynse and James Miller

Plate Notes by James Miller (plates start on p 221)

1 MARY SCOTT: Untitled (quoting Irigaray, Paley, image V. Burgin)

Represented here in an outline reminiscent of Robert Mapplethorpe's photographic studies of black nudes (though with the colours of figure and ground reversed) is the erotic male body as object of aesthetic worship. Fragments of polemical discourse in the first person express the artist's physical disgust at aestheticized pornography, and at the same time transform the male body into a page where her own feminist text ('what isn't said') is articulated by its absence.

2 WENDY COAD: *Going*

The intrusive but unthreatening presence of two black African women, the erotic contours of their 'exotic' bodies displayed without shame or social discomfort, represents a fantastic transportation and recontextualization of 'The Other' from its usual site of extreme marginality (the Third World) into the centre of patriarchal power and imperialist culture (the First World symbolized by a room in the White House). The women seem to be contemplating, in a languid unwarlike way, the possibility of occupying the empty seat of power visible through the open doorway.

3 ED PIEN: *Self Portrait*

The racist cliché that all non-white faces 'look alike' is vividly deconstructed in this restlessly shifting series of self-portraits. The act of self-representation (which is also what's represented here) reveals not only the multitudinousness of the self but also the particular difficulties faced by an 'other' self in constructing an identity within the grid of imperialist discourse. Racism, which pervades much official AIDS discourse, perpetuates a notion of the abject body of the slave as dehumanized because homogeneous, and inferior because dependent on the will of the master. The master's body, by contrast, is perceived as intrinsically valuable precisely because it is individualized. Self-representation becomes in this play of images an act of self-empowerment.

4 GERARD PÄS: *The Living Meridian #1*

At first glance this figure looks like a body in torment under the brutally objectifying and anatomizing gaze of Western medicine. Has the body become merely a specimen for scientific control, like a dead butterfly pinned down for display or dissection? The pins, however, trace out a mystical route of healing – the meridian lines on the maze-like acupuncture diagrams developed by Chinese medicine – which offers not only an implicit critique of the Cartesian mind-body dualism but also an explicit encouragement to the sick (especially persons with AIDS) to seek alternative treatments when conventional healing methods fail. The copper background of the piece symbolizes the cosmos as a conductive field of healing energies.

5 JOHN BROWN: *Human Head #7*

Scraped and wiped away here are the personalized features and polished surfaces of the conventional portrait bust, which for many centuries in Western art has served as a metonymy for the body as a classical aesthetic whole in a state of rational governance and immortal health. Revealed beneath the idealistic imagery of the painterly past is a frightening corpse-like shadow that silently cries out for a soul, or some animating creative force, to re-present the body subjectively in opposition to its deathly transformation into an icon of aesthetic transcendence.

6 SUSAN DAY: *Handicap Access Bathroom*

Set into a wall of the washroom at the Embassy Cultural House is a large tiled image of an elderly woman, nude, shrunken, painfully twisted, glimpsed from a disorienting angle as she struggles to get into or out of her wheelchair next to a bathtub. This permanent installation translates its site into a private meditation chamber where the viewer is invited to contemplate the social marginalization of the physically disabled from an empathetic position of physical intimacy and vulnerability.

7 LEON GOLUB: *'Interrogation' I* (detail)

A scene from Foucault's worst nightmare of totalitarian discipline and punishment, this graphic image of torture presents the nude male body (strung up like butchered meat) not only as a site for political oppression and dehumanization but also as an ironic symbol of policed desire. With a single stroke of his club the body-harnessed, black-booted torturer fetishizes his victim, turns him into an object of sadistic desire, while forcing him to conform to the sexually repressive dictates of the state. The viewer becomes an accessory to the crime, if not an accomplice in it, simply by viewing it from a detached position of safety outside the frame.

8 NANCY SPERO: *Ballad-Brecht-Gestapo photo*

The victimization of women as political prisoners and erotic captives within male-driven, male-dictated regimes is literally embodied in the bound figure of a nude female martyr, Marie Sanders, whose 'history' is bitterly recounted in the text of Brecht's ballad of 'The Jew's Whore.' The fragmentary state of the text – it seems to have been pieced together from scraps as if it had been shredded by the authorities and recovered by the artist as evidence of their crime – is reflected in the fragmentation of Marie's body in the lower right corner. As Monika Gagnon points out in her article for this volume (see pp 53–64), the female body, like that of the gay male PWA, is a text on which patriarchy constantly inscribes its fascistic fantasies of control.

9 STEPHEN ANDREWS: *How to Plant Tree #5: Midwife* (excerpt)

If this dream-like drawing of a fragmenting and metamorphosing male nude is construed as a Jungian allegory of homoerotic desire and gay identity-formation in the Age of AIDS, the figure seen from above at the top may represent the Shadow – a vague presence casting a phobic influence over the genital region of the 'fallen' and 'inverted' man. But for this baleful presence, suggesting the shadow of death, the Animus informing the upper body of the main figure would be in a strong and flourishing state akin to the proverbial oak tree before it was toppled by the storm.

10 SHEILA BUTLER: *Blind Swimmer*

The psychoanalytic construct of the body as an external screen that reveals (and at times defensively conceals) the conflictual dynamics of internal processes is suggested in this image of a fully clothed man standing in a defensive attitude beside a pool. If the pool represents the subconscious, as it often does in dreams, then the foreshortened nude figure swimming in it may be taken as an image of the man's submerged feminine self, or perhaps, in classical Freudian terms, the repressed erotic energies of the Id. The male Ego, failing to confront the Other, stands in apprehensive uncertainty about her power and his own. Perhaps he has been 'unseated' by forces from without as well – the feminist challenge to his authority, for instance, or the erotophobia stirred up by the epidemic.

11 GREG CURNOE: *Organic Pigments (Origin and Applications)*

Enigmatic in an oracular sense, the text in this piece predicts the irrepressibleness of the liberating artistic impulse under the disciplining constraints imposed by socialization within the family and the state. In the upper half a parallel is established between two kinds of 'shit-disturbers': despite the deep-seated taboo against touching excrement, the children and the Irish prisoner both satisfy their desire to protest their inferiorization. The body itself can provide the materials of art (quite literally) for those to whom society denies the right of self-expression. The text in the lower half implicitly opposes the excremental art of the oppressed with the socially approved products of the dominant culture. Ironically, the pigment 'Indian Yellow' (symbolizing the privileged art materials of the oppressors) is itself derived from the excrement of a tortured and inferiorized body.

12 ANDY FABO: *Encyclopedia of Experience* (excerpt)

The flaming eye and the satellite dish are recurrent symbols in the regenerative iconography of Fabo's AIDS books (see David White's article in this volume, pp 65–88). The meaning of these talismanic images is complex and cumulative, depending in part on what lies beneath them. Here they are superimposed on engineering diagrams from a book on the textile industry, which suggests that we should read them against the cultural background of the Industrial Revolution. The monstrous cyclopean eye may represent the surveillance system of the modern industrial state, which literally oversees and controls the bodies submitted to its powerful gaze (especially the erotic bodies of gay men 'exposed,' as public-health officers would say, to the virus). By contrast, the satellite dish functions in Fabo's techno-universe as a sign of triumphant communication between lovers, doctors, patients, artists, activists, the media, and the public during the AIDS crisis. One version of the dish includes the caption 'Information = Survival,' recalling the ACT UP slogan 'Silence = Death.'

1

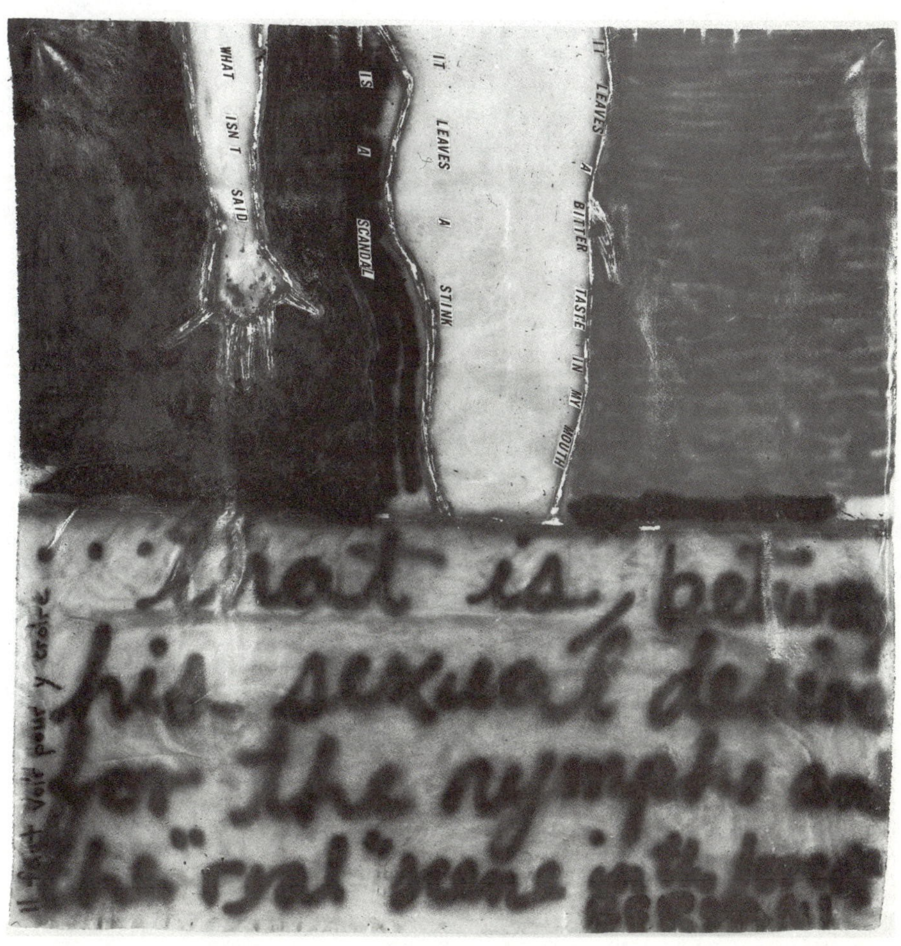
WHAT ISN T SAID
IS A SCANDAL
IT LEAVES A STINK
IT LEAVES A BITTER TASTE IN MY MOUTH
Il faut voir pour y croire

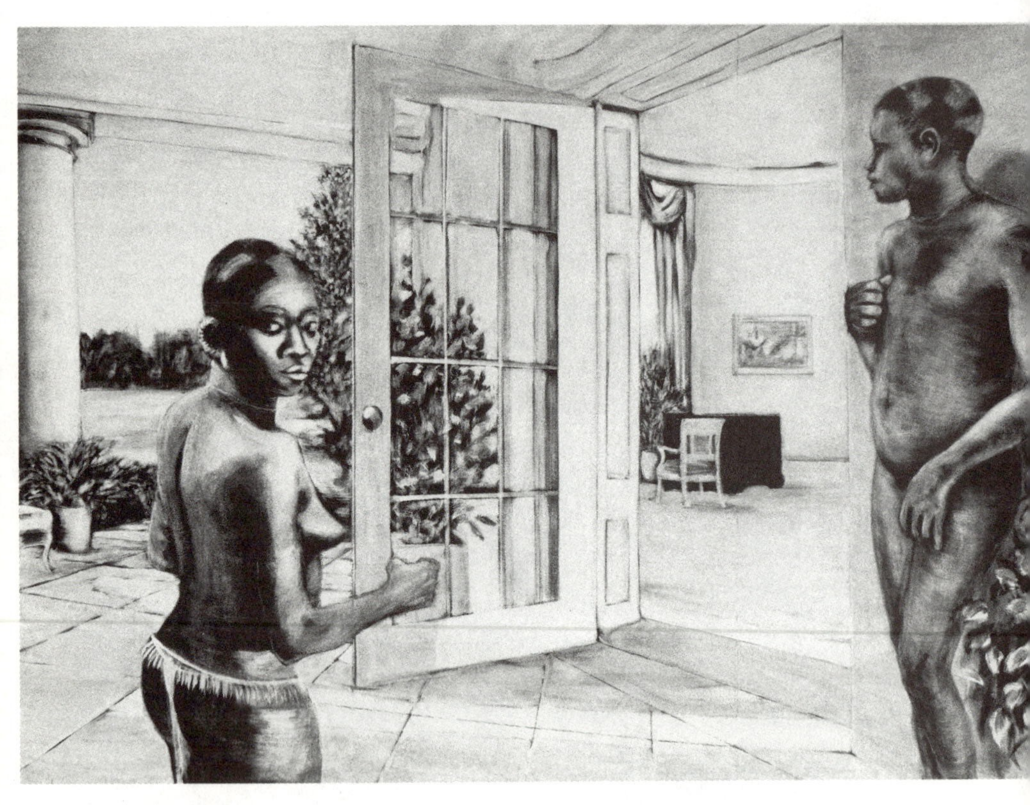

2

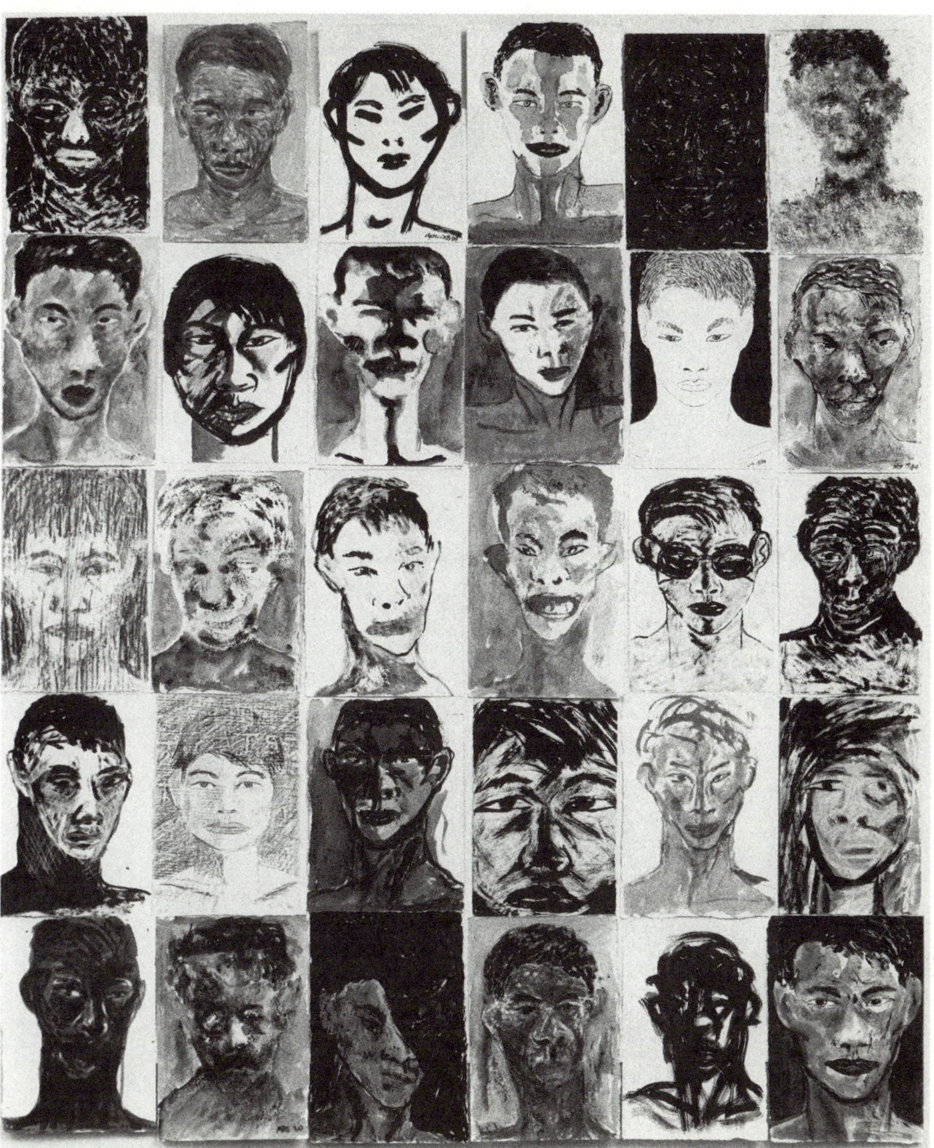

3

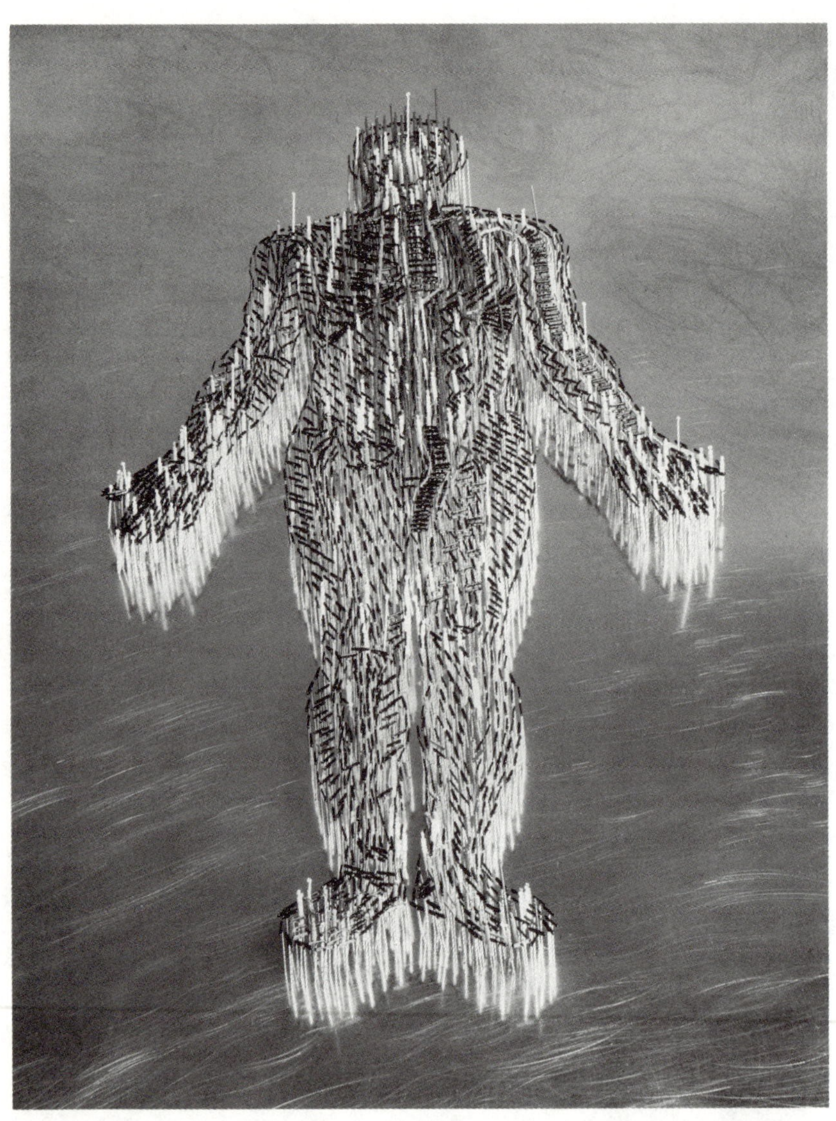

4

5

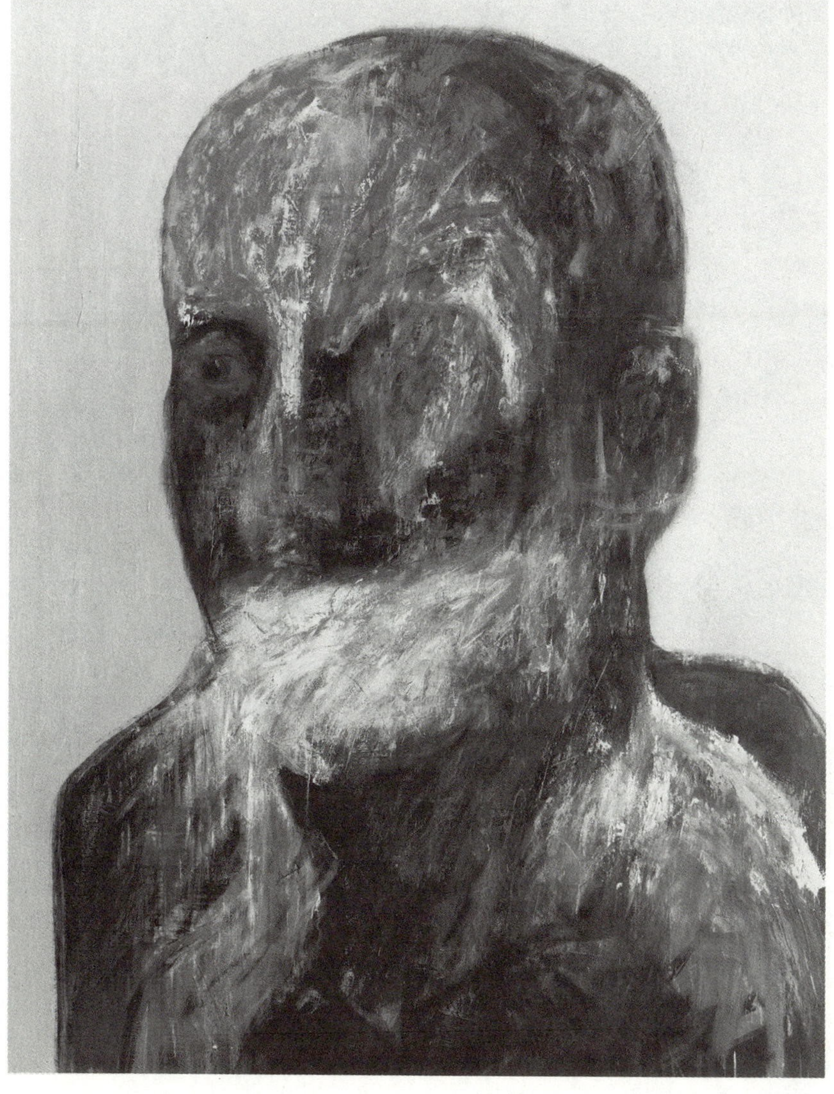

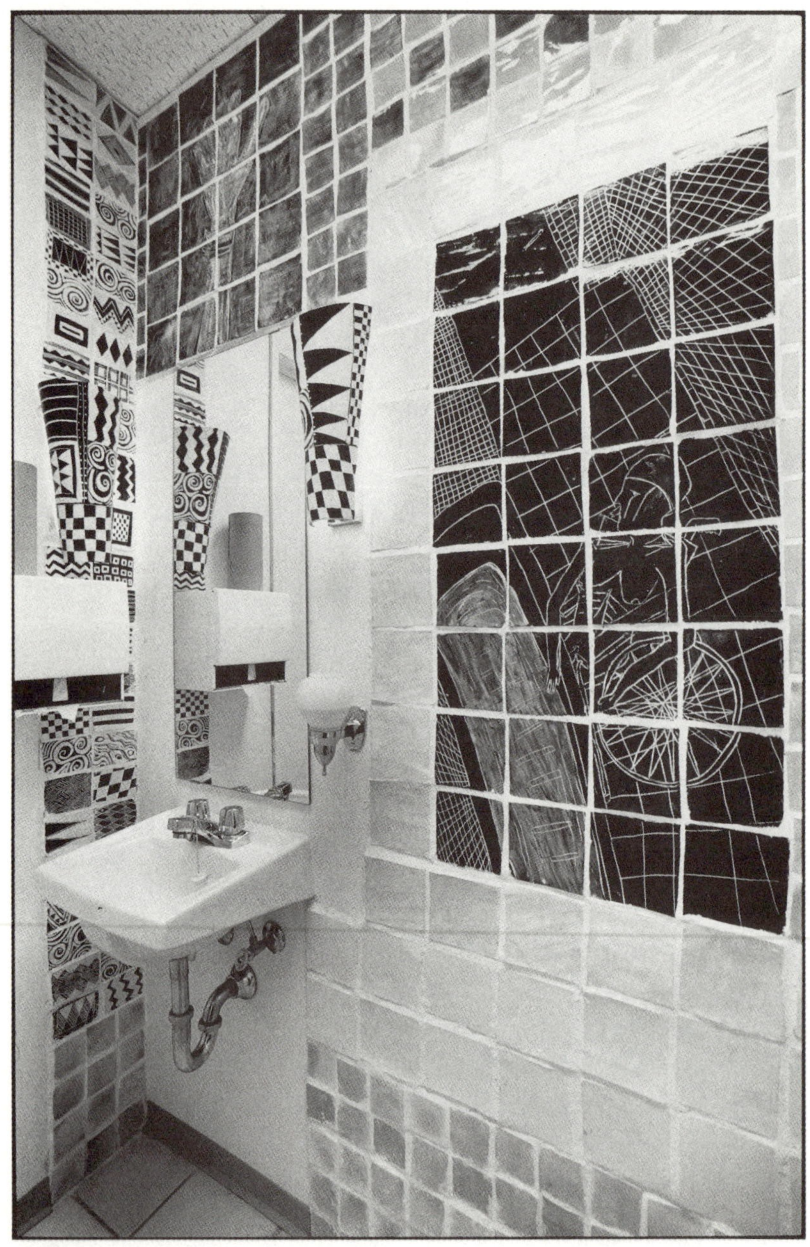

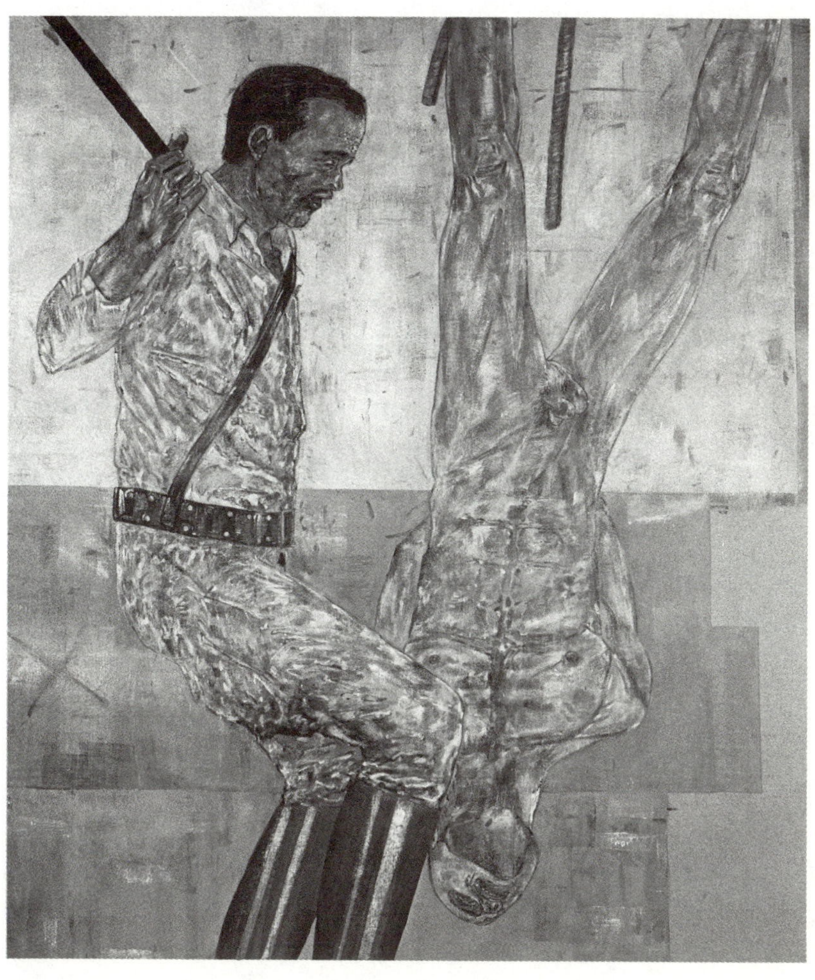

7

8

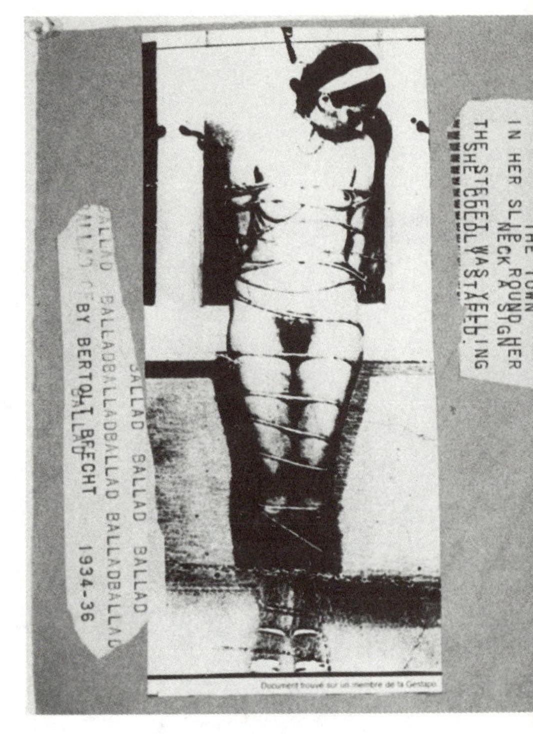
BALLAD BALLAD BALLAD
BALLADBALLADBALLAD BALLADBALLAD
BY BERTOLT BRECHT 1934-36
Document trouvé sur un membre de la Gestapo

OF MARIE SANDERS, THE JEW'S WHORE

EMBERG THEY MADE A LAW
CH MANY A WOMAN WEPT WHO'D
N BED WITH THE WRONG MAN.
PRICE IS RISING FOR BUTCHER'S MEAT..
DRUMMING IS NOW AT ITS HEIGHT.
ALIVE, IF THEY ARE COMING DOWN OUR STREET
L BE TONIGHT.'

SANDERS, YOUR LOVER'S
S TOO BLACK.
UR ADVICE, AND DON'T YOU BE TO HIM
OU WERE YESTERDAY.
PRICE IS RISING FOR BUTCHER'S MEAT.
DRUMMING NOW IS AT ITS HEIGHT.
ALIVE, IF THEY ARE COMING DOWN
OUR STREET
L BE TONIGHT.'

R GIVE ME THE LATCHKEY
N'T BE SO BAD
OON S THE SAME AS EVER.'.
E PRICE IS RISING FOR
BUTCHER S MEAT.
DRUMMING NOW IS AT ITS
HEIGHT.
ALIVE, IF THEY ARE COM
DOWN OUR STREET
LL BE TONIGHT.'

4
ONE MORNING, CLOSE ON NINE
SHE WAS DRIVEN THROUGH THE TOWN
IN HER SLIP, ROUND HER NECK A SIGN
... HER HAIR ALL SHAVEN
THE STREET WAS YELLING. SHE
COLDLY STARED.
'THE PRICE IS RISING FOR BUTCHER'S
MEAT.
AND STREICHER'S SPEAKING TONIGHT.
GOD ALIVE, IF WE'D AN EAR TO HEAR
HIS SPEECH
WE WOULD START TO MAKE SENSE OF
OUR PLIGHT.'

BY BERTOLT BRECHT
1934-36

BALLAD OF MARIE SANDERS.
THE JEW'S WHORE

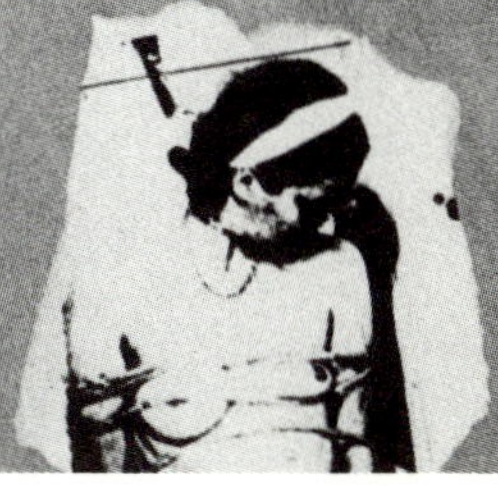

9

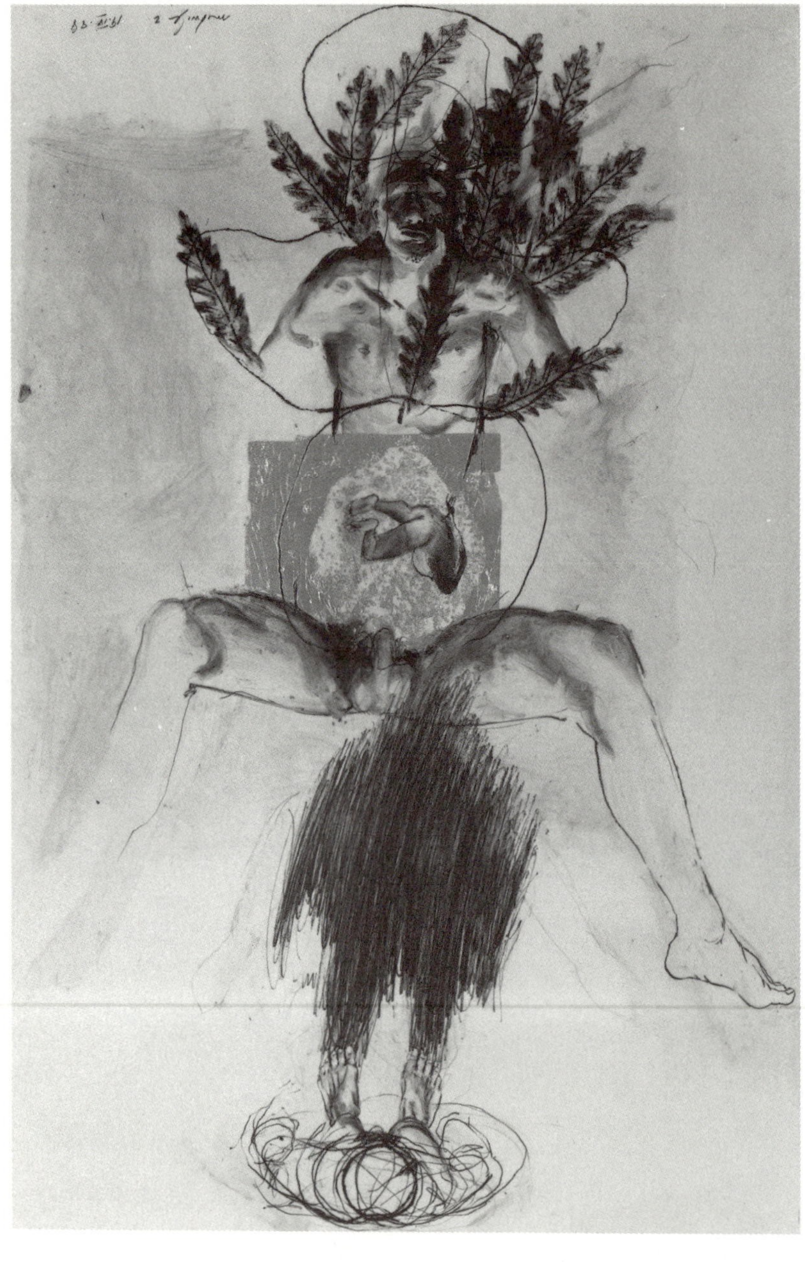

10

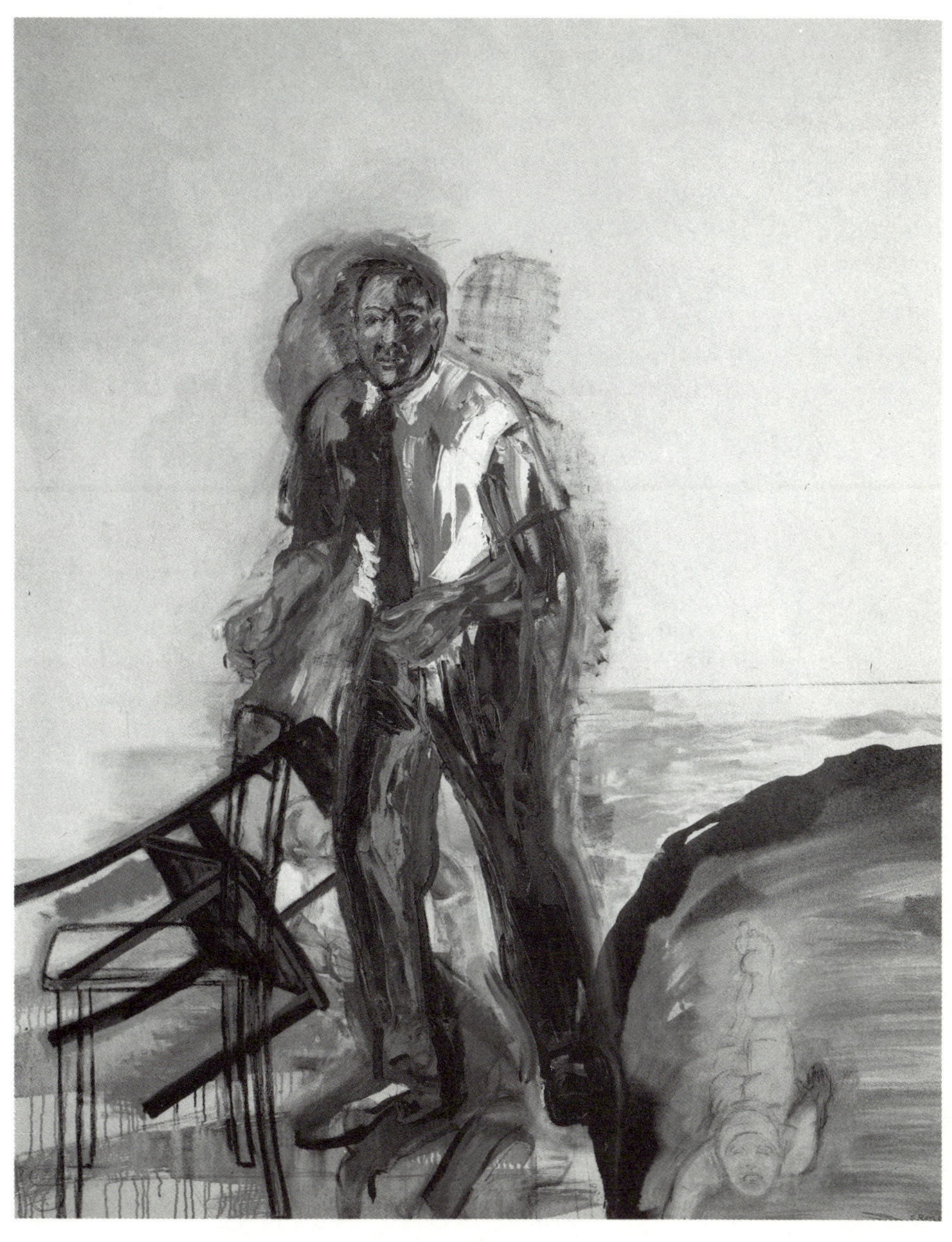

11

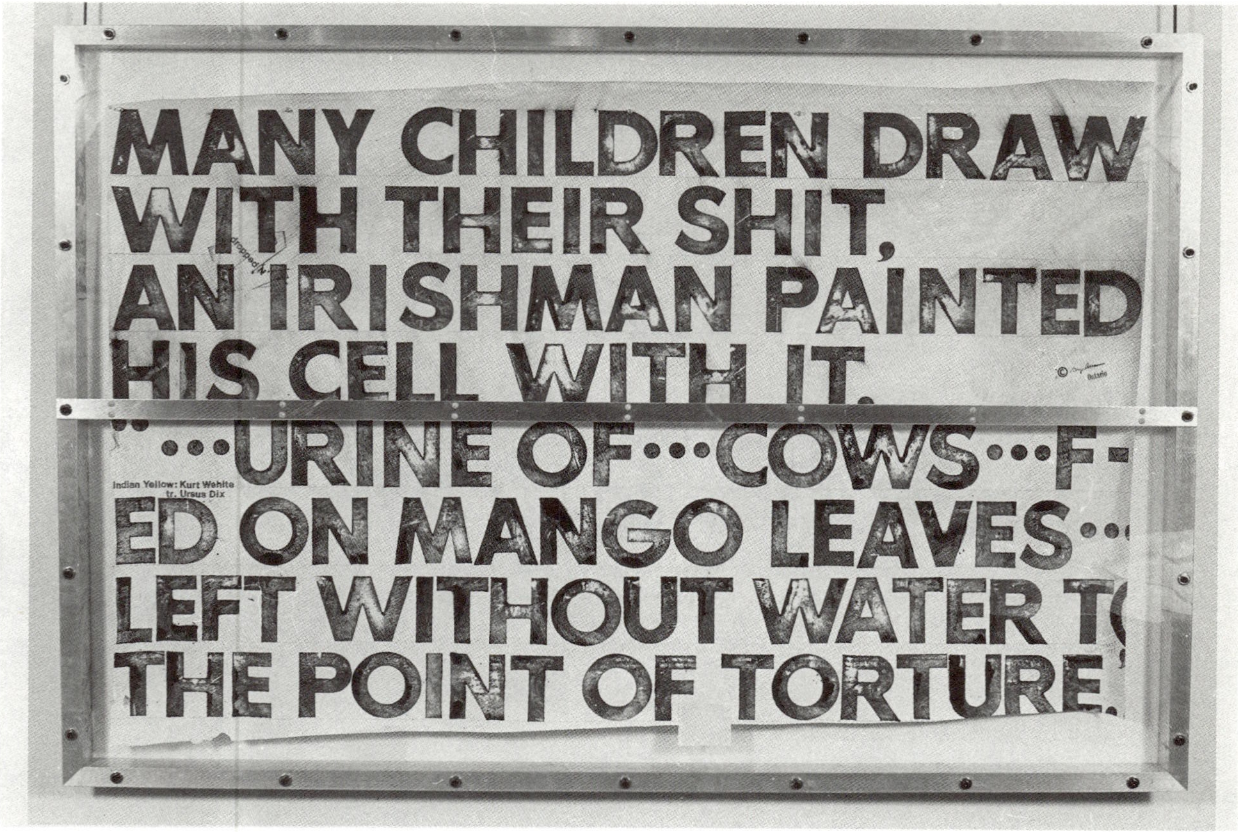

MANY CHILDREN DRAW
WITH THEIR SHIT,
AN IRISHMAN PAINTED
HIS CELL WITH IT.
"...URINE OF...COWS...F-
ED ON MANGO LEAVES...
LEFT WITHOUT WATER TO
THE POINT OF TORTURE."

dropped N

Indian Yellow: Kurt Wehlte
tr. Ursus Dix

12

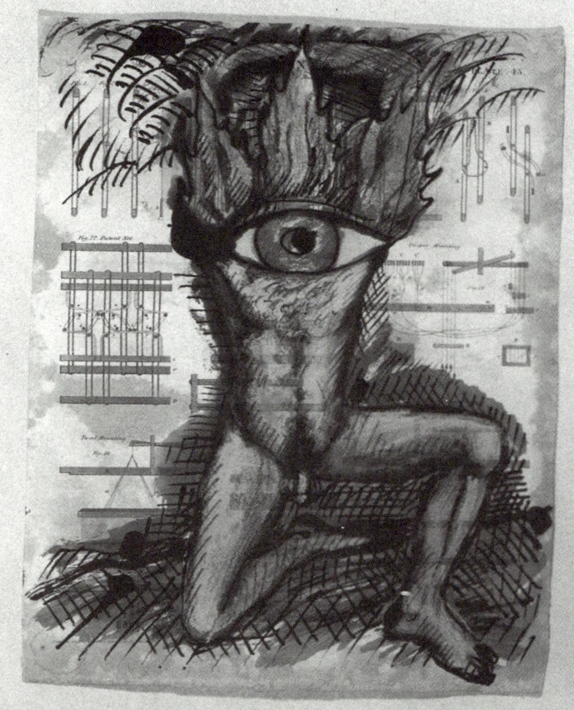

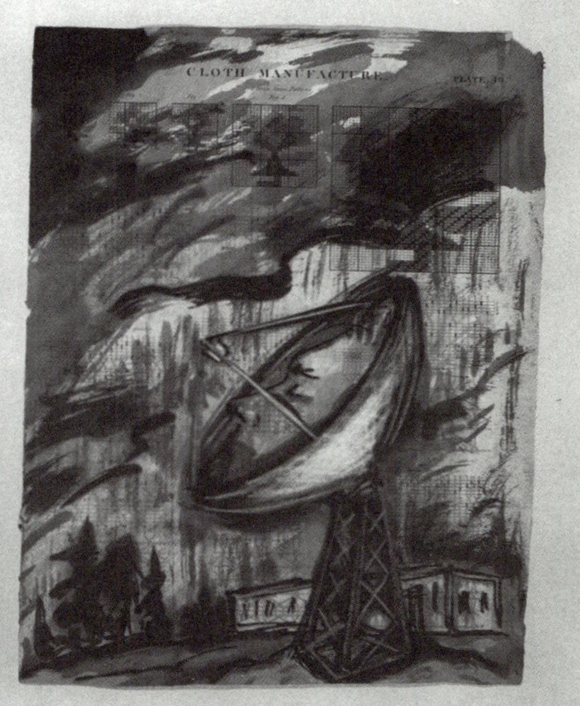

'John': *London Free Press*, 1 April 1988

DAHLIA REICH

photographs by Susan Bradnam

This story is John's choice.

It took three difficult years, but the decision was his.

He knows it may have repercussions for the rest of his life. He knows he may be shunned or suffer cruel discrimination. He's heard the horror stories.

Yet the 25-year-old London student is convinced his decision is the right one. He's counting on it.

John has AIDS related complex (ARC), now considered the early signs of the deadly disease. He can say it out loud now. He wants people to know and in London, he's the first.

'I want to help the person behind me face less discrimination, more understanding. In terms of me needing to tell my story, not to tell it would be such a waste.'

John Gordon is putting his name and face to an epidemic so controversial that fear of the public's reaction has forced those with the disease in Southwestern Ontario to remain silent or speak only under a cloak of anonymity.

For three years after discovering he had been in contact with the virus, John did the same. At that point, there were no symptoms but he was worried about losing his job, about friends staying away out of fear.

Silence = Death

An outspoken member of London's gay community, John often gave talks on homosexuality but when questions arose about AIDS, fear clouded his spirit of gay liberation.

'That would be part of the story I wouldn't tell. It always bothered me that there was a part I still didn't feel comfortable sharing.'

The diagnosis of ARC in November changed things. At a Toronto workshop to help those with ARC, AIDS, or positive antibodies to the virus emotionally deal with the problem, someone handed John a button that read 'Silence = Death.'

'I thought, there's your answer. This is the answer.'

Appearing more gaunt than he did three years ago, John's trusting and gentle manner, small build and easy laugh elicit a protective instinct. At the same time, he calmly insists his story is not about death and dying.

'I don't want people to feel sorry for me. I'm going to triumph over this. I'm going to do everything in my power and I'm not going to die. ARC hasn't given me a death sentence. The only thing I want to come out of this is public education.'

The third-born of four boys, John knew he was different at age 10.

'Guys were giggling about girls and I wasn't doing that. Through adolescence, I had crushes on boys that I had to keep to myself. I thought something was wrong with me. It wasn't until I was 19 did I meet someone who said he was gay.'

Now a fourth-year social work student at King's College, John refers to much of his high school years as an 'emotional hell' when he was forced to endure the taunting and verbal abuse of suspecting classmates.

'The older I got, the clearer it became but I would repress and deny it.'

After much suffering, John at 20 was ready to tell family and friends he was gay. He came out of the closet. AIDS and the hysteria it has generated, he said, closed the door once again.

'I didn't come out of the first closet to go into a second. Remaining in the dark goes against my principles. It just seems to add to the mysteriousness people perceive about homosexuality.'

The diagnosis of ARC and its potentially deadly ramifications came as a shock to John. Although he had all the symptoms – severe weight loss, diarrhoea, and fever which brought intense night sweats and chills – he thought they were related to an intestinal problem.

He lost 27 pounds in six weeks to weigh in at a scant 125 pounds when the final diagnosis was made.

John made a trip home to Toronto to tell his mother.

'That was the end of it for me,' recalled Grace Gordon quietly. 'I've climbed many, many difficult mountains in my life. This is the most difficult.'

A close bond exists between John and his mother who is also his best friend and a constant source of support. John's father died of cancer when he was four.

Grace remembers the day three years ago when her son told her he had antibodies to the human immunodeficiency virus (HIV), the virus that may cause AIDS. He had been exposed to the virus through a sexual contact that can't be traced.

'Fear gripped me all over. It was overwhelming for a while but I'm a person who believes in positive thinking and action. Eventually, I was able to come to grips with it.'

It has taken longer with the diagnosis of ARC. John is constantly in her thoughts. She breaks down in tears and is embraced by her son when she admits fear of losing him weighs most heavily on her mind. The love between them is untouched by the news.

'We've battled many battles together and I feel this is just another one. We're going through a rough period right now but in two months, I'll be on the positive track. From there, there will be no looking at the negative.'

Since learning of John's condition, Grace has helped establish, through the AIDS Committee of Toronto, a support group for mothers in similar situations.

Therapy Helps

'Society is pointing a finger at us, a morality finger in judgment. The government hasn't taken the bull by the horns and said "look, there are people dying out there and more are going to die if we don't do something." You feel you're going through so much, why should you have that finger pointed at you. There's a feeling like you've got a cement wall around you. There are no doors and no windows. It just feels that's where society wants to put you, surrounded by that cement wall ... There is so much fear out there, so much ignorance.'

From wanting to use his social work degree to work with children, John now wants to counsel those affected by AIDS. His plans for the future are concrete yet strangely at odds with the will the young man has already prepared and signed.

'I don't want to die, don't get me wrong. I decided long ago that I'm going to live until 100 because I like three-digit numbers. I just think that we have to face realities. If I go on to get AIDS and it takes my life,

I don't want anyone to be burdened with all that death brings with it.'

In his will, John has divided what little he owns between friends and family and has specified how the funeral service should be conducted. He wants his illness to be talked about openly.

'I want the reception to be a big bash. I want people to celebrate my life.'

Living on a tight student budget, John struggles with expenses brought about by his condition. Although outwardly healthy, he takes drugs he will need indefinitely to control candida or 'thrush,' a yeast infection in his throat.

He was recently approved by the ministry of community and social services to receive a disability pension. It covers prescription drugs but not alternative AIDS therapies that haven't been approved. A food supplement called AL 721 has helped some AIDS patients but costs about $300 a month – an impossibility on a budget of $542 a month.

John will try anything. He takes a wide assortment of vitamins, and avoids stress and fatigue that can be deadly to someone whose immune system is suppressed.

In one pocket, John always carries a much-fingered crystal. He calls it his security stone. To those who believe, crystals redirect positive energy into the person's inner being. 'I know it's bizarre. I still don't understand all the theory. I use it because it reminds me to be strong, that I'm not alone.'

He's not alone. A tight circle of friends surrounds John and he leans on them heavily. Among them is a Toronto support group which includes John in their sessions through a speaker phone.

There are other outlets. John has turned to Trager therapy, a type of massage offered free by Randy Herald of London to people with AIDS, ARC or positive antibodies.

The therapy works on the premise that stress is retained in certain parts of the body depending on the person. The massage relieves those areas and teaches the subconscious to let go of the harmful holding patterns.

Finger Pointing

John leaves the sessions energized, revitalized but at the same time relaxed. The therapy, he says, makes the regular doctor visits and the uncertainty of what the next test will find a little easier to handle. It makes the space-like and antiseptic atmosphere of the dentist's office a touch less intimidating.

One such visit came in February. It takes dental staff at Victoria Hospital – the only place John could find that would take him as a patient – one hour to prepare for his arrival.

Every nook and cranny is covered with plastic sheets from the chairs to the paper towel dispenser. It is John, in jeans and a sweater, who looks exposed and vulnerable.

Despite the good natured staff whose joking manner gives life to the cold and sterile room, John says 'when I walk in here it hits me in the face. There is something wrong with me.'

By facing that reality publicly, John admits he's concerned about the reaction of those who don't know – staff at Merrymount Children's Centre where he worked two years ago, classmates at King's College. He hopes they react intelligently and with compassion.

'People with AIDS are people. With all the facts and information on the disease, that message is getting lost. They are people who have hopes and dreams – still.'

[The following expert testimony, relating the PWA's private 'trauma' to the public drama of the Endangered Family in the Age of AIDS, appeared in a 'box' in the lower left corner of the second page of the feature.]

Few Nearby Escape Trauma

Its power to destroy reaches far beyond the person with AIDS. It becomes a family affair.

That family could be friends, relatives, or a lover, says London psychotherapist Bill Rowe. Few close to the person with AIDS are untouched by its devastating emotional symptoms of anger, frustration, guilt and fear.

'The people surrounding the HIV-positive person (those who have been in contact with the AIDS virus) have a complex mix of responses,' says Rowe, who counsels those affected by AIDS, their families and friends.

'For intimates, there's fear of their own contamination and in some cases a rush to get tested.'

For a woman who learns her partner is bisexual when he tells her he has the antibodies also comes a hurtful realization that the person has been unfaithful. For both lovers and spouses, the anger associated with the diagnosis of AIDS or antibodies may be intense.

'We've seen cases where people have literally been thrown out on the street, their lives threatened.'

That anger isn't restricted to friends and family. For some homosexual men diagnosed with the antibodies, all the anxieties and insecurities he dealt with long ago in the process of coming to grips with his sexual orientation resurface. Self-loathing and doubt are not unusual.

With time, as the person remains symptom-free, the various feelings reach a plateau, 'a kind of holding pattern,' Rowe says. 'People go on. A certain quality of denial sets in. But when the symptoms occur, there's a rekindling of all the feelings that were dealt with or not dealt with earlier. There's hard clarity that this is real.'

The grief felt by a lover whose partner has AIDS may be intensified because, afraid of rejection, they can't openly mourn the person's illness. Family members of the person with AIDS may exclude the lover from any involvement in the person's care or in the mourning process after his death. This magnifies the lover's loneliness and pain.

The dreaded diagnosis may also force a family to deal, for the first time,with issues of homosexuality.

'One cannot over-estimate the impact of the stigma associated with a gay lifestyle and AIDS on the grieving process,' says Rowe in a soon-to-be published paper. 'The stigma attached to AIDS magnifies the stigma attached to a gay lifestyle.'

Families, particularly in the London area, cling to a cloak of secrecy when a relative has AIDS, Rowe adds. One family decided to forgo collecting life insurance rather than risk the cause of death being revealed in the small town where they live.

'It (the secrecy) is intense. I've met families who have talked to me about being at work and people would be making jokes about homosexuals or AIDS patients. They would have to laugh along so as not to raise suspicion and then they feel so guilty about what they just did.'

When there is such secrecy, Rowe says, 'it almost becomes a secret within the family, too. You're sitting there with an AIDS patient that people have to deal with and respond to, and it's not being talked about.'

Early counselling for families or lovers is as essential as medical care for the AIDS patient, he says. People need the facts to dispel myths about the disease. They need to talk to someone who will listen and understand.

The AIDS-Timmy: Reflections on a Cultural Niche

DAVID KINAHAN

On a Friday morning in April 1988, I sat down to breakfast with my local newspaper, the *London Free Press*, and was tantalized by a bold graphic with the word 'AIDS' superimposed over a setting sun and a headline reading 'Young Victim's Story Bid to Fight Ignorance.' The 'hook,' as media people call it, grabbed me, and I opened the paper to the feature article by London journalist Dahlia Reich on social worker John Gordon, a recent graduate of King's College (plates 55, 56, following p 239).[1] As I read it through, it struck me as a provocative example of the mainstream media's simultaneous victimization and valorization of people with AIDS (PWAs), which prompted me to look further into the popular representation of the syndrome as an invariably fatal disease of the young. Reich's translation of Gordon into a celebrity-victim reminded me of what happened to an acquaintance of mine, London artist Gerard Päs, who was afflicted in his youth by a virus and a publicity campaign.

As a toddler Gerard Päs fell ill with polio, which left him with a withered leg. In 1965, at age ten, he was chosen to be the Easter Seal's poster-child and rechristened in public as 'Timmy.' As he himself puts it, he ceased to be Gerard when the 'Timmy' label was thrust upon him: people continued to call him Timmy years after his rise to fame as a model handicapped child. Well-intentioned philanthropic groups held him up as the perfect example of a Victorian moral type, the hapless yet cheery young victim who humbly teaches patience and charity to all around him, and in their appeal to society to 'help

Timmy,' the sponsors of the campaign only revealed an inherent weakness in the very structure and conception of the society to which they appealed. The Gerard within Timmy grew up angry and confused, expressed his defiant individuality by 'going punk,' and turned his experience as a physically and socially handicapped person into performance art and mixed-media works embodying his criticism of prevailing social constructions of the human body (such as 'The Living Meridian,' reproduced in this volume in 'Portfolio Two,' plate 4). Could John Gordon, I wondered, be fitting into a cultural niche established for him in Canadian popular culture by the success of the Timmy campaign?

The Timmy role is not a new cultural phenomenon. In 1947, the Canadian chapter of the Easter Seal Society made a public-relations decision to use a child with polio in its public fund-raising campaign. This was the first instance of a poster-child campaign that continues today and has been adopted by many other charitable organizations. Each year a new representative is chosen, and this child appears on billboards, public-transport advertisements, and at all media events related to the organization. Presumably in the interests of anonymity and 'product recognition,' the directors of the Easter Seal poster-child campaign chose to name each year's lucky boy 'Timmy' – or, recently, in the case of a lucky girl, 'Tammy.' Alexandra Adams, a PR officer at the Easter Seal Society's head office in Toronto, confirmed my suspicion that the choice of the name 'Timmy' was prompted by its sentimental associations with the Tiny Tim character in Charles Dickens' *A Christmas Carol.*

Besides supplying the name, Dickens provided a literary prototype and moralized narrative for the Sick Child held up for public sympathy in the charity 'drives.' Tiny Tim is the tearfully absent presence at the Crachit family dinner on a mythical Christmas Yet to Come. 'Whenever we part from one another,' Bob Crachit asserts, 'I am sure we shall none of us forget poor Tiny Tim – shall we – or this first parting that there was among us.' Like Tiny Tim's brief history, the poster-child's illness and potential death are represented to all good people who peer into the magic mirror of public relations as a poignant 'family tragedy' to elicit a temporary change of heart in the Scrooges of this world.

As a model of the human spirit under duress yet still rejoicing, the Timmy is the modern secular equivalent of a Christian martyr. Martyrs are 'physically challenged,' as the PR people would say if they handled martyr accounts, but the sufferings of the Soldiers of the Cross also include the social challenge of combatting a grossly materialistic world that cannot understand the spiritual diversity of human nature, a world (in the Pauline sense) that cannot and will not accept those who fall outside the narrow construction of the 'normal' or the 'healthy.'

The Timmy is paraded before the public once a year like the children in William Blake's 'Holy Thursday,' and the voice of experience must ask the question:

> Is this a holy thing to see,
> In a rich and fruitful land,
> Babes reduced to misery,
> Fed with cold and usurous hand?
> (1–4)

The Timmy is clearly presented to the public as an image to be admired, like the statue of a saint. Yet very often in the case of a medical Timmy, the context of the saintly representation elicits condescending sympathy rather than constructive empathy. This sympathy is not completely valueless. As a fund-raising technique, the Timmy campaign inspires a great deal of lucrative guilt by appealing to the 'aren't-we-lucky' attitude as well as the 'what-the-hell-it's-tax-deductible' side of our nature. Organizations like the Easter Seal Society are presumably motivated by a strong sense of (Christian?) charity – but I doubt whether the media promoting their appeals are deeply disturbed by what happens to the real people inside the charitable caricatures, the Gerards who must struggle for decades to recover their lost selves.

The Timmy in fact only succeeds in making a special case of issues that are not special, issues that society must address and alleviate not just as isolated acts of charity but as a matter of course. 'Liberal' organizations feel the need to draw attention to people like Gerard Päs and John Gordon because the general public is otherwise unresponsive to their problems.

The three most widely publicized examples of medical Timmys in Canada are Terry Fox, Steve Fonyo, and Rick Hansen. In these men we are given examples of the human spirit in a trial by ordeal. The trial is to determine their human value, and we all admire these men as they run or wheel themselves across the Canadian landscape. But what this celebration of heroic achievement in the face of great physical challenge often does is typecast other people living with those challenges and define them as somehow inadequate if they do not live up to this representation. These men were constantly attempting to deny the hero status the media was so desirous to confer upon them. The attention of the media and the public is seen as somehow more warranted in the case of these men than in the case of those they are supposedly representing. The media and charitable institutions, defining these men as heroes (secular saints), appeal to the public to 'help make the miracle,' and by writing a fat cheque we can participate in their canonization.

I do not wish to belittle or criticize the actions of the cross-country crusades; my intention is to point out that the perceived necessity for this kind of drastic action is the result of a larger cultural myopia. Perhaps a more useful and politically active strategy would have been for Rick Hansen to pull his wheelchair off the highway at random stops, with the press gathered round, and insist on using the facilities. This hero is, after all, human, and the availability of systems adequate to accommodate him would show the country just how human we really perceive he is.

In the 1980s, with AIDS threatening the fabric of our society, the media response has been to attempt to place individuals living with this disease into the pre-existing cultural niche provided by the 'Timmy' predecessors. AIDS has provided the circumstances for the most recent example of the Timmying process with the media creation of the AIDS-Timmy. Like poliomyelitis, AIDS is the result of a viral infection, but unlike the polio virus, the human immunodeficiency virus (HIV) carries with it the West's age-old horror of venereal disease and plague. This is not to deny that people living with other 'physical challenges' are not subject to social stigmatization; they most certainly are. But PWAs face the uniquely brutal social challenge of retaining personal dignity (as well as health) in the face of constant threats on the part of the 'general population' to isolate them, banish them, in effect dehumanize them as if their lives were reducible to the dim intentionless molecular level of their immune systems.

In her pioneering article 'AIDS: Keywords,' Jan Zita Grover defines the term 'general population' as merely a polite phrase for the socially privileged term 'heterosexuals.' According to the media, public-health officials, and politicians who favour this euphemism, the general population does not include the gay and lesbian population, IV drug users, sex-industry workers, and a vast array of other members of society. It is for this reason, Grover argues, that the Reagan administration and other conservative governments can issue statements such as 'AIDS hasn't spread to the general population yet.'[2] And it is very much this ironically restrictive notion of the general population that underlies the mainstream media's conception of its target audience.

As a newspaper pitched at the general population, proclaiming the twin heterosexist ideals of family values and property values to southwestern Ontario yuppies, the *London Free Press* has devised two mutually exclusive social roles for the few gay men who stray into its pages. For years the general population has been subjected to stories about the Promiscuous Pervert whose desires must be policed in downtown washrooms; but now it can enjoy tales rivalling these in human interests – heart-warming fables about the meek and mild Mama's Boy, who, though not quite normal, is really quite a sweet child.

In Dahlia Reich's utterly uncontroversial article for the *Free Press*, John Gordon came out of the closet – again. Not as a gay man (he had done that several years ago in the usual way) but as a gay PWA. When he walked out of the AIDS closet, it was into a role already prepared for him in mainstream-media discourse aimed at the general population. By putting 'his name and face to the controversial disease,' as his front-page billing put it, he became London's first gay AIDS-Timmy.

The object of the Timmying process in Gordon's case was to present the *Free Press* readers with a very palatable image of the Mama's Boy – who just happened to be gay – struggling with the physical and social challenges of the syndrome. In large print over the title of the article, Reich (or the headliner at the press) quotes Gordon as a 'victim' not of AIDS itself but of its less-threatening relative ARC: 'I want to help the person behind me face less discrimination, more understanding. In terms of me needing to tell my story, not to tell it would be such a waste.' Who is this 'person behind me'? Surely he meant any PWA who comes after him, as if he were the forerunner and herald of a vast parade of imminent victims. Yet his haunting phrase suggests, unwittingly, the real John Gordon behind the media mask of the AIDS-Timmy, the gay man who just happens to be seropositive. So is it really his story that gets told, or an AIDS update of *A Christmas Carol*?

Gordon's goal in publicizing his life with AIDS is to increase 'public awareness' in the hope of eliminating the (inevitably assumed) public stigmatization resulting from his dual 'diagnosis' of homosexuality and HIV infection, which are of course inseparable aspects of his AIDS-related complex. But for the public educational process to occur, Gordon and Reich must mediate their representation of the gay PWA to make him as safe as possible to the demographic norm of the paper's readers.

Reich's description of Gordon is the first step in the Timmying process. 'Appearing more gaunt than he did three years ago,' she observes, 'John's trusting and gentle manner, small build and easy laugh elicit a protective instinct.' Gordon is thus cast in the role of a child whose vulnerability awakens a maternal instinct. He is further infantilized by the accompanying photographs of him and his mother. Reclining at her side, or in her fond protective embrace, he appears to confirm the pop-psychological belief that homosexuality results from 'arrested development' or some failure in the 'normal sexual maturation process' caused by an overbearing Mom. This regressive neo-Freudian image is given further support by the photograph of Gordon and his doctor. Shirtless, skinny, his feet dangling from the examination table, the poor little victim appears especially innocuous as he is literally towered over by Dr Fred Pattison.

Gordon insists that his story is not about death and dying, but in this respect he is clearly at odds with the reporter. *Her* story is about death and dying. That Gordon has prepared a will is mentioned three times in the article, and Reich sees this preparation as 'strangely at odds' with his plans for the future (A6). She draws attention to Gordon's mother's fears of his death, and quotes a long passage by Gordon himself on his preparations for that end. Blocked off from the article itself are large-print quotations of John's friends' ruminations on his imminent absence. 'It hurts,' one friend remarks. 'There's a sense of loss, the loss of possibilities. That's what strikes me the most. I'll miss him' (A6). Reich's choice to call attention to this future state further locates Gordon in the victim role. Like Dickens' 'poor Tiny Tim,' Gordon is represented sentimentally (or fearfully) as an absent presence in a time yet to come. The sick-child role into which Gordon has been placed sets him before the reader as an object to be pitied.

In a curious juxtaposition of imagery, the sick-child role exists in combination with an image of Gordon as someone to be feared. The text of the article frames a picture of Gordon lying in the dentist's chair surrounded by gloved, masked, and gowned dental workers. Reich points out that 'it takes staff at Victoria Hospital – the only place John could find that would take him as a patient – one hour to prepare for his arrival. Every nook and cranny is covered with plastic sheets from the chairs to the paper towel dispenser' (A6). Despite Reich's attempt to assert that it is Gordon who 'looks exposed and vulnerable' (A6), the image presented portrays Gordon as a powerful contagion. In 'AIDS: Keywords,' Jan Grover considers the victim position within which the media so often wishes to place PWAs: 'Fear and pity are the emotions raised by the victim, and, as we know, these emotions are less than useless for dealing actively with serious issues.

Fear and pity are aroused in order ultimately to be cathartically disposed of, to enable the passive spectator of the AIDS "spectacle" to remain passive, and eventually to distance him- or herself from the scapegoated object of fear and pity' (29). The goal of Gordon's public coming-out, 'to fight ignorance' (front-page headline), seems to be lost in the victim status within which he is represented.

In *Policing Desire: Pornography, AIDS, and the Media,*[3] Simon Watney argues that 'we must refuse, absolutely, to inhabit the immensely convenient role of the "victim," which has been so generously dug to contain us like a mass grave' (147). Nowhere in her article does Reich talk about the actual difficulty of transmission of the virus. The article is socially critical at certain points, but the criticism is not supported by information that could potentially correct misconceptions. The misconceptions are instead implicitly supported.

I do not wish to dismiss this article as useless; it is not. The social criticism that it does provide is accurate and pointed, but it exists only as an unsupported subtext dwarfed by the larger concentration on Gordon as victim. On the positive side, Gordon as PWA is never shown as isolated. Of the six photographs in the article, five of them show Gordon with other people. But the settings of the photographs, placing Gordon in a passive, infantilized context, detract from the potential benefit of showing a PWA in community situations.

As an important addendum, since the publication of Reich's article and a follow-up article on Gordon and AZT, Gordon contacted the *London Free Press*, informing them of the negative connotations of the term 'victim' in AIDS-related discourse. The paper promised Gordon that they would not use the term in the future, and published an ombudsman's report on the issue of the terminology. It is this kind of important cultural activism that acceptance of the Timmy role makes difficult. Unfortunately, the promise that Gordon's activism elicited from the *London Free Press* did not extend itself to the paper's use of syndicated news sources, and 'victim' continues to be a common term for the PWA in these stories.

When a humanitarian organization or the media give attention to a specific cause such as poliomyelitis, cancer, or AIDS, as mediated through a 'representative,' they identify that person with the disease. The person becomes defined, even christened, by his or her physical challenge. One of the many difficulties of this process is that the image is very often not self-defined, but articulated through particular ideological perspectives. The Timmy figure becomes locked in this limiting definition and is at the mercy of the representational process.

Silence may indeed equal death, as ACT UP proclaims, but certain types of self-expression can function in an equally fatal manner. Cindy Patton asserts that 'AIDS represents a unique assault on the newly emerging sexual identity and community [of gay men and lesbians],'[4] and the Timmy role does nothing to counter this assault. The Timmy, whether as victim, hero, or martyr, is too easily manipulated to fit the ideological stance of the mediating body. Now, more than ever, PWAs must be aware of the dangers and limitations of representation, and must insist on being in control of their own images.

NOTES

1 Dahlia Reich 'John: Young Victim's Story Bid to Fight Ignorance' *London Free Press* 1 April 1988, A1, A6, A7
2 Jan Zita Grover 'AIDS: Keywords' in *AIDS: Cultural Analysis / Cultural Activism* ed Douglas Crimp (Cambridge, MA: MIT Press 1988) 23
3 Minneapolis: University of Minnesota Press 1987
4 Cindy Patton *Sex and Germs: The Politics of AIDS* (Boston: South End Press 1985) 120

'A Fair Representation of His Feelings': A Reply to David Kinahan

DAHLIA REICH

The critical analysis of the John Gordon article, which appeared in the *London Free Press*, both surprised and distressed me. As the reporter who wrote the story, I'm amazed so much was read into the article that was not only unintentional but, in my view, simply not there.

The analysis is evidence that individuals truly see, or in this case read, what they want. There are likely as many views on the article as there are reviewers. I can only give you my perceptions, which, since I wrote the article, convey the intention behind it.

I asked to contribute to this collection of comments on the AIDS issue because I feel strongly that an academic analysis of a newspaper article cannot be done fairly or accurately without some understanding or knowledge of how a newspaper is put together. That lack of understanding is evident in some of the comments of Kinahan.

Of newspaper writing, it's important to keep in mind that reporters do not have time to produce the calculated type of work described by Kinahan in his review. Secondly, the reporter's written word is not final. Headlines, layout, and editing are done by a team of people, all of whom have a hand in shaping and presenting a story. The reporter has limited control over the final product.

This brings me to my criticisms of the review.

Victim Perception

Kinahan's attack on the word 'victim' was justified. It's important to note, however, that the word appeared in a sub-headline written by an editor. It was not a word I chose. In fact, when I saw the proofs (before the article appeared) I vehemently argued against it. I lost the battle for reasons still not clear to me. One poor excuse used by the editor was that 'victim' was shorter than 'person with ARC.' In the newspaper world, brevity is all important, sometimes to the detriment of the story. Editors can make some bad decisions. In my opinion, this was one of them.

As the *Free Press* medical reporter writing on numerous illnesses and disease, I never use the word victim.

Mama's-Boy Perception

I find it very peculiar that the reviewer felt John was presented as a 'Mama's Boy.' It's as if Kinahan is attempting to fit the article into pre-existing theories, whether applicable or not.

The purpose of the article was to present John in a realistic light. John is very close to his mother. The photographs and references to his mother were meant to portray that closeness, which is an important part of John's life. The pictures were real, not staged. The comments were real. Rather than portraying John as a weak child, that part of the article showed a wonderfully strong relationship between him and his mother.

The photographer and I visited with the pair for several hours and the photographs precisely convey that meeting during which John lay on the couch next to his mother, who chatted about her feelings. The photographs present the scenes that were there – not created, not forced.

Similarly, my description of John as more gaunt than three years ago was also precise. Kinahan goes on to be critical of the description of John as trusting and gentle with a small build and easy laugh, which elicit a protective response.

The intention was to paint a picture of John as he appears to others. The comparison of his weight shows the physical effect AIDS has had on him. The other comments were simply to provide a glimpse of John that can't be gleaned from the photographs. Granted, the descriptions are subjective and perhaps others would describe John differently.

But also subjective is whether the description casts John into the role of a child. I don't think it does. It casts John into the role of a human being, no different from anyone else. The public tends to lose sight of the fact that people affected by AIDS are just that, normal people. The description was meant to enhance the portrayal of the human element of AIDS.

As mentioned, anything can be fit into a theory if an attempt is made to do so. It appears that elements from the article are being stretched to comply with the theories.

Photographs

Words, or in this case photos, can strike people differently. I can only present alternative impressions evoked by the photographs.

1. John and the doctor. It was a regular medical check-up for John, not staged. If the doctor towers over John, it's because the doctor actually towers over John. Everyone feels and looks vulnerable when sitting on an examination table. The same scene takes place in every doctor's office. Because this scene involves AIDS, Kinahan has read 'victim' into the image. The purpose of the photo was to portray the part of John's life that involves frequent doctor visits. As with all AIDS patients, the medical system for John has become an important part of daily life.

2. In the dentist's office. If the picture presents John as a 'powerful contagion,' that's because some people who encounter John obviously see him as such. There's no denying that AIDS elicits fear. The picture is indeed powerful but its power comes from a startling reality – people, including the medical profession, are worried about their exposure to those with AIDS. The dentist scene says it without words. This is what AIDS people face. John faces it with every dental check-up.

Death and Dying

Yes, there was a juxtaposition. Perhaps it should have been more clearly highlighted so as not to appear as a contradiction, but it was there. The article was not meant to be about death and dying, so says John, yet it was repeatedly raised by John himself as well as his mother.

It wasn't a topic I pushed or sought from John. It came out, it was on his mind, it was on his mother's mind. The prospect of death certainly loomed for John. Perhaps that juxtaposition is a phenomenon common to many AIDS patients trying not to let thoughts of death occupy their thoughts as they carry on living. With John, those thoughts were acknowledged.

Kinahan says that the references to death again present John as a victim. Perhaps that's true. In any context, death elicits pity. It's not exclusive to the AIDS issue.

Logo

Although I had no input into the logo used with John's story, I have asked the designer what it represented. Contrary to Kinahan's comments, it was not a setting sun, nor was there any intention to signify death. In fact, it wasn't a sun at all but a generic light source. The purpose was to cast a shadow as AIDS has on the lives of so many.

Transmission

The purpose of the article was to profile John, not to present the technical, medical side of AIDS. The *Free Press* had focused on AIDS transmission numerous times prior to the John article. In fact, a three-part series dealing strictly with AIDS education appeared shortly before John's article. The raison d'être of a newspaper is to present new information, not to repeat the facts in every article. The AIDS issue has been carefully handled by the *Free Press* to ensure the facts reach the public. It continues to do so.

Conclusion

Perhaps there's another way to look at the presentation of AIDS in the media. In the John Gordon article, there was no intention to create the impression that people with AIDS are weak, victims, or people to be pitied. It aimed simply at presenting John in a realistic light and the AIDS issue as it exists for him. I think it did that. It provided a glimpse of real life involving a difficult topic.

If there is a sense that AIDS patients are prevalently portrayed as victims to be pitied, perhaps it's because writers take their cues from those with AIDS.

John obviously felt he had a story to tell, that AIDS has had an impact on his life. The final question should go to him. How does he really feel about what's happening to him? I should add that John had no problem, other than the use of the word victim in the sub-headline, with the story. In fact, he told me he found it to be a fair representation of his feelings and life and it elicited only positive responses from friends as well as strangers. John's opinion was the true test of the article.

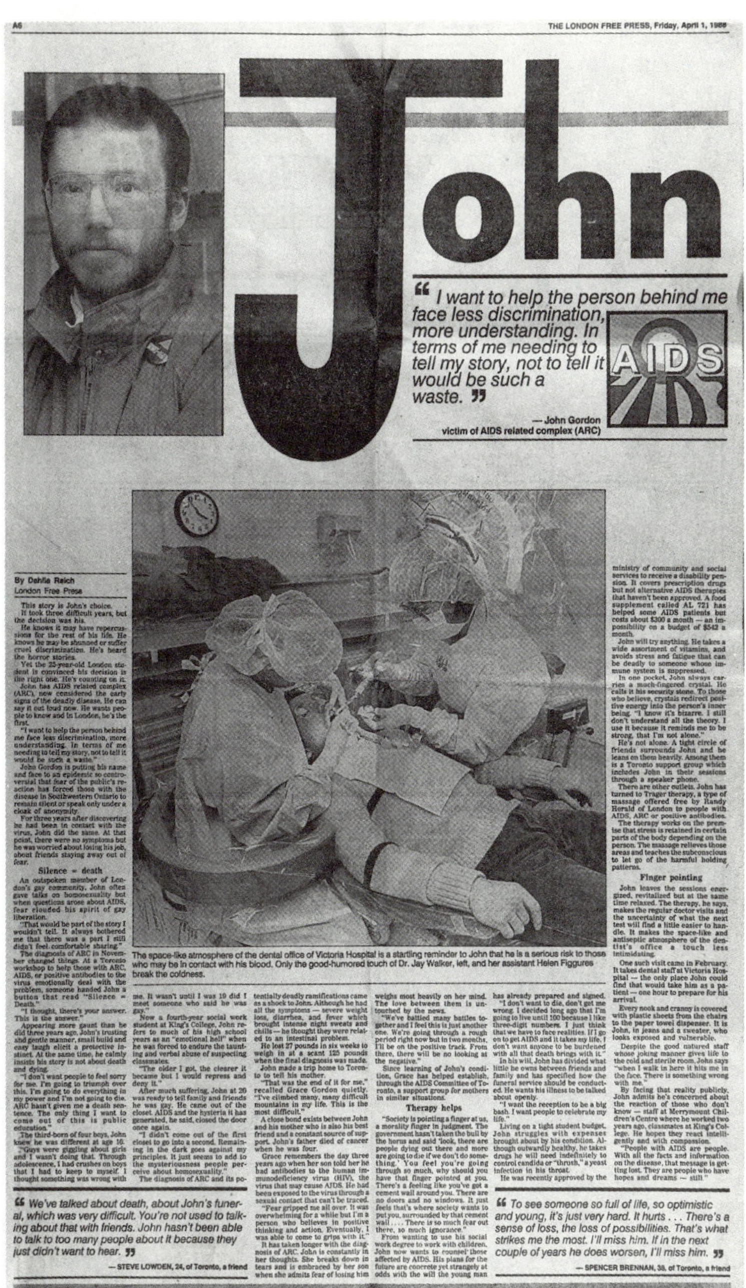

A6 THE LONDON FREE PRESS, Friday, April 1, 1988

John

"I want to help the person behind me face less discrimination, more understanding. In terms of me needing to tell my story, not to tell it would be such a waste."

— John Gordon
victim of AIDS related complex (ARC)

The space-like atmosphere of the dental office of Victoria Hospital is a startling reminder to John that he is a serious risk to those who may be in contact with his blood. Only the good-humored touch of Dr. Jay Walker, left, and her assistant Helen Figgures break the coldness.

By Dahlia Reich
London Free Press

This story is John's choice.

It took three difficult years, but the decision was his.

He knows it may have repercussions for the rest of his life. He knows he may be shunned or suffer cruel discrimination. He's heard the horror stories.

Yet the 25-year-old London student is convinced his decision is the right one. He's counting on it.

John has AIDS related complex (ARC), now considered the early signs of the deadly disease. He can say it out loud now. He wants people to know and in London, he's the first.

"I want to help the person behind me face less discrimination, more understanding. In terms of me needing to tell my story, not to tell it would be such a waste."

John Gordon is putting his name and face to an epidemic so controversial that fear of the public's reaction has forced those with the disease in Southwestern Ontario to remain silent or speak only under a cloak of anonymity.

For three years after discovering he had been in contact with the virus, John did the same. At that point, there were no symptoms but he was worried about losing his job, about friends staying away out of fear.

Silence = death

An outspoken member of London's gay community, John often gave talks on homosexuality but when questions arose about AIDS, fear clouded his spirit of gay liberation.

"That would be part of the story I wouldn't tell. It always bothered me that there was a part I still didn't feel comfortable sharing."

The diagnosis of ARC in November changed things. At a Toronto workshop to help those with ARC, AIDS, or positive antibodies to the virus emotionally deal with the problem, someone handed John a button that read "Silence = Death."

"I thought, there's your answer. This is the answer."

Appearing more gaunt than he did three years ago, John's trusting and gentle manner, small build and easy laugh elicit a protective instinct. At the same time, he calmly insists his story is not about death and dying.

"I don't want people to feel sorry for me. I'm going to triumph over this. I'm going to do everything in my power and I'm not going to die. ARC hasn't given me a death sentence. The only thing I want to come out of this is public education."

The third-born of four boys, John knew he was different at age 10.

"Guys were giggling about girls and I wasn't doing that. Through adolescence, I had crushes on boys that I had to keep to myself. I thought something was wrong with me. It wasn't until I was 19 did I meet someone who said he was gay."

Now a *fourth-year* social work student at King's College, John refers to much of his high school years as an "emotional hell" when he was forced to endure the taunting and verbal abuse of suspecting classmates.

"The older I got, the clearer it became but I would repress and deny it."

After much suffering, John at 20 was ready to tell family and friends he was gay. He came out of the closet. AIDS and the hysteria it has generated, he said, closed the door once again.

"I didn't come out of the first closet to go into a second. Remaining in the dark goes against my principles. It just seems to add to the mysteriousness people perceive about homosexuality."

The diagnosis of ARC and its potentially deadly ramifications came as a shock to John. Although he had all the symptoms — severe weight loss, diarrhea, and fever which brought intense night sweats and chills — he thought they were related to an intestinal problem.

He lost 27 pounds in six weeks to weigh in at a scant 125 pounds when the final diagnosis was made.

John made a trip home to Toronto to tell his mother.

"That was the end of it for me," recalled Grace Gordon quietly. "I've climbed many, many difficult mountains in my life. This is the most difficult."

A close bond exists between John and his mother who is also his best friend and a constant source of support. John's father died of cancer when he was four.

Grace remembers the day three years ago when her son told her he had antibodies to the human immunodeficiency virus (HIV), the virus that may cause AIDS. He had been exposed to the virus through a sexual contact that can't be traced.

"Fear gripped me all over. It was overwhelming for a while but I'm a person who believes in positive thinking and action. Eventually, I was able to come to grips with it."

It has taken longer with the diagnosis of ARC. John is constantly in her thoughts. She breaks down in tears and is embraced by her son when she admits fear of losing him weighs most heavily on her mind. The love between them is untouched by the news.

"We've battled many battles together and I feel this is just another one. We're going through a rough period right now but in two months, I'll be on the positive track. From there, there will be no looking at the negative."

Since learning of John's condition, Grace has helped establish, through the AIDS Committee of Toronto, a support group for mothers in similar situations.

Therapy helps

"Society is pointing a finger at us, a morality finger in judgment. The government hasn't taken the bull by the horns and said 'look, there are people dying out there and more are going to die if we don't do something.' You feel you're going through so much, why should you have that finger pointed at you. There's a feeling like you've got a cement wall around you. There are no doors and no windows. It just feels that's where society wants to put you, surrounded by that cement wall . . . There is so much fear out there, so much ignorance."

From wanting to use his social work degree to work with children, John now wants to counsel those affected by AIDS. His plans for the future are concrete yet strangely at odds with the will the young man has already prepared and signed.

"I don't want to die, don't get me wrong. I decided long ago that I'm going to live until 100 because I like three-digit numbers. I just think that we have to face realities. If I go on to get AIDS and it takes my life, I don't want anyone to be burdened with all that death brings with it."

In his will, John has divided what little he owns between friends and family and has specified how the funeral service should be conducted. He wants his illness to be talked about openly.

"I want the reception to be a big bash. I want people to celebrate my life."

Living on a tight student budget, John struggles with expenses brought about by his condition. Although outwardly healthy, he takes drugs he will need indefinitely to control candida or "thrush," a yeast infection in his throat.

He was recently approved by the ministry of community and social services to receive a disability pension. It covers prescription drugs but not alternative AIDS therapies that haven't been approved. A food supplement called AL 721 has helped some AIDS patients but costs about $300 a month — an impossibility on a budget of $542 a month.

John will try anything. He takes a wide assortment of vitamins, and avoids stress and fatigue that can be deadly to someone whose immune system is suppressed.

In one pocket, John always carries a much-fingered crystal. He calls it his security stone. To those who believe, crystals redirect positive energy into the person's inner being. "I know it's bizarre. I still don't understand all the theory. I use it because it reminds me to be strong, that I'm not alone."

He's not alone. A tight circle of friends surrounds John and he leans on them heavily. Among them is a Toronto support group which includes John in their sessions through a speaker phone.

There are other outlets. John has turned to Trager therapy, a type of massage offered free by Randy Herald of London to people with AIDS, ARC or positive antibodies.

The therapy works on the premise that stress is retained in certain parts of the body depending on the person. The massage relieves those areas and teaches the subconscious to let go of the harmful holding patterns.

Finger pointing

John leaves the sessions energized, revitalized but at the same time relaxed. The therapy, he says, makes the regular doctor visits and the uncertainty of what the next test will find a little easier to handle. It makes the space-like and antiseptic atmosphere of the dentist's office a touch less intimidating.

One such visit came in February. It takes dental staff at Victoria Hospital — the only place John could find that would take him as a patient — one hour to prepare for his arrival.

Every nook and cranny is covered with plastic sheets from the chairs to the paper towel dispenser. It is John, in jeans and a sweater, who looks exposed and vulnerable.

Despite the good natured staff whose joking manner gives life to the cold and sterile room, John says "when I walk in here it hits me in the face. There is something wrong with me."

By facing that reality publicly, John admits he's concerned about the reaction of those who don't know — staff at Merrymount Children's Centre where he worked two years ago, classmates at King's College. He hopes they react intelligently and with compassion.

"People with AIDS are people. With all the facts and information on the disease, that message is getting lost. They are people who have hopes and dreams — still."

"We've talked about death, about John's funeral, which was very difficult. You're not used to talking about that with friends. John hasn't been able to talk to too many people about it because they just didn't want to hear."

— STEVE LOWDEN, 24, of Toronto, a friend

"To see someone so full of life, so optimistic and young, it's just very hard. It hurts . . . There's a sense of loss, the loss of possibilities. That's what strikes me the most. I'll miss him. If in the next couple of years he does worsen, I'll miss him."

— SPENCER BRENNAN, 38, of Toronto, a friend

55 Layout for first page of John Gordon article, *London Free Press* (1 April 1988). Story Dahlia Reich, photography Susan Bradnam

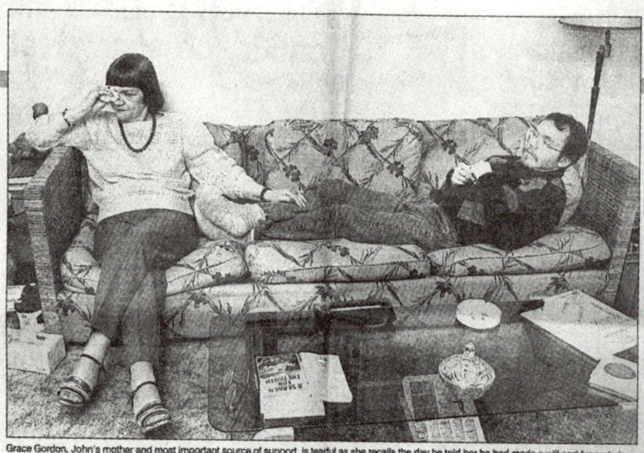

Grace Gordon, John's mother and most important source of support, is tearful as she recalls the day he told her he had made a will and funeral plans.

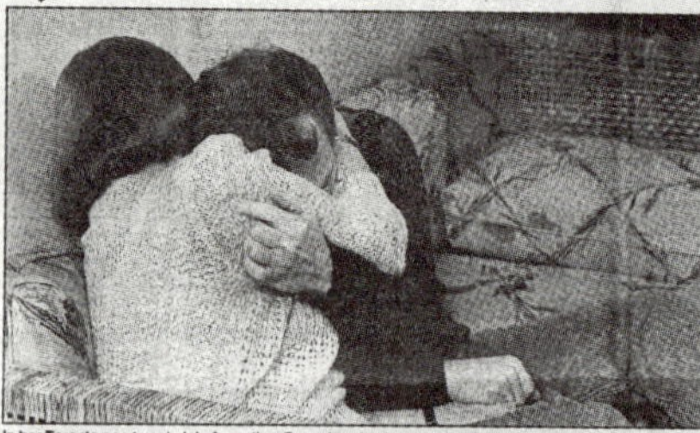

In her Toronto apartment, John's mother Grace breaks down and embraces her son when she tells him for the first time her greatest fear is losing him. Clutched in his hand is the crystal he carries for strength.

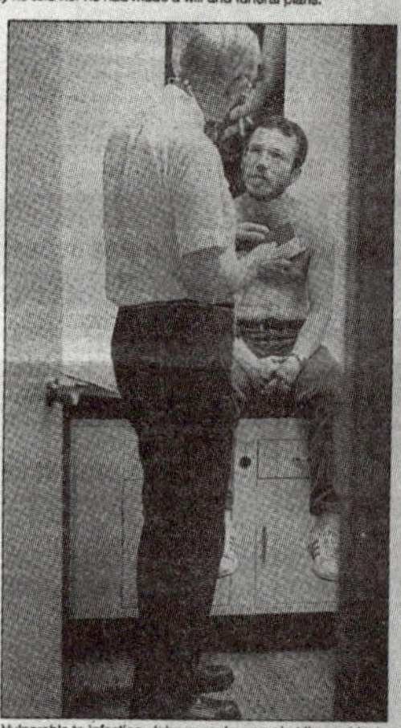

Vulnerable to infection, John never knows what the next test will find and makes regular trips to Dr. Fred Pattison, head of student health services at the University of Western Ontario.

“People distance themselves from John because they know he's gay and because he has ARC. I treat John as I would treat any close friend with a serious illness. It's hard to think he may die, because he has so much to offer.”

— LIANA LOWENSTEIN, 22, of London, a friend

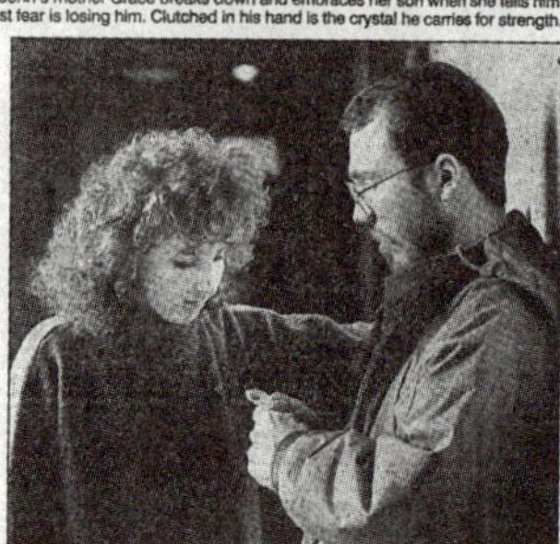

In the halls of King's College, John confides in Liana Lowestein, 22, a close friend about the crystal that reminds him he is not alone in his battle.

Photos by Susan Bradnam
Stories by Dahlia Reich
London Free Press

Few nearby escape trauma

Its power to destroy reaches far beyond the person with AIDS. It becomes a family affair.

That family could be friends, relatives or a lover, says London psychotherapist Bill Rowe. Few close to the person with AIDS are untouched by its devastating emotional symptoms of anger, frustration, guilt and fear.

"The people surrounding the HIV-positive person (those who have been in contact with the AIDS virus) have a complex mix of responses," says Rowe, who counsels those affected by AIDS, their families and friends.

"For intimates, there's fear of their own contamination and in some cases a rush to get tested."

For a woman who learns her partner is bisexual when he tells her he has the antibodies also comes a hurtful realization that the person has been unfaithful. For both lovers and spouses, the anger associated with the diagnosis of AIDS or antibodies may be intense.

"We've seen cases where people have literally been thrown out on the street, their lives threatened."

That anger isn't restricted to friends and family. For some homosexual men diagnosed with the antibodies, all the anxieties and insecurities he dealt with long ago in the process of coming to grips with his sexual orientation resurface. Self-loathing and doubt are not unusual.

With time, as the person remains symptom-free, the various feelings reach a plateau "a kind of holding pattern," Rowe says. "People go on. A certain quality of denial sets in. But when the symptoms occur, there's a rekindling of all the feelings that were dealt with or not dealt with earlier. There's hard clarity that this is real."

The grief felt by a lover whose partner has AIDS may be intensified because, afraid of rejection, they can't openly mourn the person's illness. Family members of the person with AIDS may exclude the lover from any involvement in the person's care or in the mourning process after his death. This magnifies the lover's loneliness and pain.

The dreaded diagnosis may also force a family to deal, for the first time, with issues of homosexuality.

"One cannot over-estimate the impact of the stigma associated with a gay lifestyle and AIDS on the grieving process," says Rowe in a soon-to-be published paper. "The stigma attached to AIDS magnifies the stigma attached to a gay lifestyle."

Families, particularly in the London area, cling to a cloak of secrecy when a relative has AIDS, Rowe adds. One family decided to forgo collecting life insurance rather than risk the cause of death being revealed in the small town where they live.

"It (the secrecy) is intense. I've met families who have talked to me about being at work and people would be making jokes about homosexuals or AIDS patients. They would have to laugh along so as not to raise suspicion and then they feel so guilty about what they just did."

When there is such secrecy, Rowe says, "it almost becomes a secret within the family, too. You're sitting there with an AIDS patient that people have to deal with and respond to, and it's not being talked about."

Early counselling for families or lovers is as essential as medical care for the AIDS patient, he says. People need the facts to dispel myths about the disease. They need to talk to someone who will listen and understand.

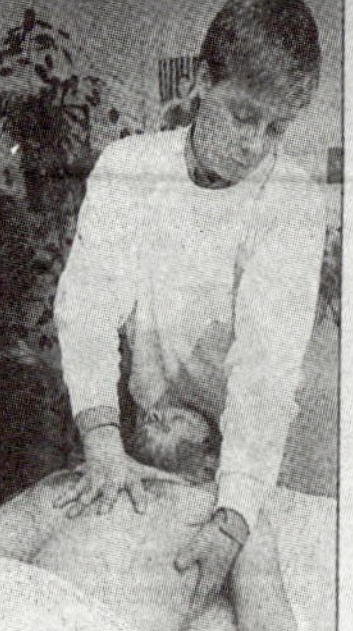

Trager therapy, a type of massage that relieves stress, helps John cope with the emotional strain of his condition. Randy Herald of London donates his time and therapy to those affected by AIDS.

AIDS

Acquired immune deficiency syndrome is an infectious disease transmitted through the exchange of body fluids, either through sexual contact or contact with infected blood. The disease cripples the body's immune system, leaving the person vulnerable to certain types of infections and cancer.

ARC

AIDS related complex is characterized by severe weight loss, diarrhea, chronic weakness, prolonged fever and other symptoms now considered early sign of AIDS. Although John Gordon has recovered from most of those symptoms, it is likely he will go on to have AIDS.

Although homosexual and bisexual men account for most of the AIDS cases in Canada, the disease can affect anyone — men and women, young and old.

56 Layout for second page of John Gordon article, *London Free Press*

57 T-shirt with malicious parody of insecticide logo and slogan ('RAID kills bugs dead'), on sale in Grand Bend, Ontario, 1989

57

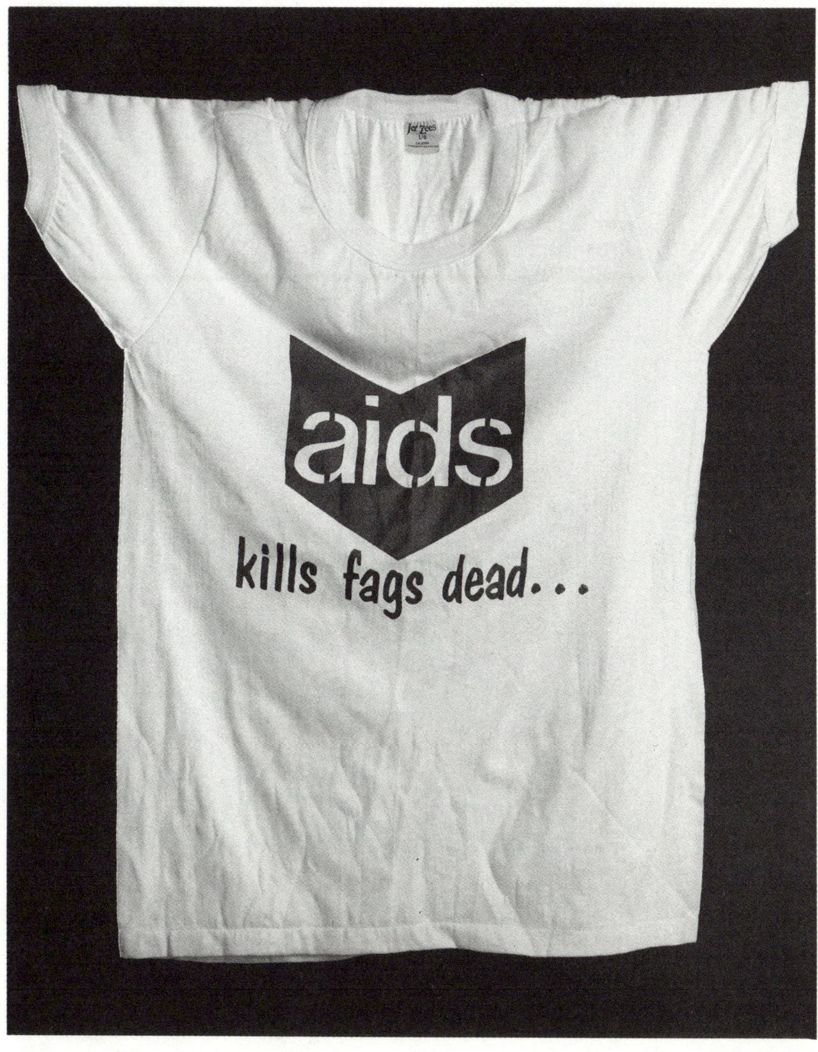

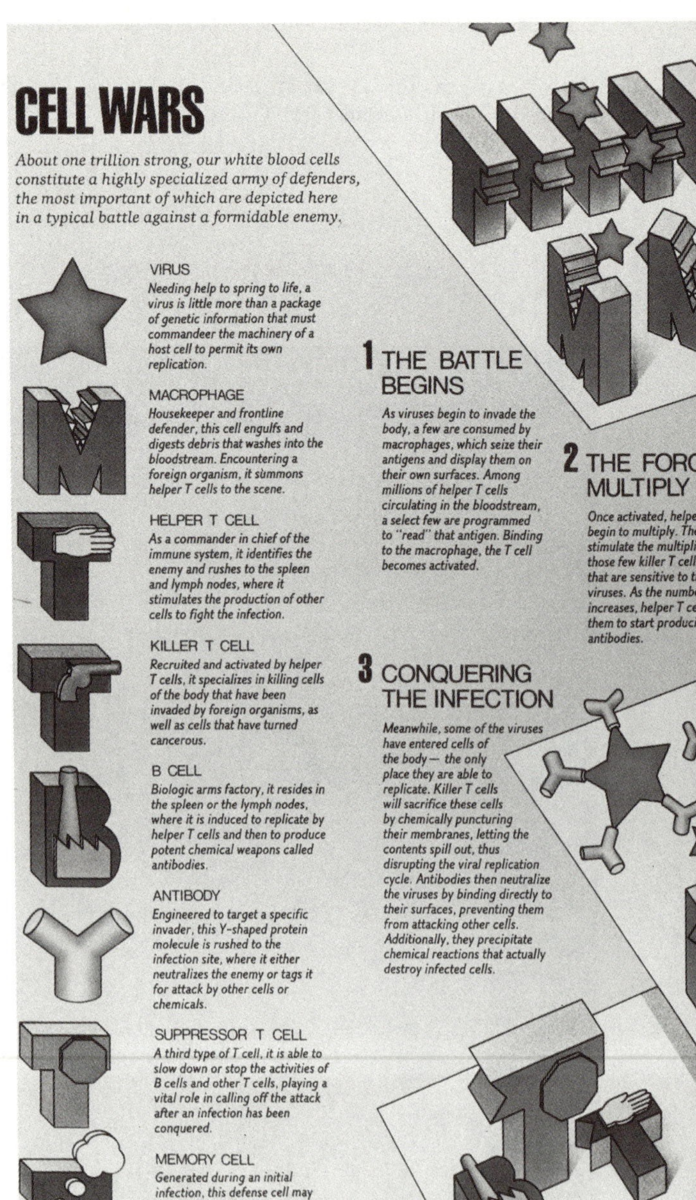

CELL WARS
About one trillion strong, our white blood cells constitute a highly specialized army of defenders, the most important of which are depicted here in a typical battle against a formidable enemy.
VIRUS
Needing help to spring to life, a virus is little more than a package of genetic information that must commandeer the machinery of a host cell to permit its own replication.
MACROPHAGE
Housekeeper and frontline defender, this cell engulfs and digests debris that washes into the bloodstream. Encountering a foreign organism, it summons helper T cells to the scene.
HELPER T CELL
As a commander in chief of the immune system, it identifies the enemy and rushes to the spleen and lymph nodes, where it stimulates the production of other cells to fight the infection.
KILLER T CELL
Recruited and activated by helper T cells, it specializes in killing cells of the body that have been invaded by foreign organisms, as well as cells that have turned cancerous.
B CELL
Biologic arms factory, it resides in the spleen or the lymph nodes, where it is induced to replicate by helper T cells and then to produce potent chemical weapons called antibodies.
ANTIBODY
Engineered to target a specific invader, this Y-shaped protein molecule is rushed to the infection site, where it either neutralizes the enemy or tags it for attack by other cells or chemicals.
SUPPRESSOR T CELL
A third type of T cell, it is able to slow down or stop the activities of B cells and other T cells, playing a vital role in calling off the attack after an infection has been conquered.
MEMORY CELL
Generated during an initial infection, this defense cell may circulate in the blood or lymph for years, enabling the body to respond more quickly to subsequent infections.
1 THE BATTLE BEGINS
As viruses begin to invade the body, a few are consumed by macrophages, which seize their antigens and display them on their own surfaces. Among millions of helper T cells circulating in the bloodstream, a select few are programmed to "read" that antigen. Binding to the macrophage, the T cell becomes activated.
2 THE FORC
MULTIPLY
Once activated, helper
begin to multiply. They
stimulate the multiplic
those few killer T cells
that are sensitive to the
viruses. As the number
increases, helper T cell
them to start producin
antibodies.
3 CONQUERING THE INFECTION
Meanwhile, some of the viruses have entered cells of the body — the only place they are able to replicate. Killer T cells will sacrifice these cells by chemically puncturing their membranes, letting the contents spill out, thus disrupting the viral replication cycle. Antibodies then neutralize the viruses by binding directly to their surfaces, preventing them from attacking other cells. Additionally, they precipitate chemical reactions that actually destroy infected cells.

58 'Cell Wars,' diagrams by Allen Carroll and Dale Glasgow, for 'Our Immune System: The Wars Within,' *National Geographic* 169:6 (June 1986) 708–9

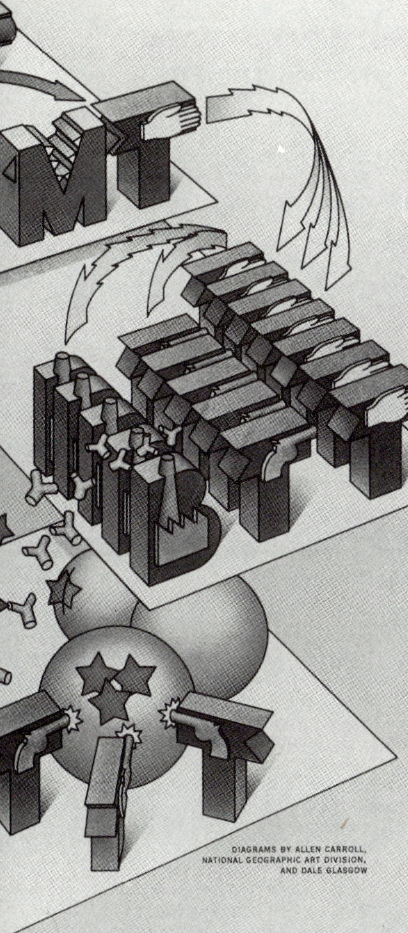

DIAGRAMS BY ALLEN CARROLL, NATIONAL GEOGRAPHIC ART DIVISION, AND DALE GLASGOW

A miracle of evolution, the human immune system is not controlled by any central organ, such as the brain. Rather it has developed to function as a kind of biologic democracy, wherein the individual members achieve their ends through an information network of awesome scope. Accounting for one percent of the body's 100 trillion cells, these defender white blood cells arise in the bone marrow. They fall into three groups: the phagocytes, or "cell eaters," of which the stalwart macrophage is one, and two kinds of lymphocytes, called T and B cells. All share one common objective: to identify and destroy all substances, living and inert, that are not part of the human body, that are "not self." These include human cancer cells, which have turned from self to nonself, friend to foe.

There are four critical phases to each immune response: recognition of the enemy, amplification of defenses, attack, and slowdown. Each immune response is a unique local sequence of events, shaped by the nature of the enemies. Chemical toxins and a multitude of inert environmental substances, such as asbestos and smoke particles, are normally attacked only by phagocytes. Organic invaders enlist the full range of immune responses. Besides viruses, these include single-celled bacteria, protozoa, and fungi, as well as a host of multicelled worms called helminths. Many of these enemies have evolved devious methods to escape detection. The viruses that cause influenza and the common cold, for example, constantly mutate, changing their fingerprints. The AIDS virus, most insidious of all, employs a range of strategies, including hiding out in healthy cells. What makes it fatal is its ability to invade and kill helper T cells, thereby short-circuiting the entire immune response.

4 CALLING A TRUCE

As the infection is contained, suppressor T cells halt the entire range of immune responses, preventing them from spiraling out of control. Memory T and B cells are left in the blood and lymphatic system, ready to move quickly should the same virus once again invade the body.

59 A plug for panic sex: Swiss AIDS-Foundation poster ('Always fuck with a condom,' 1989) showing how to get a charge out of fellatio without getting sperm in your mouth

59

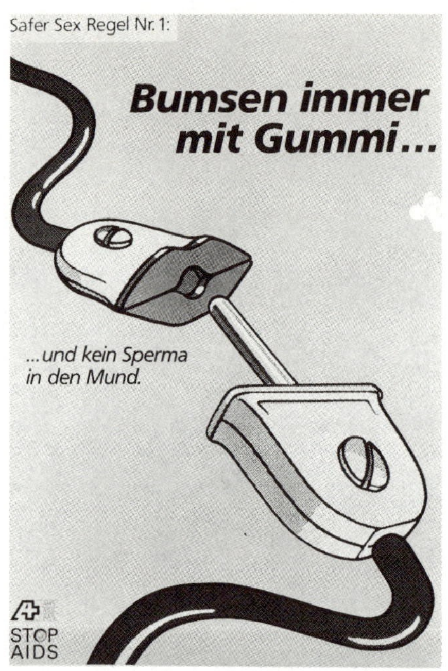

60

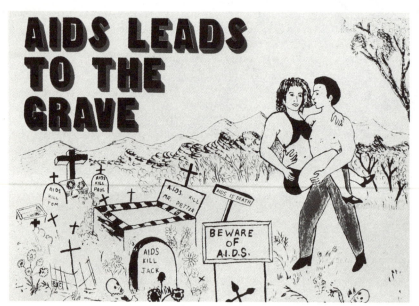

60 A bed for sacrificial sex: St Lucia Ministry of Health poster (c. 1989) showing where you can dig up a date in the British West Indies

'aids kills fags dead ...': Cultural Activism in Grand Bend

JOHN GORDON AND CLARENCE CROSSMAN

EDITOR'S NOTE: The following informal case study presents an example of successful AIDS activism conducted at a local level against a particularly hateful representation of gay PWAs as annoying insects easily exterminated by bourgeois holiday-makers with the application of a common household pesticide. Through a trick of language, the coincidental chiming of a brand-name ('Raid') with an acronym ('AIDS') and a common noun ('bugs') with a common insult ('fags'), acquired immunodeficiency syndrome is symbolically identified with the pesticide known to millions of TV viewers as the remorseless Übermensch of bug sprays, the mighty cannister that not only kills bugs but 'kills bugs DEAD.' Only exterminating angels and wrathful deities can get away with that redundancy. To kill is human; to kill dead, divine.

The dehumanizing identification of bugs and fags is surely not coincidental: it betrays, as cruel ethnic jokes often do, a fascistic wish on the part of a majority (uninfected heterosexual middle-class consumers) to exert control over a socially inferiorized yet demonically threatening minority (men doubly infected with gayness and HIV) through the exercise of supreme technological power. The Final Solution in an aerosol can: what could be more convenient?

AIDS is thus deviously imagined and casually advocated by those who would laugh at this complex pun – and there are those who would laugh at it, alas, without ever recognizing their latent complicity with the Nazi proponents of Zyklon B – as a simple tool for solving the complex social problems produced or exacerbated by the epidemic. Representing AIDS as the new Holocaust is no laughing matter to the many gay activists who proudly wear ACT UP's pink triangle into the political fray in memory of the homosexuals forced to wear such a device in the Nazi extermination camps. Pink triangles can routinely be found on the lapels of the two authors of this study.

So what's in a bad pun? The stimulus for determined cultural activism, as John Gordon reveals in section one: his account of the Grand Bend T-shirt challenge is an edited transcript of his moving presentation at the 'Representing AIDS' conference delivered on 10 November, 1988 at the University of Western Ontario, London, Canada. In the second section, Clarence Crossman, his colleague at the AIDS Committee of London, presents some general reflections on AIDS activism prompted by the narrative.

The Grand Bend T-Shirt Challenge

The AIDS Committee of London received a telephone call in June 1988 from a concerned citizen who had been in Grand Bend, a village on Lake Huron with a large and popular beach, and had seen a T-shirt at a booth where many T-shirts are sold. There were two washrooms on either side of this booth, and the T-shirt was hanging on display (plate 57, following p 239). The T-shirt was a take-off on the Raid insecticide logo (a black shield) and slogan ('Raid kills bugs dead'). On and beneath a similar shield, which came in a variety of colours, the T-shirt bore the message: 'aids kills fags dead ...' The obvious implication is that gay men (and presumably lesbians) are vermin or bugs that can and should be exterminated. The woman who called was hoping that the AIDS Committee of London, a community-based organization with a mandate for education, support, and advocacy, could do something about the shirt.

We began to investigate what legal recourse was available to us to have the T-shirt removed. As a gay man and a person living with AIDS I experienced both hurt and anger at hearing that such a T-shirt was being sold. Using my anger as fuel for energy, I immediately contacted a number of people. I first called a lawyer, who supports the committee's work, to ask her opinion on what kind of legal action we could take. I thought that perhaps legislation prohibiting hate literature might be of use to us. The lawyer informed me that, since the hate-literature legislation was too vague, that approach would not be useful to us. She did offer to investigate our options further. My next step was to call the Ontario Human Rights Commission. I spoke to Mr Walter Burns, who informed me that the Ontario Human Rights Code covered housing, employment, contracts, and services, none of which was denied to an Ontario citizen in this instance. Therefore he would not be able to put a case together for us. But he also believed that the T-shirt violated the spirit of the code if not its letter. He was supportive of our wish to approach the owner of the booth, encouraged us to inform the owner that the selling of this T-shirt violated the spirit of the code, and wanted to know the results of our efforts. Later he called me back to confirm that any action they could take would be very limited, but stated he was checking out every option for action on their part because he found the T-shirt so offensive.

I next called London city hall because of an experience of a friend of mine in Toronto, who was verbally and physically harassed by a cashier in a variety store where he was attempting to buy a gay magazine. This friend had gone to Toronto city hall to inquire about the possibility of revoking the vendor's licence for that variety store. He was successful in having the licence revoked. Remembering this incident, I thought that it was an option worth investigating in our situation. If such action could be taken we would present the possibility to the booth owner as an incentive to remove the T-shirt. I was directed by London city hall to the Grand Bend village council clerk, who informed me that such action might be a possibility and it would be best for me to make a presentation to the Grand Bend village council. So I immediately had our concern entered as an agenda item for the next village council meeting. I emphasized that I did not wish the council to take any action to warn the vendor before we could confront him or her personally with our concern.

We also had to 'claim our turf' with a reporter, a friend of mine, whom I had informed of the T-shirt over lunch and who wanted to immediately investigate the selling of the shirt. We were concerned that a reporter's investigation could possibly tip off the vendor, who might cover up the action of selling the T-shirt before we could actually obtain one, and before we could explain directly to the vendor our reasons for taking offence at the T-shirt and enlist whatever legal support we could find. I agreed with the appropriateness of the reporter going with a photographer to take pictures of the T-shirt for sale, and she agreed to let us proceed with whatever action we could, keeping her informed of developments. This negotiation was not achieved without some tension and feelings of awkwardness.

At the next staff meeting of the AIDS Committee of London we confirmed the activist plans we had been discussing. We would buy a T-shirt, obtain a receipt, and confront the vendor. If he or she refused to cooperate in removing the T-shirt we would organize a demonstration. We would seek support for the demonstration from the committee's volunteers, members of the Homophile Association of London Ontario – the largest gay and lesbian organization in town and very supportive of our work – and any other friends and supporters we could muster.

I first went to Grand Bend on a Wednesday, with a friend accompanying me for support, only to find that the booth was closed. With another friend, who is also HIV-positive, I returned to Grand Bend on Saturday when the beach is much busier. The T-shirt was hanging in the booth. I remember feeling so angry and hurt by the sight that I was not able to go up to the booth to purchase the shirt. Although it was also difficult for him to do, my friend purchased the T-shirt for $17.00, plus tax. He chatted with the sales clerk, who informed him that they had already sold four of those T-shirts that day.

Because the shirt's hateful message had such an emotional impact on us, and because we were keyed up to fulfil our activist plans, we were in fact a bit paranoid, and locked the purchased shirt in the trunk of our car. We wanted to foil any ideas of stealing the shirt back from us.

We tnen returned to the booth to obtain a receipt and to find out where the booth owner was at that moment. The receipt described the purchase as an '"AIDS" T-shirt.' We were directed to a store in the village; I agreed with my friend that I would go in alone. After going through about four people, I finally met the owner of the store and booth, whose name was Nick.

I introduced myself: 'My name is John Gordon. I am a person with AIDS and I am a gay man. I have just seen this offensive T-shirt hanging up in the booth on the beach, saying "aids kills fags dead."' I told him it was sending out a seriously false message, not only in identifying AIDS with gay men but also in stating that gay men should be exterminated like vermin. I informed him that selling the shirt violated the spirit of the Ontario Human Rights Code and requested that he remove it immediately and permanently because it was so offensive to me and other persons with AIDS.

He responded: 'What are you getting so upset about? It's just a gimmick. We sold all of them last year.'

I got angry: 'Just a gimmick? It's not just a gimmick to me as a person with AIDS; it's not just a gimmick to my family or the brothers and sisters of persons with AIDS who come on the weekend to use the beach and see this kind of T-shirt.' I reminded him that it violated the spirit of the code and became insistent that he take the shirt down.

He finally said: 'Well it's just a gimmick, but if it violates the code, of course I will remove it.'

I then gave my card and explained that I was a counsellor at the AIDS Committee of London, thanked him for promising to remove the shirt and then warned him that people would be checking all summer to make sure that the product did not go back up on sale some time later. When I shook his hand I realized that I was trembling.

When I left the store, my friend and I drove around to the front of the beach where the shirt had been sold, and in the five minutes that it took us to get back to the booth, the T-shirt was gone.

Although our initial activist efforts were successful, we were left with mixed feelings. Obviously we felt relief and gratification that our mission had been achieved. There was a certain sense of empowerment from confronting the vendor and enlisting his cooperation. However the hurt and anger remained to some degree and was reactivated in other AIDS Committee staff when they saw and held the T-shirt. We also acknowledged to each other with somewhat sheepish laughter that we were disappointed that we did not need to organize a demonstration. We had anticipated that such an act would have been both an emotional release and a valuable coalescing of those people involved with AIDS, in the London area, with activist leanings. One staff member had pleaded that we wait for him and not schedule the demonstration for a period of time when he had to be out of town. We were already thinking up slogans for placards and chants, including 'AIDS Jokes Are Not Funny' and 'Hate Kills Canada Dead!'

We also did not trust someone who saw the T-shirt only as a profit-making sales gimmick, and decided to continue with our plans to make a presentation to the Grand Bend village council. Preceding our presentation at the council meeting was a presentation from their public-health unit, outlining an AIDS-prevention education campaign planned for the beach that summer. One council member wanted to know why AIDS education was happening on their beach since AIDS was a gay disease. A motion of support was passed but met with some resistance.

I was accompanied by Betty Anne Thomas, executive director of the AIDS Committee of London, who introduced herself and introduced me, including the fact that I was a person with AIDS. Then she described the T-shirt that had been for sale and held it up for the council members to see.

We demanded that the village council see that the T-shirt remained off the shelf by having one of the village councillors go down to the business and inform the owner that it was the council's wish that this T-shirt never be sold again, and if it was sold again that his vendor's licence would be revoked by the council. Betty Anne introduced our concerns and I presented the 'human impact' dimension of the story. I described how angry and offended I was by this product, which was hurtful to persons with AIDS, their loved ones, and caring residents of Grand Bend. I repeated the fact that it was within their jurisdiction to revoke the merchant's vendor's licence. The council members appeared to be overwhelmed with our presentation. Their main concern was to minimize the negative reflection on Grand Bend. They asked questions in a businesslike yet empathetic manner, and once the presentation and questions were finished, one councillor jumped practically out of his chair and volunteered to go down the next morning and talk to the shop owner to make sure that our demands were met. The council passed a motion unanimously in support of our requests.

Throughout the summer various people checked the sales booth on the beach to make sure that the garment was not for sale again. To our knowledge it was not available for the rest of the summer. We felt we had achieved significant success, in that we did get the T-shirt removed and obtained support for our concern about it. It does not appear, however, that we were successful in making the vendor understand the reasons why we found the T-shirt so offensive, and inexcusable as a gimmick. We certainly received no apology. The *London Free Press* published a brief article. Apparently when the vendor was being interviewed he tried to persuade the reporter not to bother with the story because he saw it as not really newsworthy.

We were also unsuccessful in identifying where and by whom the product was made and distributed, so we could not stop its sale elsewhere. If we had been able to locate the producer, we would have attempted to enlist the support of Johnson & Johnson, the manufacturers of Raid, to disassociate themselves from the parody of their slogan and logo and threaten any appropriate legal action against the borrowers.

The AIDS Committee of London was officially involved in this activist venture because our mandate lists advocacy as one of our program goals. The staff and board of directors perceive advocacy on behalf of individuals who are unfairly treated or on behalf of HIV-infected persons and their loved ones as a group as crucial to the effectiveness of a community-based AIDS service organization.

My personal motivation comes from the solidarity I feel with other people with AIDS and the urge I feel to act on behalf of them all when confronted with such an offensive set of circumstances. Such advocacy is also a fulfilment of my values and vocation as a social worker. I have been profoundly influenced by my mother's example. She has been a forthright activist in the women's movement and the labour movement. It is a joke in my family that I was born in a committee room.

So I was exposed to activism from an early age. All of those factors in my life impel me to do what I can to prevent such offensiveness from happening or reoccurring. Certainly people with AIDS and people affected by AIDS in any way have enough trauma to deal with without having to confront this kind of abuse. So I would most definitely take such action again, and, in fact, am assisting a client of mine who was fired from his job for being HIV-infected and is seeking legal redress through the Ontario Human Rights Code.

The *London Free Press* described me in a headline recently as an 'AIDS victim,' a phrase that drives me absolutely crazy. I choose to be called a 'person with AIDS,' and am pursuing my concerns with the reporter who wrote the story, the newspaper's ombudsman, and the editorial staff. In fact, in my most recent contact with the *Free Press*, concerning my retelling of this incident, I informed the reporter that I would not speak to him unless he would assure me that he would not use the word 'victim' in reference to me. I did receive that assurance.[1]

John Gordon

Reflections on AIDS Activism and Advocacy

It is generally expected that the purpose of a community-based AIDS service organization involves education and support services. It is perhaps less obvious, and therefore needs to be emphasized, that actions of advocacy such as the intervention narrated above are also a crucial part of community-based AIDS work. Advocacy, on behalf of individuals and groups experiencing injustice because of AIDS, is one of the program goals for the AIDS Committee of London, as submitted to the AIDS Section of the Ontario Ministry of Health, the committee's major funding source. The goal is fulfilled by such activities as referrals to the Ontario Human Rights Commission, direct intervention into discriminatory situations, demonstrations and other forms of public protest, enlisting media coverage, and lobbying various levels of government and other decision makers. It is apparent to most community-based AIDS workers that other goals, such as education or support services, cannot be adequately fulfilled without an advocacy dimension. Effective education would need to challenge prejudice and engender compassion. Effective support would facilitate restitution where possible.

The instance of discrimination outlined above is not an isolated incident. In south-western Ontario and throughout Canada, people affected by HIV and AIDS in a variety of ways are regularly treated unequally and unfairly. The following examples of discrimination in the London area are selected to illustrate their diversity:

- A man was fired from his food-service job after his employer was informed by a spiteful third party that the man was HIV-antibody positive.
- A woman quit her job as a dental assistant because the dentist for whom she worked was rumoured to be gay and have AIDS; she met a patient of the dentist's on the street and urged her not to continue as his patient.
- A person with AIDS was asked by a disability-pension bureaucrat how long he intended to live because other people with AIDS for whom he had processed pension claims had died within three months and it had not been worth his while to do the work.
- The AIDS Committee of London was refused office space by a property-management company whose president told a third party that there was no way he was going to rent to 'those AIDS people.'
- A dental hygienist made arrangements with the receptionist staff in a dental clinic to inform her of any patients that were likely to be gay; because she came from a rural area she believed the other women would be more experienced than she at identifying gay men and she wanted to be warned so that she could question them about their HIV-antibody status.
- A man was verbally harassed and threatened by a co-worker who suspected him of being gay, while his supervisor, in an effort to find out his HIV-antibody status, returned phone calls that were left as personal messages for him.
- Some husbands have ordered their wives who are nurses not to work with people with AIDS.
- Some physicians renting offices in a medical building opposed the establishment of an HIV clinic in the building because the clients would break into their offices to steal drugs and needles and would have sex in the elevators.
- An inmate in a detention centre was required to clean phones, showers, and beds after he used them in a manner that was both unnecessary and humiliating; the guards were 'not taking any chances.'
- A car-repair shop posts and after-hours sign that reads: 'Guarded by pit bull with AIDS.'

Some of these instances were successfully referred to the Ontario Human Rights Commission, some were successfully challenged by AIDS Committee of London staff intervention, some issues were not pursued because the victim feared public disclosure or further abuse, and some have yet to be pursued because of the overwhelming demands on AIDS workers.

Sharing the marginalization of people affected by AIDS can come as a shock to many social-service staff or volunteers who have moved into AIDS organizations from other kinds of social-service agencies. Having a theoretical understanding of AIDS-related discrimination is usually not enough preparation for the emotional impact of such a hurtful reality. Initially, most do not expect to experience discrimination themselves simply because they are involved in AIDS-related work. Yet many people they encounter no longer view them with respect or gratitude because of the service work they do. Instead, they are often shunned or ridiculed, and acquaintances react to them with fear, anger, or discomfort.

The AIDS workers (paid staff or volunteers) who are best prepared to deal with the discrimination that they and the people they help experience are generally those who have already been involved in some kind of social-change organization or activity and bring that experience and analysis to their AIDS-related tasks. Predominant among such people are gay and lesbian activists. It has been a natural extension of the activist and community-development work of many lesbian and gay liberationists to become involved in, and often to initiate, AIDS service organizations. The community for which they have worked was the one first affected by HIV and AIDS in North America, while medical, social-service, and governmental establishments have been slow to respond to the epidemic.

Ironically, in Canada and particularly in Ontario, involvement in community-based AIDS service organizations has meant access to the funding of operating expenses, salaries, and other resources and to an increased perception of validity that are not easily gained by gay and lesbian activists. It is worthwhile noting that without the political analysis and self-reflection that comes with social-change activity, gay men and lesbians are no more prepared to deal with the emotional fallout of AIDS-related discrimination than are non-gay people. Gay men and lesbians who have not been involved in gay-liberationist activities or reflection, but have been personally touched by HIV or AIDS in some way, and are thereby motivated to contribute to some form of

AIDS-related service, can find the participation in discrimination related to AIDS as devastating as any other well-meaning individual would who lacks an analytical perspective.

It would be a mistake, however, to perceive seasoned activism as devoid of emotional involvement. One dimension of intense activism is passion, which has been described as a combination of moral outrage and yearning for the very best for oneself and others. Activism is best understood as involving self-reflection, political analysis, and emotional motivation. For example, John Gordon describes using his anger at the T-shirt slogan as 'fuel for energy' in order to take action. Many people who have become involved in some form of AIDS-related work without any sense of that work being a form of social change have been moved by their intense emotional reaction to AIDS-related injustice toward social and political analysis as a basis for their work. The Grand Bend incident illustrates that AIDS activism can be deeply personal at the same time as it is corporate and public.

The presentation of the Grand Bend case study has resulted in some interesting discussions as to whether the advocacy involved was gay activism or AIDS activism. These comments are written from the perspective that in this case the two forms of activism are inseparable as are the two forms of bigotry, and that the inseparability of AIDS-phobia and homophobia is true of most cases of AIDS-related discrimination that occur in North America.

An anecdotal report of nursing care in London, Ontario, further illustrates the point. Some years ago the first person with AIDS to be admitted to a particular hospital ward reportedly inspired high fear in the nursing staff about their risk of being infected with HIV. Because of their fear of the patient the level of nursing care, patient contact, and compassion was dramatically reduced. Some time later a second person with AIDS was admitted to the ward, but the nurses were emphatically less afraid of contracting HIV from this patient and the quality of their care, contact, and compassion markedly improved. When questioned about the reason for the marked difference in attitude and behaviour in relation to the two people with AIDS, it became evident that the nurses were less afraid of the second person, not because they already had experience caring for a person with AIDS, but because the second person was a haemophiliac and the first person was a gay man. Studies of attitudes and behaviour of hospital staff toward people with AIDS support this anecdote by demonstrating a high correlation between fear of HIV infection from patients and homophobia.[2]

It is important to state that the quality of nursing care in London,

Ontario, for people with AIDS is generally exemplary at this time. Current informal observation of nursing staff in south-western Ontario matches another of the studies' conclusions: the hospital staff most fearful of working with people with AIDS are usually the ones who have had little or no experience providing such care. Personal interaction with a person with AIDS is one of the most effective ways to dispel AIDS-phobia. Homophobia is generally reduced as well, although it is a more tenacious attitude. Nurses have been easiest to assess in reference to attitude and behaviour; however, it can be assumed that the same attitude and behaviour patterns would be true of most people.

The conclusion can be drawn, therefore, that effective AIDS activism must contain a simultaneous challenge to AIDS discrimination and to homophobia. Even heterosexuals can and do experience discrimination that entails homophobia. Any person suspected of being HIV-infected or of being sympathetic toward people with HIV or AIDS can be suspected of being homosexual. Ryan White, the haemophiliac adolescent featured in *People* magazine, was accused by some of being homosexual even during his early teens because of his AIDS diagnosis.[3] Comprehensive civil- and human-rights protection is an important tool in gaining some form of restitution in cases of AIDS-related discrimination, as well as in preventing such discrimination from occurring in the first place.

The Ontario Human Rights Code is a good model: protection against discrimination is provided both on the basis of sexual orientation and on the basis of disability or illness. The code provides protection in the areas of employment, rental accommodation, education, medical care, and any provision of goods, facilities, or services including union and business contracts. It offers protection against firing, demotion, or eviction; against refusal of job, rental accommodation, or other business, medical, or education services; and against harassment, mandatory testing, and breaking of confidentiality. The disability/illness protection applies to people having HIV infection or AIDS, suspected of having HIV infection or AIDS, or associated with people with HIV infection or AIDS. The sexual-orientation protection applies to people known to be gay or lesbian, suspected of being gay or lesbian, or associated with gay men and lesbians. It is equally a violation of the code to discriminate against someone on the basis of heterosexuality. Restitution includes such measures as cash settlements, reinstatement, or written promises that discrimination will cease.

The Ontario Human Rights Code has limitations, however. Curiously, when the amendment to the code to include sexual orientation as grounds for protection against discrimination was passed in December 1986, protection from harassment about sexual orientation was specifically omitted from the amendment. Also, elementary- and secondary-school teachers are explicitly excluded from employment protection in reference to sexual orientation.

There are people who cannot avail themselves of the protection the code offers because they cannot provide enough evidence for the complaint to stand. Others may have a conclusive case of discrimination but are afraid of public disclosure in the process or of future ramifications, and therefore do not lodge a complaint. The code is not completely useless for such people, however. The moral suasion of the code is significant. For example, after being informed by John Gordon that the selling of the T-shirt violated the spirit of the code, the booth owner relented and removed the merchandise.

Public education about the code's protection can act as a deterrent to some potential discriminators. The Coalition for Lesbian and Gay Rights in Ontario has established a liaison committee with the Commission that provides advice on education and enforcement issues concerning sexual orientation and HIV/AIDS. Spreading the word that, according to the Ontario government, discrimination on the basis of sexual orientation and HIV status is not acceptable will have a censuring impact on discriminatory attitudes and behaviours. The success of the Grand Bend T-shirt challenge was not complete without media coverage and other public-education efforts that conveyed the message that it is no longer socially acceptable to discriminate on the basis of sexual orientation or health status. If the 'novelty' vendors of the world are not easily persuaded that their attitudes and behaviour are hurtful and prejudicial, it is still possible to pressure them into curtailing their discriminatory actions. Another equally important education task is informing people affected by HIV and AIDS in any way that they do have legal recourse against discrimination, as indicated in the Ontario Human Rights Commission's flyer 'AIDS and the Human Rights Code: Know Your Rights' (see appendix to this article).

Concern about reverse-discrimination that prevents citizens' freedom of expression and action and results in censorship deserves careful consideration. Simple disagreement with a message or offence taken to a message would not be sufficient grounds for suppressing that message without serious curtailment of freedom of expression. As Walter Burns, the Commission staff member, pointed out to John Gordon, this particular incident was not covered by the letter of the code because it was not the kind of discriminatory act that denied an

Ontario citizen (or group of Ontario citizens) specific services or opportunities such as employment, promotion, or accommodation. Quite specific grounds need to be used for challenging an action of a more general nature believed to be discriminatory. The following criteria are offered for the reader's consideration: a message that makes malicious statements about a category of people, with potential to be harmful to them, and without an opportunity for witnesses to have equal access to a response from the people referred to in the message, could be deemed appropriate to suppress.

The Canadian AIDS Society, the coalition of over forty community-based AIDS service organizations across Canada, has been involved in a variety of activist efforts aimed at federal and provincial governments. One significant activist project for the fall of 1989 was to provide input into the formation of a National AIDS Strategy. The Society stated emphatically in its brief 'Working Together: Towards a National AIDS Strategy in Canada' that protection against discrimination on the basis of sexual orientation and HIV status needs to be a part of the human-rights legislation of the federal government and of every province and territory.[4] Manitoba, Ontario, Quebec, and the Yukon are the only provinces and territory that provide protection on the basis of sexual orientation as of December 1989.

The opportunities for and varieties of AIDS activism are immense. The action focused on the T-shirt booth in Grand Bend is offered for reflection as a concrete example that is both deeply personal for John Gordon and an effective fulfilment of the mandate of the AIDS Committee of London. It entails careful strategy, cooperative effort, and intense emotional involvement. It entails an assertion and affirmation of human dignity.

Clarence Crossman

APPENDIX

AIDS AND THE HUMAN RIGHTS CODE KNOW YOUR RIGHTS

The Ontario Human Rights Code prohibits discrimination against people with HIV (Human Immunodeficiency Virus). This includes all those who have ARC (AIDS-Related Complex), AIDS or who have tested positive for HIV, whether they show symptoms or not. The Code also prohibits discrimination against people who are *believed* to have HIV, as well as those who associate with them.

- If you have been denied a job, dismissed or demoted because you have AIDS/ARC/HIV, or because someone thinks you do, and you can still do that job;
- If you have been required to undergo HIV-antibody testing at an employment medical or have been asked whether you have AIDS, ARC or HIV at an employment interview;
- If you have been denied accommodation because you have, or are believed to have, AIDS/ARC/HIV;
- If you have been denied service by a store, restaurant, theatre, club, government agency, insurance company, hospital, dentist's or doctor's office, or other such provider of services, goods and facilities because you have, or are believed to have, AIDS/ARC/HIV;
- If you or your child have been denied permission to attend school because you or he or she have, or are believed to have, AIDS/ARC/HIV, or if you or your child have been asked to take a HIV-antibody test as a condition of admission;
- If you have been harassed at work by your superiors or co-workers, or by your landlord, building superintendent or other tenants in your building, because you have, or are believed to have, AIDS/ARC/HIV;

get in touch with the nearest office of the Ontario Human Rights Commission, or phone (416) 965-6841. You may be able to file a complaint. You have a right to be protected against discrimination because you have, or are believed to have, AIDS/ARC/HIV. You do not need a lawyer or have to pay a fee to anyone in order to file a complaint.

> [This statement on AIDS-related discrimination is put forth by the Ontario Human Rights Commission (400 University Ave., Toronto, Ontario M7A 2R9).]

NOTES

1 Dahlia Reich 'AIDS Group Complains: Shirt Pulled from Shelf' *London Free Press* (23 June 1988)

2 See J.H. Pleck, L. O'Donnell, C. O'Donnell, and J. Snarey 'AIDS-Phobia, Contact with AIDS, and AIDS-related Job Stress in Hospital Workers' *Journal of Homosexuality* 15, no. 3/4 (1988) 41–54. See also L. M. Pomerance and J. J. Shields 'Factors Associated with Hospital Workers' Reactions to the Treatment of Persons with AIDS' *AIDS Education and Prevention* 1, no. 3 (1989) 184–93.

3 J. Friedman and D. Van Biema 'AIDS: A Diary of the Plague in America' *People* 3 Aug 1987, 61

4 'Working Together: Towards a National AIDS Strategy in Canada' Canadian AIDS Society, first submission, 19 Sept 1989, 51, 54

'Fighting spirit remains in 29-year-old victim': *London Free Press*, 8 July 1991

DAHLIA REICH

There's a spirit in John Gordon that won't fade. It disappears now and then but it always returns, strong and determined, again and again.

Clothes hanging on his thin frame, John answered the door Saturday with the same smile with which he has greeted every opportunity to tell people who he is and why his story is important.

It's been just over three years since the first signs of AIDS became apparent in a now battle-weary 29-year-old who learned he had antibodies to the virus, indicating he had been in contact with it, in 1985. He went public in a *Free Press* article in April, 1988, becoming the first person with AIDS in Southwestern Ontario to put his name and face to the controversial disease.

Now that disease has taken its toll. Twice in the last four months, John thought he was about to die. In February, radiation treatment for cancer inside his mouth left a mass of painful blisters that made eating or even drinking water agony. 'I was wasting away to nothing.'

He recovered from that ordeal to come down with a bacterial infection that ravaged his body, also nearly killing him.

Yet he recounts these incidents in the matter-of-fact way he has always talked about AIDS. Now weighing just 116 pounds at 5′5″, he points out how the purple spots of Kaposi's sarcoma, a rare cancer common among AIDS sufferers, have spread from his eyebrow to his scalp. He explains that the myriad pill bottles stacked in a large basket are needed to combat tension headaches, depression, panic attacks, seizures, a chronic throat infection, nausea and the bacterial infection.

John is not always matter of fact. These days, he admits, he hasn't come to grips with his fear of dying. 'I've discovered that I'm still afraid of death.'

And the tears come when he thinks about how his lover, Cliff, who cares for him in the apartment they share, and his mother, who makes frequent trips to London from Toronto, will cope if he dies.

He also admits that the fighting spirit he had hoped would help him live to a ripe old age becomes eroded at times. 'But it's still there. It always comes back when I'm feeling well. I still have a strong will to live. I don't want to die. I'm not ready to die.'

Also intact is his hope for a cure, and despite the ups and downs of his health, John goes about living as fully as possible. He had to give up his counsellor position at the AIDS Committee of London, but he volunteers for the federal NDP [New Democratic Party], marched in Toronto's Gay and Lesbian Pride Parade, and is planning a camping trip. His message to the public is also unchanged.

'The people living with AIDS are people, human beings that require everyone's compassion and understanding, not discrimination and hatred.'

AIDS in the Novel: Getting It Straight

JAMES MILLER

The Novel of Social Criticism has an honoured place in our literature, a place secured for it by Charles Dickens at the height of the Age of Progress. Now, in the regressive 'Age of AIDS,' as Masters and Johnson are urging heterosexuals to label our era, we find a worthy (if unlikely) successor to Dickens in gay journalist Randy Shilts.[1] Shilts has artfully mated *Hard Times* with *Oliver Twist* to produce a symphonic opus of public oppression and private suffering, *And the Band Played On.*

'This book is a work of journalism,' he insists. 'There has been no fictionalization.' Oh, no? 'For purposes of narrative flow,' he warns us, 'I reconstruct scenes, recount conversations and occasionally attribute observations to people with such phrases as "he thought" or "she felt."'[2] Despite this disclaimer, his flowing narrative of 'politics, people, and the AIDS epidemic' closely adheres to the chronicle structure and bourgeois moral code of its great Victorian prototypes, as Douglas Crimp and other hostile reviewers have pointed out.[3] That Shilts seems to have mistaken his novel for the Facts in no way undermines his right to be hailed as one of the great contemporary masters of straight middle-class fiction.

The skill with which he has woven a thousand plots together into a coherent cautionary tale set in a sleazy slum-world writhing with green monkeys, bicentennial sailors, and exotic bathhouse bugs quite dazzles me. I marvel at his Dickensian talent for vivid caricature, villains being his great specialty. Uriah Heep is a mere parasite compared to his unctuously self-advancing Robert Gallo, and Fagin a minor skinflint next to Mayor Ed Koch. Madame DeFarge is surely outdone in evil banality by Margaret Heckler, and all the sluts in Oliver Twist's London pale by comparison with San Francisco's Sisters of Perpetual Indulgence – Sister Boom-Boom, Sister Missionary Position, Sister Vicious Power Hungry Bitch, and that sinister neo-Victorian, Sister Florence Nightmare.

Viler than all these political villains and unholy sisters, however, is Shilts's nightmarish personification of motiveless malignity – Patient Zero. If HIV had a human face, a pretty face, it would look like Patient Zero's. There is no character in Dickens even remotely like him. He is a truly original creation of Shilts's homophobic imagination, a Bad Fairy out of Walt Disney, the sort of *National Enquirer* alien that inquiring minds don't want to know.

What's more, he's a Canadian alien: his weird extraterrestrial name was Gaetan Dugas, we learn, and he hailed from the remote snow-bound planet of Quebec via Air Canada. I still shudder – whether with voyeuristic pleasure or zero-at-the-bone fright I can't tell – whenever I recall the lurid bathhouse scene where Patient Zero exchanges bodily fluids with a Castro Street clone and then cackles vampirically as he reveals his fulminant lesions: 'I've got gay cancer ... I'm going to die and so are you.'[4] That scene is enough to set anyone straight about gay sex.

While gays get AIDS exclusively from sex in *And the Band Played On*, straights get it from blood – bad gay blood – transfused into their innocent veins by doctors who have all graduated from the Foucault School of Medical Despotism. You would think that gays and straights die of AIDS in much the same way, however different their modes of infection, but in Shilts's fictive world the death scenes of gays contrast sharply with those of straights in narrative tone and allegorical significance.

Consider for instance the death scene of gay psychotherapist Gary Walsh, a good Catholic boy from Iowa who had chucked 'guilt' from his vocabulary when he came out in San Francisco. Only a few years ago, in August 1981, Gary had been flashing his 'wicked smile' through the cruising crowds in the Castro, which Shilts, with theological éclat, describes as 'the biggest sexual candy store God ever invented.'[5] God presumably also invented HIV to teach Gary a lesson about sin and death: a bitter pill to swallow even with a candy coating. When death comes to him, in February 1984, he has been translated by AIDS into a saint of postsexuality, a pure essence devoid of body, a transcendent psyche glowing in the ruins of the former libertine. This metamorphosis was evident to his friends, reports Shilts with a knowledge of divinity rare among journalists: '[Gary's old friend] Lu Chaikin had always loved Gary, even when he was willful, self-centred, and sometimes defensive, because she saw the essence of Gary Walsh, and she saw that it was good.' Lu evidently has what medieval Catholics called 'discretio spirituum,' the ability to perceive spiritual essences. Recollections of Genesis colour her medieval perception of Gary's spirit: 'This essence explained why Gary had devoted his career to helping others accept and integrate themselves ... In the year since his AIDS diagnosis, Lu had watched adversity transform her friend. The pretensions of personality had dropped away, layer by layer, until that altruistic essence was all that remained.'[6] This makes AIDS sound like the latest California dietary therapy: yes, folks, watch those unsightly layers of personality melt away as you slim down to your altruistic essence!

'Gary had forgotten the hurts of his Catholic childhood and the abuses he had suffered as a gay man,' Shilts reports, as if these were mental fringe benefits of the AIDS diet plan: 'He now offered his friends unconditional love. People came away from conversations with Gary like pilgrims leaving a holy shrine.' They were evidently witnessing the birth of the latest California cult: 'Lu wasn't sure whether Gary knew the effect he was having on others. She wasn't sure whether he understood that, finally, he had become totally himself and that he was very beautiful.' A California apotheosis, if ever there was one!

'After all the friends and relatives had left, Lu went back into Gary's room and tried to express again what she had tried to tell Gary before. Gary smiled his mischievous grin and interrupted her. "I got it, I finally got it," he said.' What he got along with AIDS, evidently, was Acquired Immanent Divinity Syndrome:

> 'I *am* love and light,' [he declared], 'and I transform people by just being who I am.'
>
> Gary recited the words carefully, like a schoolchild who had struggled hard to master a difficult lesson. Lu broke down and started weeping.[7]

Who wouldn't lapse from steely Scepticism at the sight of such transfigured beauty, the ultimate fulfilment of the California dream of being a 'together person'?

The miraculous rejuvenation of Gary, his return to the love and light of childhood, is a triumph of late Romantic crypto-Christian allegorizing. The 'difficult lesson' Gary had mastered was the Pelagian insight that sex in the Fallen World was thoroughly evil, and that AIDS alone, the most ascetic of therapies, could redeem his depraved spirit from the darkness of carnality. With an unapologetic burst of Dickensian sentimentality, Shilts has effectively rewritten the death of Little Nell as the death of Little Nellie.

Counterpointed with the exquisite suffering of Gary Walsh is the excruciating agony of Frances Borchelt, a feisty yet family-loving San Francisco matron whom Shilts presents as the paradigmatic straight victimized by the Plague. Frances, married for forty-one years to feisty yet family-loving Bob Borchelt, contracted AIDS in August 1983 through a blood transfusion administered to her without her knowledge during minor hip surgery – surgery she underwent, of course, for purely family reasons. Her son was getting married that October and she wanted to be strong enough to dance at his wedding reception.

This social detail would hardly be worth noting (even as journalistic human interest) if it did not highlight Shilts's allegorical agenda, which is to expose through symbolic types and actions the Plague's pernicious attack on bourgeois family values and to reveal the gay community's viral subversion of mainstream American social order. There is a time to mourn and a time to dance, we're told in the Bible, but in Shilts we're taught that all dancing stops for straights with the coming of HIV. Gays of course dance like crazy all through the Plague, and all through the novel, but never on nice family occasions. They writhe and bop to the death-rattley beat of disco on the dance floor of Desire. As the inexorable band plays on, Patient Zero leads the denizens of the Castro in a frenzied marathon of dirty dancing.

Dancers from *that* dance are not clean until they experience a ritual purification of carnality through AIDS. Even then they do not come close to the godly cleanliness of Mrs Borchelt, whom Shilts portrays as a 'clean freak' before and even after her operation: 'She was always cleaning. Every morning she'd dust. It seemed she washed her hands twenty times a day.' Frances' feisty yet family-loving daughter Cathy 'joked that they'd bury her with a can of Mop 'n Glow.'[8]

I wonder whether they did: it would have been the perfect symbol of her neo-Pelagian consumerist ethos. Cathy's little joke takes on enormous significance in the context of Shilts's allegory of the Too Too Sullied Flesh. Dear Old Mom, in her uninfected state, has to be imagined as 'pure' for social, economic, and moral reasons; socially, because she is the nucleus of the straight nuclear family threatened by the gay virus; economically, because the multi-billion-dollar cleanser industry that has mopped and glowed its way into her TV consciousness would soon fold if Frances and her ilk died in droves; and morally, because the Plague would not seem so dirty and diabolical to Shilts's (mostly) straight Middle American Book-of-the-Month Club readers if it only attacked Sister Vicious Power Hungry Bitch and the already unclean, already demonically possessed gay community.

'When pressed,' as Shilts coyly puts it, 'Frances admitted she was just one of those people who didn't like the idea of germs.'[9] Shilts, I suspect, is one of those people too – not just because germs bring nasty diseases for which Johnson & Johnson supplies no convenient household remedy, but because the *idea* of germs carries with it the idea of a contaminated and contaminating gayness that regressive moralists like Shilts (who may hate himself for belonging to the germ family) simply cannot resist.

While Gary Walsh turns into pure spirit on his deathbed, Mother Frances turns into pure body. She becomes a spiritless lump of putrescent corporeality, a 'messa damnata,' next to whose agonies the Sacred Sorrows of Gary seem like minor female trouble. We are spared none of the horrifying physical details in the Borchelt case as we are in the many others Shilts reports – partly because Frances had no mental life to speak of during her long career as Mrs Clean, but mainly because it was our author's latent misogynist plan to transform her ravaged body into a *tableau mourant,* a *nature morte,* representing Sister Florence's worst nightmares about the corruptibility of the Flesh, the dreaded Female Flesh.

Hepatitis, night sweats, thrush, pneumocystis pneumonia, bronchial pneumonia, lymphadenopathy, mastitis, idiopathic thrombocytopenic purpura – Frances gets everything on the CDC checklist of AIDS-related illnesses with the exception of Kaposi's sarcoma, the lesion of honour, the gay stigmata. The straight counterpart of this cancerous skin condition is the non-cancerous rash celebrated for decades in American patent medicine ads as 'the heartbreak of psoriasis.' Needless to say, when Frances gets psoriasis, she gets a spectacularly heartbreaking case: itchy red patches cover her body from top to toe, transforming her into a prurient spectacle of social degradation. Cathy begins to suspect that Mom might be slipping into something 'very removed from her life'[10] – namely the underworld of gay guignol horrors. If getting AIDS gay means turning into Light and Love, getting AIDS straight must mean the reverse: a loathsome metamorphosis into darkness and dreck.

'I feel like a leper!' Frances feistily exclaims, echoing recurrent TV commentary on the social alienation of the infected.[11] In a medieval allegory of salvation her biblical simile would have transfigured her into a type of Christ or a vessel for grace or figure of 'humilitas,' that paradoxical Christian virtue through which the human spirit proudly rises from the dark 'humus' or dust of mortality towards the Light. In a postmodern allegory of cultural dissolution we might expect the leper simile to imply the alienation of the panic-stricken Self from the hyper-real world of media imagery. But the allegory we discover as the band plays on is neither medieval nor postmodern, neither Christian nor Krokerite. Its reference is to the neo-Victorian familialism and materialism of conservative American life in the 1980s. Shilts invites us to view Frances' 'leprosy' as a shocking affront to the dignity of the consuming materfamilias whose antiseptic body is identified in an endless stream of commercials with the fortifying ingredients, extra-strength formulas, and charismatic cleansing powers of the products she ingests, sprays on, pours out, mops up. Her body functions as a screen on which we view a mini-series on the AIDS crisis as a crisis of faith in the heroic hygienics of American capitalism.

Shilts cannot leave her body alone. He must expose it to us again and again, its repulsiveness increasing each time we view it. We are finally forced to imagine it naked, to see it through Cathy's aesthetically appalled eyes, as the figure-conscious daughter helps her mother into the shower after yet another attack of psoriasis. 'She was staggered at her mother's appearance,' reports Shilts from inside Cathy's narrow soul: 'Frances had shrunk to ninety-eight pounds. Her tailbone protruded from her baggy skin.'[12]

The Naked Truth is thus revealed to us in a surprising 'epopteia' in the mystery temple of cleanliness, the hospital shower stall. Frances, once a tough old bird, now the proverbial ninety-eight-pound weakling, has become a baggy-skinned embarrassment to her own family because she has failed to keep up 'appearances' – especially the appearance of wifely invincibility, that clean look of cosmetic perfection, maintained by all the fantasy women in American soap operas and cleanser commercials. *Their* world is insulated from the ravages of time and HIV. Hers, surprise, is not.

Since Cathy is fictively mind-linked with Shilts, she is momentarily able to see the Age of AIDS through the Holocaustic gaze of Shilts's culture-hero, Larry Kramer. Gazing at the Maternal Body with the sort of primal horror formerly reserved for young Fred Nemishes in the throes of expensive Oedipal angst, Cathy thinks her mother looks 'like the pictures of concentration camp victims she had seen in World War II books.'[13] The Maternal Body is thus textualized and read as if it were a Time-Life coffee-table book on Nazi atrocities at Dachau and Auschwitz: it is (like Shilts's own book) both a ghastly sign of the dark side of human nature and a glossy product of contemporary bourgeois culture. Frances is victimized by the Holocaust metaphor so that even her feisty personality is purged away in the end. Just as the Jews in Dachau became the numbers branded on their arms, so she will become a mere CDC statistic in the *Morbidity and Mortality Weekly Report*.

Though Shilts tries hard to present a coldly clinical picture of Mrs Borchelt's bodily decline, a wrenching sentimentality too deep for laughs overcomes him (even him, the objective reporter, the stern social critic!) at the pathetic denouement of her tale. The final atrocity committed against her in the concentration camp of the Body is not blindness – as it is for instance in *Borrowed Time*, Paul Monette's novelization of Rog Horwitz's long AIDS journey into night.[14] Nor is the last straw the onset of AIDS dementia, though Frances, having lost both her mind and her sight, is reported to have conducted pitiful conversations with an imaginary friend before she was thankfully put on a respirator. Her frantic mutterings are the straight world's counterpoint to the pretentiously serene Platonic dialogues Paul Monette reads to poor bored Rog during their final months together.

'Why am I sick?' cries Frances through her pulmonary mucus, right on cue, as if the aged Donna Reed were cast as Job addressing God *de profundis*. But no answer comes back to her from the whirlwind – not even Robert Gallo's insane answer that green monkeys are to blame for the whole mess. God has evidently abandoned her in the end. She's just a body after all: no soul worth saving.

These reconstructed facts are sad enough, as AIDS fictions go, but there's sadder still. The final indignity Frances must suffer is an act of desecration so profoundly symbolic within the familialist context of the allegory that it makes even her imaginary burial with a can of Mop 'n Glow seem trite by comparison. 'Frances,' reports Shilts, 'had been adamant that she did not want to be buried with her wedding rings. As her body began to fill with fluids and bloat, Cathy decided it was time to remove them. However, her mother's fingers were already so swollen, the hospital had to call custodians to cut the plain bands of white gold from her fingers. After that, Frances's muttering stopped.'[15] What more can she possibly say? Her voice must be hushed when she loses her wedding bands, the golden tokens of her wifely essence in the Great Chain of Patriarchal Being. Without them she ceases to exist as herself: she literally passes out of the novel at this point – a bloated travesty of her former self. Gays, of course, go out ethereally slim.

The cutting of her wedding bands can be viewed as a grotesque parody of elective surgery, a nightmare operation performed by hospital janitors terrified (no doubt) by the bodily fluids that might spurt out of the patient during their hack-job. But this is not how Shilts presents the scene. The cutting of the rings sentimentally symbolizes the ultimate threat AIDS poses to America in his fiction: the dissolution of monogamous heterosexual union, the social bond that was supposed to be America's ring of protection against the Alien Virus.

Inherent in the intractable heterosexist discourse of the Novel of Social Criticism is a tendency to construct and moralize an etiology of human suffering. Money, or power, or sex, or slavery, or industry, or the Strange Virus of Unknown Origin becomes the root of all evil, and we are summoned back to the poison tree to taste the bitter fruit of matrimonial experience in the fallen world. Marriages have a short half-life in the Novel of Social Criticism, even though its 'realistic' or 'journalistic' form ironically promotes the nostalgic fantasy that we should *all* end up like a Dickensian heroine marrying into a good healthy family, preferably of old stock, with lots and lots of money.

In view of its familialist stratagems I cannot think that the Novel of Social Criticism will do any of us (except Shilts) much good in the Age of AIDS. I suspect that Shilts is making lots and lots of money out of his *succès de scandale* by feeding his straight and some of his gay readers exactly what they want: large dollops of guilt. I also fear that novelists who follow his successful lead will actually do more harm than good in moralizing about the causes of the various epidemics consuming us today – fundamentalist vengeance, heterosexist hysteria, liberal hypocrisy, media confusion, Nazi-bunker hedonism, not to mention HIV infection – simply because their retrospective causal speculations distract us from the crucial issue of how to end the Plague.

At best the Novel of Social Criticism alerts the straight white middle-class 'general public' to what they already half suspect and subliminally fear about the evils lurking in 'their' society. At worst such fiction serves to reinforce prevailing Victorian pieties about family life and family values by subjecting readers to allegorical shock treatments – sudden jolts of high-intensity socio-religious symbolism – that effectively paralyse the critical faculties of the brain, black out all sane distinctions between reality and its perceptual constructs or fictive re-creations, and induce insanely clear instant-replay visions of the old Manichaean battle between the Clean and the Corrupted, the Fit and the Fallen.

Shilts is easy enough to trash, though chucking his large tome into the garbage may be painful for those who've sacrificed forty bucks for the hard-cover edition. Before he writes the inevitable sequel to *And the Band Played On* – which will have to be called *The Boys in the Band Strike Back* – I think we should seriously ask ourselves whether novels have any constructive role to play in ending the AIDS crisis or at least in undoing the damage done in the Age of Shilts. Is there, I wonder, a good replacement for AIDS fiction in the gloomy Shiltsian vein? Or are we doomed to endless soon-to-be-TV-movie variations on the neo-Dickensian themes approved for 'general audiences' by the censors of bourgeois tastes and morals?

Gloom and Doom are in such abundant supply these days that it's probably hubristic of me to propose, in an optimistic mood, the invention of a new kind of AIDS fiction. Creative writers will just have to bear with me in my speculations about its anti-Shiltsian form and Watneyesque stratagems. I'm really a destructive writer, I confess, and that's why such a proposal (coming from me) is likely to sound absurd. I suppose it also sounds absurd to profess an interest in prophetic literary criticism, a hitherto uncharted realm of the discipline. But since literary critics have recently muscled in on the creative process, I'm going to assume creative powers and have a go at imagining what the novel might do to defy the Gloom and Doom.

Since the act of naming is often the first step in bringing the named into being, I shall start by proposing a name for this new kind of AIDS fiction. I christen it the 'Novel of Cultural Activism.'

In the Winter 1987 issue of *October*, Crimp distinguished the usual roles played by art in the AIDS crisis from what he called 'an engaged, activist aesthetic practice.' These usual roles – art as advertisement, art as memorial, art as commodity – have become usual largely because they are constantly sanctioned by mainstream-media coverage of the 'cultural side' of the epidemic, a side usually presented as quite separate from the 'medical or scientific side' (which of course it is not). The supposed separateness of the cultural side has led to its being widely perceived as a relatively powerless namby-pamby adjunct to the macho high-tech enterprise of Robert Gallo, whose big-game hunt for the microscopic source of all our woe has led him over the snows of Kilimanjaro to the lairs of the Green Monkey.

In theory, an engaged, activist aesthetic practice such as Crimp advocates extends the heroic energy of the medico-scientific enterprise, which stages its fund-raising triumphs in the ultra-straight Man's World of 'public life,' into the languishing art world, which stages its Liz Taylored fund-raising galas in the lavender limelight of private anguish. In theory, their extension of activist power will have several amazing results. First, artists will cease to be passive wimps on the sidelines or in the cemeteries of the epidemic: they will 'act up' outside the conventional boundaries of the fantasy world of retrograde bourgeois art, invading spaces in the real world of hospitals, shopping centres, city halls, public washrooms, and other haunts of the unsuspecting general public. Second, general-public types who normally wouldn't set foot in a gallery for fear of catching 'gay plague' from doorknobs, toilet seats, and other pieces of found art, will be exposed to the harsh politics of the crisis through artistic mediations on their home ground. And most amazing of all, art, predicts Crimp, will actually start to fight AIDS and even to 'save lives' – an agenda currently defined and monopolized by medical science.[16]

While Crimp locates the rare products of cultural-activist aesthetic practice mainly in the domain of the visual arts – for instance, in New York's New Museum of Contemporary Art where members of ACT UP displayed their shocking 'Let the Record Show ...' installation with its celebrated neon 'Silence = Death' sign – I can see no reason, at a theoretical level, why cultural activism should not be extended into the much wider public domain of the verbal arts. Indeed, if Silence truly equals Death in the AIDS crisis, then might not the obverse be true? Words, lots of words, the fighting words of a Novel of Cultural Activism, might equal Life if the readers of such a work were collectively engaged with the novelist in attacking prejudicial allegories of the epidemic, addressing the social and spiritual needs of PWAs, altering rigid ideological attitudes towards sex, death, and the body, and acting up against governmental indifference to specific life-and-death issues like the restrictive testing of pentamidine.

None of the AIDS novels I have read (they're all American) would qualify as a model for the Novel of Cultural Activism, and I know of none yet published, in any country or language, that could be hailed as the verbal counterpart of the 'Silence = Death' installation in New York City. Predictably, most AIDS fiction functions like the usual kinds of AIDS art – as instruction, memorial, or commodity.

Instructional novels like Paul Reed's *Facing It* (1984) turn PWAs into talking symptoms of physical and social decline: 'Hi, my name is Andy: I'm Reed's cute case-book victim of AIDS. See my lesions, feel my swollen glands, chart my weight loss, watch my gay lifestyle deteriorate.' The psychological horrors of coming out, in Andy's case, are replayed as the physical horrors of breaking out. When KS starts its malignant spread over his body, it acts as an outward and visible sign of the emotional lesions fulminating in his soul, bringing to the surface, as it were, the cancerous outrage and resentment he feels towards his cruelly homophobic father.[17] Strung out along Reed's thin story-line of father-son conflict (perhaps the *only* story-line in gay fiction to date) are heavy excerpts from the *Morbidity and Mortality Weekly Report*, which, with its stern commentary on 'promiscuity,' provides an ironic patriarchal gloss on the gay myth of the Prodigal Son who's never welcomed home. The plotting of instructional novels is invariably soap-operatic: the Hung and the Restless wind up in General Hospital where stubborn parents reject their dying children, and clever doctor's wives outsmart wicked closet cases in the research-grant game.

Closet cases are replaced by basket cases in memorial AIDS fiction, which is designed to lament the obvious fact that life's a bitch – a vicious power-hungry bitch – for good gays and bad gays alike who are caught in the immunosuppressive Dance of Death. AIDS memoirs like Paul Monette's *Borrowed Time* (1988) and memorializing novels like Christopher Davis' *Valley of the Shadow* (1988) have basically the same inverted *Bildungsroman* plot: the great expectations of a sensitive artistic youth in the fifties, who becomes a liberated stud in the sixties, who settles down as a successful gay professional in the seventies, are suddenly dashed when he becomes an AIDS 'victim' in the eighties.[18] While Davis simply turns his victim into an obit on the last page of his novel, Monette can't let poor Rog rest in peace until he has tearily translated his beloved friend into an immortal Greek hero on an ancient monument: a preposterous metamorphosis considering Rog's blandly yuppie identity as an LA lawyer who liked Haagen Dazs and old Joan Collins movies.

The absolute nadir of AIDS fiction as pure fund-raising commodity was reached by a fantasy novelette entitled *The Swan Prince*, which hit the New York bookstores in the fall of 1987. Conceived by Mikhail Baryshnikov, it parodies in fashion-mag style the tragic romance plot of *Swan Lake*. 'The book,' coos *Life* magazine, 'stars Mikhail's body luscious, a bevy of would-be seductresses and enough feathers to smother the Bolshoi's corps de ballet. This Prince Siegfried disdains dames and swoons over swans, but profit, not art, was the motive – the proceeds will go to the American Foundation for AIDS Research.'[19] As if that justified its flip travesty of Eros and Thanatos in the Age of AIDS!

For $16.95 you get not only the story of Siegfried's cygno-erotic perversions but also several glamour pix of Mikhail's body – including one that shows the Swan Prince decadently martyred in the style of St Sebastian with swan quills instead of arrows. A sacrilegious gay idol since Sodoma painted him in the Renaissance, Sebastian has recently regained something of his traditional religious status as the patron saint of plague victims: it takes no great leap of faith to see a resemblance between the tormented body of the young male martyr (the Christian West's original embodiment of Imminent Divinity Syndrome) and the tormented body of a young male PWA. Shilts, for instance, made this hagiographic leap in the tale of Gary Walsh.

But what is Baryshnikov doing here? Obviously cock-teasing for charity: as the studied saint or sainted stud of American Ballet Theatre, he's the unattainable straight sex symbol for gay balletomanes to drool over with a clear conscience as they prepare for their next AIDS benefit or memorial service. Drooling over the romantic prince stripped of his dance belt and leotards is a safe-sex practice, after all. So too is laughing at the possibility that straights might just get 'it' as bad as gays and suffer as much, and that's just what Mikhail himself is doing in this pernicious send-up of the crisis. As a super-straight who has playfully placed himself in the symbolic position of a gay victim of the epidemic, he is shamelessly mocking the real agonies of PWAs who are forced to play out the insufferably passive martyr role demanded of them by prevailing fictions of victimization.

Our hypothetical Novel of Cultural Activism should counteract these fictions by representing PWAs as actively engaged, along with their lovers and friends and families, in the struggle to end the epidemic. It should have as its central figure a cultural activist whose agenda (whatever that might be) will provide the main impetus for the plot by opposing the agendas of fatalistic governments and fundamentalist bigots. It should also amplify the voices of PWAs so that they can be heard above the din of safe-sex pedagogues, weeping elegists, and glamorous fund-raisers.

Several AIDS novels already do this on a small scale. In Armistead Maupin's *Babycakes*, for instance, gay hero Michael Tolliver refuses to succumb to viral melancholia and erotophobic passivity after his lover Jon dies of AIDS and leaves him HIV-positive: he deals with his grief by working as a volunteer at the Castro Street AIDS hot line, by introducing his straight friend Brian to the wonders of safer sex, and, most provocatively, by looking for a new lover.[20]

Novelist Robert Ferro, who died of AIDS in 1988, wrote his last work

Second Son from the viewpoint of a PWA who releases himself from his own and his family's paralysing fear of death through a passionate eleventh-hour love affair with another PWA.[21] Significantly, neither Michael Tolliver, nor Ferro's alter ego, Mark Valerian, dies like a martyr at the end of the story. In fact, they don't die at all. They're still kicking when their stories close, as if the mere potential for a sequel in an AIDS novel were a *grand défi* to the disease.

If the Novel of Cultural Activism is to have any politically engaging impact on the general public, it must show that straights are not insulated from the disease by sexual practice or cultural privilege. It must represent straight PWAs coping with the epidemic, and working towards its end, alongside gays, so that channels of empathy may be established between the larger and smaller community of readers. Armistead Maupin tried to open up such channels in *Significant Others* by having his straight hero Brian suffer the early symptoms of AIDS (night sweats, fevers, fatigue) for two hundred suspenseful pages before his test turns out negative.[22]

Sharon Mayes in her 1987 novel *Immune* went a step further than Maupin by returning a positive test result to her femme fatale heroine, Dr Suzanne Keller, whose career as an AIDS researcher in San Francisco burns out when she encounters the new bogeyman of AIDS fictions: Ivan the Bisexual. Like everyone else in San Francisco, Ivan's a psychotherapist with a new diet plan (his answer to Suzanne's woes: a shot of smack before, during, and after meals). Before falling into Ivan's chilling clutches, Suzanne was *almost* happy in the warm embrace of Dr Chris Alterberg, an engorged and tingling virologist with whom she had throbbing sex all up and down the coast of California and Mexico.

In a flashback to this affair Mayes portrays Suzanne as a Vicious Power Hungry Bitch in Venus drag rising from the tempest-tossed waves of women's erotica. Suzanne doesn't just go to the beach. She has symbolic intercourse with the Ocean, communing with the luminous forces of heterosexual Nature against the dark backdrop of the Gay Plague. 'She jumped up and down like an enraptured little girl,' gushes Mayes, 'then picked up a long rubbery piece of seaweed. Three inches across and twelve feet long with a bulbous head on one end, it looked like a gigantic penis from the sea.' Once again sexism rears its unprotected head! But does this deter our heroine? Of course not. No dong from Erica Jong can compare with the gigantic penis from the sea: 'She wrapped it around her legs, then her waist until the round head sat on her shoulder caressing her neck. She walked back to [her lover Chris] and kissed the head of the seaweed that wound around her. "You are a princess of the sea, [he said,] ... a timeless creature." He tugged at the seaweed, unwrapping her ceremoniously, slowly. His body ached to bc inside her. His penis stood out larger than he'd ever remembered it, the colour more purple, the tip more swollen and glistening.'[23] What Chris evidently needs is a gigantic condom from the sea, but none washes up on shore. Meanwhile, Suzanne's crimson nipples 'beckoned to him ... pursed into succulent, sun-dried tomatoes.' A true California gourmet touch.

I recommend *Immune* for a good laugh, but as a serious attempt to foreground the Plague in heterosexual erotic consciousness it fails in the end because its heroine fails to overcome her hostility towards her gay patients. 'This AIDS situation is getting heavy,' she writes in her diary. 'Sometimes I want to strangle the patients. I'm so enraged this is happening. It's giving sex a very bad name.'[24] When she learns about her own seropositive status and realizes that she's been spreading the virus to half the straight population of northern California, she promptly takes her sun-dried nipples back to Father Neptune and drowns herself in San Francisco Bay. Her suicide is an ironic confirmation – since it was provoked by a reluctance to tell her lovers about her infection – that silence does indeed equal death.

NOTES

1 Only when 'heterosexual behavior' has to change in response to AIDS do we enter a new 'Age,' as William H. Masters, Virginia E. Johnson, and Robert C. Kolodny suggest in *Crisis: Heterosexual Behavior in the Age of AIDS* (New York: Grove Press 1988). For Masters, Johnson, and Kolodny, apparently, AIDS only became a 'crisis' (ie a historical calamity requiring political intervention) when it began to affect heterosexuals. It was just this attitude that led to the Reagan administration's scandalous indifference to the AIDS crisis from 1981 until the death of 'straight' role model Rock Hudson in 1985, argues Randy Shilts in *And the Band Played On: Politics, People, and the AIDS Epidemic* (New York: St Martin's Press 1987).

2 Shilts 'Notes on Sources' in *And the Band Played On* 607

3 Douglas Crimp 'How to Have Promiscuity in an Epidemic' in *October* 43, ed Douglas Crimp (Winter 1987) 238–46. I am indebted to Crimp for pointing out the 'conventional novelistic fashion' in which Shilts's chronicle was written to please straight middle-class readers (pp 244–5).

4 Shilts 'Too Much Blood' *And the Band Played On* 165. Shilts unapol-

ogetically admits that 'rumors' were his source for this sensational story. So much for objective reportage.

5 Shilts 'Ambush Poppers' *And the Band Played On* 89
6 Shilts 'The Feast of the Hearts, Part II' *And the Band Played On* 424–5
7 Ibid 425. For further discussion of this passage in the light of martyrological discourse, see James Miller 'Acquired Immanent Divinity Syndrome' in *Perspectives on AIDS: Ethical and Social Issues* ed Christine Overall and William P. Zion (Toronto: Oxford University Press 1991) 55–74
8 Shilts 'Politics' *And the Band Played On* 364–5
9 Ibid 365
10 Shilts 'Prisoners' *And the Band Played On* 411
11 Shilts 'Exiles' *And the Band Played On* 520
12 Ibid 520–1
13 Ibid 521. Fred Nemish is the gay anti-hero in Larry Kramer's novel *Faggots* (New York: Random House 1978).
14 On Rog's herpetic blindness and Platonic consolations, see Paul Monette *Borrowed Time: An AIDS Memoir* (San Diego, New York, London: Harcourt Brace Jovanovich 1988) 249–51, 317.
15 Shilts 'Acceptance' *And the Band Played On* 567
16 Crimp 'AIDS: Cultural Analysis / Cultural Activism' 7
17 Paul Reed *Facing It: A Novel of A.I.D.S.* (San Francisco: Gay Sunshine Press 1984) 173–4
18 Christopher Davis *Valley of the Shadow* (New York: St Martin's Press 1988). As the title of his novel indicates, Davis sets his fictional memoir within the redemptive context of traditional Christian eschatology. Eschewing the anti-gay discourse of Christian redemption, Monette, by contrast, turns to the late nineteenth-century rhetoric of Golden Age classicism to translate his memories of Rog into Greek tragedy: eg 'Perhaps the world is always full of portents, as the oracle maintained it was, in every flight of birds that passes. The only thing we could do to hold the fates at bay was to keep our own world full to the brim, or that at least is how I read the magic of that summer's end' (*Borrowed Time* 24).
19 For the photograph of Baryshnikov as Sebastian, see 'For the Birds' *Life* (October 1987) 89. The photograph was taken for *The Swan Prince: A Fairy Tale*, text by Peter Anastos, photography by Arthur Elgort (Bantam).
20 Armistead Maupin *Babycakes* (New York: Harper & Row 1984)
21 Robert Ferro *Second Son* (New York: Crown 1988)
22 Maupin *Significant Others* (New York: Harper & Row 1987)
23 Sharon Mayes *Immune* (St Paul: New Rivers Press 1987) 53
24 Ibid 169

Cell Wars: Military Metaphors and the Crisis of Authority in the AIDS Epidemic

BRIAN PATTON

In *Illness as Metaphor*, Susan Sontag argues against the widespread tendency to invest disease with metaphorical significance. 'Nothing,' she contends, 'is more punitive than to give a disease a meaning – that meaning being invariably a moralistic one.'[1] Her objection to the use of illness as metaphor is that it is 'punitive'; modern disease metaphors, she says, are 'cheap shots'[2] that stigmatize and demoralize those who must live with actual diseases. Speaking on behalf of the diseased as a victimized group, Sontag sets out to right a wrong by urging us to detach the reality of illness from the myths and 'false' representations surrounding it.

The central point of her argument is that 'illness is *not* a metaphor, and that the most truthful way of regarding illness – and the healthiest way of being ill – is one most purified of, most resistant to, metaphoric thinking.'[3] While Sontag is certainly correct in her assertion that the process of investing a disease with moral significance is potentially damaging to those who have the disease, and her desire to draw attention to this problem and to rectify it is undoubtedly admirable, the remedy that she offers is, unfortunately, highly problematic. Where are we to look for this 'most truthful way of regarding illness' that she proposes? Without relying upon metaphors, how can we think about illness at all?

The modern disease that provides a focus for Sontag's essay is cancer, with tuberculosis serving as a historical reference point. Recently, however, she has focused her attention on the AIDS epidemic.

This new syndrome, she says in *AIDS and Its Metaphors*, 'has helped to divest cancer of its aura of shame, of the unspeakable.' Although the nature of the disease and hence the nature of the metaphors differ, the problem and the proposed solution are similar: 'With this illness, one that elicits so much guilt and shame, the effort to detach it from loaded meanings and misleading metaphors seems particularly liberating, even consoling.'[4] With regard to the important role of metaphor in the language of disease, however, *AIDS and Its Metaphors* takes a much more pragmatic view than its predecessor. The book begins with an acknowledgment of the inevitability of metaphor: 'Of course, one cannot think without metaphors. But that does not mean there aren't some metaphors we might well abstain from or try to retire.'[5] In *AIDS and Its Metaphors* Sontag challenges the particular metaphors she views as pernicious.

Sontag's change in strategy – from urging us to seek 'the most truthful way of regarding illness' in *Illness as Metaphor* to suggesting in *AIDS and Its Metaphors* that we retire the more destructive metaphors – acknowledges that a truthful way of regarding illness is not available to us. While popular belief would perhaps suggest that ultimately we have recourse to 'the facts' (scientific data, research findings, information untainted by subjective interpretation), the AIDS epidemic has shown us time and again that such a belief is naïve: science is ultimately as value-laden as any other discipline and its 'facts' are no closer to Absolute Truth than are the most metaphorical (and hence moralistic) visions of sickness and health. Indeed, the epidemic has brought into question the validity of a binary opposition between truthful and untruthful representations of disease.

In his introduction to *AIDS: Cultural Analysis / Cultural Activism*, Douglas Crimp announces that he takes as a starting point François Delaporte's assertion that '"disease" does not exist,' and that one cannot therefore '"develop beliefs" about it or "respond" to it.' We can only know AIDS, he insists, as a construct: 'AIDS does not exist apart from the practices that conceptualize it, represent it, and respond to it. We know AIDS only in and through those practices. This assertion does not contest the existence of viruses, antibodies, infections, or transmission routes. Least of all does it contest the reality of illness, suffering, and death. What it *does* contest is the notion that there is an underlying reality of AIDS upon which are constructed the representations, or the culture, or the politics of AIDS.'[6] Crimp's contention that there is no essential, graspable 'AIDS' underlying all the *mis*representations clearly represents a challenge to Sontag's earlier line of argument.

To the extent that we can know it at all, he suggests, illness *is* metaphor.

The findings of Paula Treichler underscore the fact that the attempt to detach illness from its misrepresentations is bound to be more difficult than one would perhaps wish. A reliance upon scientific facts as a means of escaping from the process of representation would require us to have faith in science as the totally rational provider of solid, testable representations of the world. Yet Treichler's examination of the multiplicity of meanings that have been generated around AIDS leads her to conclude that there are in fact *two* epidemics, the second being 'an epidemic of meanings or signification'[7] – an epidemic that rages even within that fortress of 'facts,' the ivory tower of empirical science.

Treichler's analysis reveals the seductive manner in which biomedical discourse works to conceal from the uninitiated 'general public' the myths and biases inherent in the scientist's representations. 'Scientific and medical discourses,' she notes, 'have traditions through which the semantic epidemic as well as the biological one is controlled, and these may disguise contradiction and irrationality.'[8] Thus, by invoking our faith in the essential truth of the facts discovered by means of scientific inquiry, the scientist is able to present himself as an authority whose findings and deductions lie outside the process of representation in some domain of verifiable truth. However, Treichler goes on to provide abundant instances in biomedical discourse of the 'semantic legerdemain about AIDS'[9] that permeates popular discourses. The myths propagated by science are perhaps less easily recognized as such, but they are none the less there. Authority, the power over or title to influence the opinions of others, does not derive solely from special knowledge. It also inheres in particular ways of constructing the world through language or, to borrow the Foucauldian phrase, in particular 'modes of discourse.'

The predominant image upon which numerous commentators have relied as a means of conceptualizing HIV and its effects on the immune system metaphorically is war. More specifically, AIDS has repeatedly been figured in terms of postmodern warfare: HIV is portrayed as the ultimate terrorist, the 'Abu Nidal of viruses,'[10] who wreaks havoc from within, reducing the once-perfect order of the immune system to utter chaos. The use of such a metaphor to provide some understanding of the virus and its effects merits some consideration. Clearly, some sort of model is necessary to our understanding of events that take place at a microscopic level, and the military metaphor that suggests a body under siege appears a 'natural' choice to this end. But of course it is not.

The seeming transparency of the military metaphor is in fact a product of its familiarity. Sontag notes that the military metaphor became widespread in medical discourse towards the end of the nineteenth century, when bacteria were identified as agents of disease. 'But talk of siege and war to describe disease,' she continues, 'now has, with cancer, a striking literalness and authority.'[11] Because the language of warfare appears to have a similar authority when applied to the AIDS epidemic, we can with little difficulty overlook other, hidden and potentially destructive messages that are embedded in that language and are implicit within the metaphor. But the figurative war may have some very real casualties who pass unnoticed. A closer examination of the military model suggests a great deal about the political nature of biomedical discourse and the role of scientific and medical institutions as agents of social control.

In June 1986, *National Geographic* ran a lengthy feature on the immune system entitled 'The Wars Within,' which, as the title would suggest, relied heavily upon the language of warfare as a means of conceptualizing the microscopic goings-on within the human immune system: 'Besieged by a vast array of invisible enemies, the human body enlists a remarkably complex corps of internal bodyguards to battle the invaders. They can cleanse the lungs of foreign particles, rid the bloodstream of infectious microorganisms, and weed tissue of renegade cancer cells.'[12] Clearly, there is more going on here than a transparent metaphoric rendering of biological fact. The body becomes a nation under siege, calling up its 'internal bodyguards' to combat 'foreign invaders' and 'renegades'; its goal is to restore its untainted purity, to 'cleanse' itself of the 'foreign' particles. This model of the immune system is simultaneously a political allegory of national purity.

The political nature of this allegory is extended and further clarified in the accompanying diagram (plate 58, following p 239), whose title – 'Cell Wars' – clearly echoes the popular name given to one of former U.S. president Ronald Reagan's pet projects, the Strategic Defense Initiative – namely, 'Star Wars.' The nature of the society under siege is spelled out in the accompanying explanatory gloss. 'A miracle of evolution,' we are told, 'the human immune system is not controlled by any central organ, such as the brain. Rather, it has developed to function as a kind of *biologic democracy*, wherein the individual members achieve their ends through an information network of awesome scope.'[13] Complete with its own military composed of Killer

T-cells, and an industry composed of B-cells ('Biologic arms factories'), the immune system becomes a microcosm of American society as perceived from the Right. The virus, the foreign invader who poses a threat to this miraculously evolved biologic democracy, is represented in the diagram as a red star, an appropriately duplicitous symbol. As a *star*, it complements the blue *stripes* of the helper and killer T-cells neatly aligned against a white background; as a *red* star it completes the red, white, and blue colour scheme of the diagram. It appears, in other words, to complete the pattern of the American flag. But the appearance is deceptive: the red star that appears to be an integral part of the whole is in fact the 'Red threat,' quietly subverting the whole system from within. 'Cancer,' says Sontag, 'is now in the service of a simplistic view of the world that can turn paranoid.'[14] AIDS, evidently, has been drawn into similar service. 'Cell Wars' registers a paranoia of the McCarthyesque kind.

In the context of the AIDS epidemic, where the vast majority of deaths (in Western countries) has thus far occurred among gay men and IV drug-users – groups that are widely perceived as threats to society, or at best as marginal members of society – the notions of purity, cleansing, and subversion implicit in this instance of the military metaphor are highly significant. By imagining the body as a society, we inevitably say something about the society that we envision. The creator of 'Cell Wars' depicts a democratic society purged of a subversive communist threat. But, of course, communists are not the only subversives waiting to crawl out from under the bed. Cindy Patton has noted that the rhetoric of certain extreme factions of the American New Right often elides homosexuality with communism under the rubric of subversion. 'Even today,' she says, 'some rightist groups claim that homosexuality and even AIDS is a communist plot.'[15] Medical and military terminologies, moreover, have been used interchangeably in describing such subversive elements: 'reds and queers were alternately diseases and invasions.'[16] As the body is threatened, so too is the body politic.

Bryan Turner contends that this conflation of social illness and natural disease is a by-product of a secularized society. 'Medicine,' he argues, 'has replaced religion as the social guardian of morality. This substitution involves a "medicalization"' – and, we might add, a concurrent militarization – 'of the body and society.'[17] According to Turner, modern medicine and law have appropriated and come to dominate 'the remaining moral debris of previous generations'[18] who equated disease with sin and read sickness as a physical manifestation of a corrupt soul. Christian asceticism is in modern times preached by the medical establishment under the new guise of preventive medicine; the family doctor becomes the modern-day confessor: 'Medicine provides, as it were, a second-order moral framework – a framework which is, however, masked by the language of disease.'[19] As the new guardian of morality, the medical establishment is invested with an extraordinary amount of power – power to distinguish the healthy from the sick, the sane from the demented, the normal from the abnormal. That the medical authorities are in possession of such power underscores the importance of close and critical analyses of their models and metaphors for the body and society.

To be fair, we should keep in mind that 'Cell Wars' is clearly produced for non-specialists, perhaps for that group called the 'general public' whose existence is repeatedly affirmed in the press. *National Geographic* is a popular magazine: the same issue containing the 'Cell Wars' piece features articles on the Snow Leopard, the Tea and Sugar train in the Australian Outback, Tolstoy's Russia, and the Pacific island of Bikini. But symptoms of the 'epidemic of signification' are also in evidence in the pages of the more specialist-oriented *Scientific American*, where supposedly better-informed individuals show clear signs of infection.

In an article entitled 'The AIDS Virus,' published in that magazine in January 1987, Robert Gallo, officially one of the 'co-discoverers' of HIV, makes an appeal to his readers' faith in the authority of the scientist. He begins with a dramatic rhetorical flourish: 'It is a modern plague,' he proclaims, 'the first great pandemic of the second half of the 20th century.'[20] However, the threat of the epidemic is confronted by our guardian – the rational and authoritative scientist. Gallo goes on to describe the behaviour of the virus that is the source of the 'plague' in the familiar terms of postmodern warfare. Gallo's virus is an anarchist armed with an armalite rifle: following a latency period of uncertain length, he says, 'the virus bursts into action, reproducing itself so furiously that the new virus particles escaping from the cell riddle the cellular membrane with holes and the lymphocyte dies.'[21]

We are assured, however, that there is another war being waged, a far nobler one: the ongoing struggle of science against an anarchic, civilization-threatening nature, the war between science and the 'plague.' What's more, the 'terrible tale' of this war has a moral. Oddly enough, the moral is aimed neither at the infected nor at those at risk of infection – the usual targets of moral plagues – but rather at the scientist who has tried, perhaps, to do too much. 'In the past two decades,' he says, 'one of the fondest boasts of medical science has been the conquest of infectious disease, at least in the wealthy countries of the industrialized world. The advent of retroviruses with the capacity to cause extraordinarily complex and devastating disease has exposed that claim for what it was: hubris. Nature is never truly conquered.'[22] Gallo re-writes the AIDS epidemic as Greek tragedy, casting the scientist – himself – as Prometheus, the well-intended but overzealous tragic hero whose noble aspirations for humanity bring about his own downfall. (A person with AIDS would perhaps find Gallo's vision of his own tragic heroism a curious one under the circumstances. One wonders if he is familiar with the sufferings of Philoctetes.) Sadder but wiser, though, Science continues in its quest to maintain control. The response of scientists to the epidemic, he implies, has been so impressive as to allow for a restoration of faith in the efficacy of scientific inquiry. 'In sharp contrast to the bleak epidemiological picture of AIDS,' he reassures us, 'the accumulation of knowledge about its cause has been remarkably quick.'[23] Adopting the familiar and reassuring role of the committed but disinterested scientist, Gallo taps into the persuasive power of the biomedical institution. But this renowned authority has provided much more than the 'facts': Gallo offers a highly self-interested account of the epidemic affirming the scientist's heroic role as social guardian.

Gallo is by no means unique in his inflated sense of his own importance to civilization. The belief that the scientist is the protector of the social order is also very much in evidence in a recent book by the well-known 'sexologists,' Masters and Johnson. Ostensibly a much-needed compendium of 'some hard-hitting facts about real but generally ignored risks of infection with this insidious virus,' their *Crisis: Heterosexual Behavior in the Age of AIDS* is a veritable text-book on institutional discourse and institutional power.[24] The basic premise underlying *Crisis* is outlined in its opening words: 'Hundreds of millions of words have been written about the global epidemic of AIDS – acquired immune deficiency syndrome. Regrettably, much of what has been written has simply been incorrect.'[25] Mounting their clinical pedestal, the authors inform us that their aim is to 'point to many instances of misinformation that the general public has been fed about AIDS' – 'misinformation' that has prevented the 'general public' from thus far reaching

> the alarming conclusion that we have reached, based on our own research and studies conducted by others: contrary to claims by

> various government agencies and public health experts that infection with the AIDS virus is still largely confined to the original 'high-risk' groups (gay and bisexual men and intravenous drug users), the epidemic has clearly broken out into the broader population and is continuing, even now, to make silent inroads of infection while many maintain an attitude of complacency, not realizing that they too are at risk.[26]

Masters and Johnson are conducting a clinic in biomedical rhetoric here. The world, as they describe it, is neatly divided into categories; their audience, the unknowing 'general public,' implies its complement – the knowledgeable scientific establishment to which Masters and Johnson belong, an establishment possessed of the facts and prepared to educate the masses, thus eradicating a dangerous ignorance. But what exactly do these experts have to teach us? Included among their arsenal of 'facts' is the possibility that AIDS can be communicated via a public toilet seat! The dissemination of 'facts' such as this prompted Jonathan Mann, former director of the Global Program on AIDS at the World Health Organization, to accuse the authors of *Crisis* of an irresponsible abuse of their popular prestige.[27]

The authors also establish another category that ought to be noted here – the 'high-risk' groups that are clearly distinguished from 'the broader population.' The far-too-familiar designation 'high-risk group' is as misleading with respect to the nature of the 'risk' as it is revealing regarding the attitudes of the authors towards those individuals who are thus categorized. As Jan Zita Grover has noted, 'the aging of the epidemic has made clear the indifference of HIV to categories such as *junkie* and *faggot*. It doesn't care whether it enters the body of a nurse or a prostitute, a Senator Paul Gann or a "Patient Zero."'[28] To employ a term like 'high-risk groups' implies that gay men and IV drug users are *inherently* prone to HIV infection; it ignores the fact that the real danger lies in high-risk practices – unprotected sex with an HIV-infected partner, or sharing a needle with an HIV-infected person. The medical establishment, however, persistently uses the essentially condemnatory term. Moreover, it repeatedly suggests that gays, almost always perceived as a group outside of 'the general population,' are at risk as a result of 'the gay lifestyle.'

In a recent interview in *Omni*, Luc Montagnier, another recognized authority, responded to the question 'Why in the United States did the virus first attack homosexual men?' in the following manner: 'The AIDS virus plays the role of a lion hunting down a troop of gazelles. It will bring down only the weakest among them. Likewise the virus will kill children and adults with immune systems less strong than others.' The immune system of homosexuals is already depressed.'[29] The voice of the other official co-discoverer of HIV tells us that AIDS spread first among gay men because they are the weak gazelles of our society, whose immune systems, like those of children and unlike those of strong, heterosexual gazelles, are 'already depressed.' How, we might ask, would Montagnier's analogy explain the large numbers of cases of HIV infection among straight gazelles today, several years into the epidemic? Obviously, it cannot. Montagnier has provided us here with an example of the anti-gay bias that pervades biomedical discourse. As the new moral guardian of society, the medical establishment will inevitably oppose the sexual 'deviance' from the norm that homosexuality represents.

In spite of their protestations to the contrary – 'unless one believes that God had a particular gripe with the peoples of central Africa,' they insist, 'it is hard to look at AIDS as a form of divine retribution with a moralistic twist'[30] – Masters, Johnson, and their co-author Kolodny exhibit throughout *Crisis* an implicitly moralistic stance, of which their reference to 'high-risk groups' is only one manifestation. Their reliance upon the military metaphor to describe the activities of HIV is also revealing in this regard. 'The invasion,' they state, 'is an intriguing one that is almost like a military operation. First, the AIDS virus seeks out and identifies the T-helper cells as targets. Next, it attaches itself to the outside of the cell, from which it will launch its actual attack.'[31] Once inside the host cell, the virus produces RNA that is in turn transformed into DNA which, 'acting something like a missile, then penetrates the nucleus of the T-helper cell, which is the heart of the cell's usual operations.'[32]

This micro-level invasion of the body by HIV is paralleled by the macro-level invasion that prompted the authors to write their book – that is, the invasion of 'the AIDS virus' that 'is now running rampant in the heterosexual community.'[33] Once again, it is not merely the body, but society that is under siege, and the slippage that occurs in the authors' references to the virus and to gay or bisexual men and IV drug users creates a certain amount of confusion as to who or what the invader is. On the subject of directed blood donations, for instance, they warn that 'there are no guarantees that your closest friend, whom you trust implicitly, is not bisexual or hasn't received a tainted blood transfusion or hasn't been a "closet" IV drug user.'[34] The McCarthyesque rhetoric of this sentence elides two threats to society: the virus and the deviant. They become, in the rhetoric of Masters, Johnson, and Kolodny, one and the same. Thus the authors' assertion that the motive behind the improvement of blood-donor screening is 'to attempt to eliminate homosexual and bisexual men and IV drug abusers from the donor pool'[35] does not strike them as problematic, in spite of their insistence elsewhere that 'AIDS is not a "gay" disease. It is a viral infection that doesn't discriminate in choosing its targets.'[36] One is left wondering just what (or who) is to be 'eliminated.'

The covert anti-gay message of *Crisis* is only one indicator of the moral agenda of its authors – that is, essentially, the traditional pro-monogamy and pro-family agenda of the New Right. Of those people who have multiple sexual partners we are informed, 'because they have difficulty finding a person with whom they can form a committed, one-to-one relationship, many of them engage in casual sex as a social act.'[37] The implication is very clear: monogamy is at once the norm and the preferred state; other options are there only for those who 'have difficulty' attaining it. Not surprisingly, Masters, Johnson, and Kolodny wage their war against AIDS on another front: prostitution, which, like homosexuality, threatens to infect the rest of society. For the authors of *Crisis*, prostitutes play the role of the bogeyman in the nightmare they have dubbed 'the Age of AIDS.' Prostitution, they assert, 'has become one of the principal vectors in spreading the AIDS virus to the heterosexual world' – no longer can anyone claim that it is a 'victimless crime.'[38] Apparently immune to the actual *effects* of AIDS, prostitutes are represented in *Crisis* as uncaring and highly efficient transmitters of HIV. Of course, it is taken for granted that 'prostitutes at any price level who know they are carrying the virus do not instantly stop working as a public service gesture.'[39] How entirely unimaginable that a prostitute should be in the least concerned about the public good!

This sort of scapegoating of prostitutes in the AIDS epidemic has been challenged by Carol Leigh, a member of COYOTE (Call Off Your Old Tired Ethics), an American prostitutes' rights group.[40] The incidence of HIV infection among prostitutes, Leigh argues, is no higher than it is among women with three to five sexual partners a year. Moreover, she suggests that seropositivity among prostitutes is confined to IV drug users. Of course, Leigh is anything but a disinterested observer – her aim is to assert the authority of the prostitute over that of the medical establishment represented by Masters and Johnson – and her facts, like any others, must be handled with caution. Still, her assertions are much more convincing than the shrill and paranoid ones of the authors of *Crisis*. Who, after all, has better reason than a prostitute to practise safer sex?

The authorities to whom we look for the truth about AIDS – whether they are popularly recognized as such, like Masters and Johnson, or whether they are recognized by the biomedical establishment, as are Gallo and Montagnier – do not, cannot, speak from a vantage point that would enable them to provide us with untainted facts. Like the creator of 'Cell Wars,' these scientists engage in the process of metaphorization in order to describe the disease, and in doing so they advance their own personal and political causes. The facts come to us wrapped in an obfuscating cloud of paranoia, self-aggrandizement, and ridiculous statements regarding strong and weak gazelles.

An increasing number of people with AIDS, however, stand desperately in need of facts, truths, and authorities. The awful dilemma of the person with AIDS in the midst of this confusion is strikingly captured by Emmanuel Dreuilhe in *Mortal Embrace*, in which he recounts his own approach to living with AIDS. Dreuilhe appropriates the language of warfare – the very language that the authorities employ against him – in a desperate effort to regain control over his body, his life. In other words, he consciously attempts to turn his illness into metaphor for *therapeutic* ends. The proliferation and extension of military metaphors in *Mortal Embrace* are truly remarkable. Yet what distinguishes Dreuilhe's use of those metaphors from the other examples that we have seen is that he is aware of how and why he is using them. Here, perhaps, in the use of metaphors (including the military ones condemned by Sontag as destructive) for self-reconstruction and self-empowerment by persons with AIDS and their caregivers, lies a solution to the dilemma that arises from our recognition of the inevitability of metaphoric thinking in response to new phenomena.

Dreuilhe undertakes the writing of the diary that provides the basis for his book as an attempt to deal with the unbearable isolation that has entered into his life as a result of his lover's death from AIDS and his own illness. He views his fictionalization of himself, his life, and his disease as essential to his survival: 'As the sole protagonist in my drama, with no one to talk to anymore, for the first time in my life I began keeping a diary, from which these pages have been drawn. From then on there were two of us – again, like Anne Frank. So, eager for even more company, I repopulated my universe with the only being whom I truly missed. I conjured up a complete puppet theater, a whole barracksful of toy soldiers, a voodoo exercise that did lead, in the end, to my emergence from the burrow where I'd gone to ground.'[41]

The writing of his diary and the metaphorical militarization of his body provides Dreuilhe with a sense of control that he cannot find elsewhere. The highly mutable nature of 'the facts' in the AIDS epidemic (he describes the attempts of patients to sift through 'the apparent anarchy of commands and countermands issuing from headquarters'[42]) provides precious little assurance to the person with AIDS to whom those commands are so terribly important. The authorities fail him; so Dreuilhe seizes not only their rhetoric but their power. He becomes simultaneously his own author and his own authority.

The locus of power for Dreuilhe is not 'the facts' of science and medicine; he has been bereft of his faith in the healing powers of those institutions. Instead, he reinvests his faith in a magical, talismanic art. The writing of his book, the transformation of his disease into fiction, becomes a rite of exorcism by which 'each phrase, each metaphor will stand in for one of my lymphocytes claimed by AIDS. In my world turned upside down, writing is not only a form of therapy but also a magical exercise.'[43] The completed book, the illness made metaphor and released into the world, becomes a formula of ritual healing. Drawn into that rite are 'all those who read my words, so that they might save me.'[44] Deprived of a reassuring authority, and yet so desperately in need of one, Dreuilhe creates for himself a new authority whose power resides in mysticism and magic. Alone, by the only remaining means available to him, Dreuilhe resolves his crisis of faith.

Mortal Embrace could perhaps be described as an exercise in lunatic discourse, but to dismiss it in this manner would be to ignore the circumstances that produced it. Given those circumstances, the book is an understandable, even reasonable, response. The apparently rational discourses of the authorities – Gallo, Montagnier, and Masters and Johnson – are hardly free of irrational elements. Like Dreuilhe, these authors communicate in their writings personal, political, or ideological agendas that extend beyond their ostensible interest in presenting the 'facts' about AIDS. They differ from Dreuilhe, however, in that those agendas are not so blatantly announced – they are more implicit than explicit. Furthermore, the acknowledged authorities tend to take their own positions of authority for granted, quietly affirming them where Dreuilhe, rendered helpless by circumstance, screams out his desire for control with every paragraph. His goal is to write himself into continued existence, to create a linguistic talisman and to draw his audience into his healing ritual. Medical authorities offer Dreuilhe dubious truths that are of no positive worth to him. Given the choice between these and his own fantastic constructions, Dreuilhe sets aside the 'truth' that destroys for that which empowers.

Postscript on the Mother of All AIDS Metaphors

In the 24 June 1991 issue of *Time*, medical reporter Christine Gorman looks to one of the hardware heroes of the Gulf War for the latest symbol of the deadly and elusive AIDS virus. 'Like a Stealth fighter plane,' she muses, 'HIV may have hidden parts that do not show up on the immune system's radar screen.' A possible solution to this reconnaissance problem, suggests one military-minded immunologist, is to enhance the technical capability of the immune system to detect the viral bombers so that the body might 'mount a more effective response.'[45]

Accompanying Gorman's report on the development of a vaccine to boost the immune system after HIV infection is a diagram entitled 'The Stealth Counterattack.' Its schematic design (by *Time* artist Joe Lertola) will appear familiar to anyone who experienced the televised version of the Gulf War. Against the black background of two silhouetted human figures the AIDS virus appears in spectral white outlines as a trio of tiny triangular Stealth bombers. The immune system is represented as a bunker-like munitions factory from which tiny cartoon anti-aircraft rockets are being fired. This vision of Cell Wars is eerily similar to the Pentagon's video-game images of the bombing of Iraqi military installations.

Behind this obscenely ironic analogy lurks a collective wish (with no possibility of fulfilment) that the War on AIDS might be as swiftly and decisively 'won' as the War in the Gulf. If only America's high-tech wizardry could assure us a speedy victory over HIV! *Time*'s coverage of the preliminary results of the vaccination experiments conducted by the Walter Reed Army Institute of Research is really a celebration of America's gung-ho victory in the Gulf rather than a clarification of the Institute's complex immunological work. The Stealth bomber's current status as the epitome of elusive destructiveness is triumphantly confirmed by its metaphorical association with HIV. But the analogy, by extension, also suggests that American militarism, in its drive towards President Bush's 'New World Order,' will spread over the globe like the AIDS epidemic: an irony that would not escape the multitudes who still suffer the debilitating consequences of the bombing of Baghdad.

NOTES

1 Susan Sontag *Illness as Metaphor* (New York: Farrar, Straus and Giroux 1978) 58
2 Ibid 85
3 Ibid 3
4 Sontag *AIDS and Its Metaphors* (New York: Farrar, Straus and Giroux 1989) 94
5 Ibid 5
6 'AIDS: Cultural Analysis / Cultural Activism,' *October* 43, ed Crimp (Winter 1987) 3
7 Paula Treichler 'AIDS, Homophobia, and Biomedical Discourse: An Epidemic of Signification' in *AIDS: Cultural Analysis* ed Crimp, 32
8 Ibid 37
9 Ibid
10 Ibid 60
11 *Illness as Metaphor* 67
12 Peter Jaret 'The Wars Within' *National Geographic* 169 (1986) 702
13 Ibid 709 (emphasis mine)
14 *Illness as Metaphor* 69
15 Cindy Patton *Sex and Germs: The Politics of AIDS* (Boston: South End Press 1985) 88
16 Ibid
17 Bryan S. Turner *The Body and Society: Explorations in Social Theory* (Oxford Basil Blackwell 1984) 211
18 Ibid 213
19 Ibid 214
20 Robert Gallo 'The AIDS Virus' *Scientific American* 256.1 (January 1987) 47
21 Ibid
22 Ibid 56
23 Ibid 47. Given the terrible tale behind Gallo's terrible tale, his bid for our trust, on behalf of the biomedical establishment, is more than a little ironic. Raging in the background of the *Scientific American* article is a highly political scientific squabble that appears to be as much about self-glorification and greed as it is about 'the AIDS virus,' if Randy Shilts's account is to be believed. Shilts suggests that the 'co-discoverer' label worn by Gallo and Luc Montagnier of the Pasteur Institute is nothing more than a 'pleasant fiction' beneath which lies a veritable 'quagmire of scientific politicking' (*And the Band Played On* [New York: St Martin's Press 1987] 593, 462). Indeed, Gallo emerges as one of the arch-fiends of Shilts's melodramatic history of the epidemic – a ruthless, self-seeking nasty who apparently stole the virus from the Pasteur Institute (who had named it 'lymphadenopathy-associated virus,' or LAV) and re-named it 'human T-cell lymphotropic

virus type III,' or HTLV-III. Gallo's designation was designed to make HIV appear to be the third in a family of leukemia retroviruses discovered by himself, even though the virus was clearly unrelated to his HTLV-I and HTLV-II (in which the 'L' stood for 'leukemia' rather than 'lymphotropic'). The ensuing wars over nomenclature were intimately related to the issue of possession or, to borrow Paula Treichler's term, 'paternity' of the virus ('AIDS, Homophobia, and Biomedical Discourse' 58). Gallo's insistence, in his *Scientific American* article, on referring to HIV by *his* own designation, HTLV-III, several months after the adoption of the new term by a subcommittee of the International Committee on the Taxonomy of Viruses is part of a messy and drawn-out paternity battle. Shilts's account of that battle would shake anyone's faith in 'the scientific community.' As we come to recognize how the political squabble underlying Gallo's article is to a great extent masked by an apparently apolitical scientific discourse, the story behind the story calls into question the existence of a scientific 'community' populated by disinterested scientists.

24 William Masters, Virginia Johnson, and Robert Kolodny *Crisis: Heterosexual Behavior in the Age of AIDS* (New York: Grove 1988) viii
25 Ibid 1
26 Ibid 2
27 'AIDS Expert says Masters Irresponsible' *The Gazette* (Montreal) 9 March 1988, C7
28 Jan Zita Grover 'AIDS: Keywords' in *AIDS: Cultural Analysis* ed Crimp, 28
29 Interview with Thomas Bass in *Omni* December 1988, 132
30 *Crisis* 17
31 Ibid 18
32 Ibid
33 Ibid 7
34 Ibid 80
35 Ibid 29
36 Ibid 90
37 Ibid 66
38 Ibid 132–3, 154
39 Ibid 132
40 Carol Leigh 'Further Violations of Our Rights' in *AIDS: Cultural Analysis* ed Crimp, 177–81
41 Emmanuel Dreuilhe *Mortal Embrace: Living with AIDS* trans Linda Coverdale (New York: Hill and Wang 1988) 43
42 Ibid 45
43 Ibid 139
44 Ibid
45 Christine Gorman 'Returning Fire Against AIDS' *Time* 24 June 1991, 52

Law as an 'Art Form' Reflecting AIDS: A Challenge to the Province and Function of Law

MARGARET A. SOMERVILLE

AIDS is raising challenges to many societal institutions. The law is no exception. In doing so, AIDS is providing new insights into the province and function of law. This paper seeks to identify and to explore some of these. But, before embarking on that task, there are some preliminary points that merit articulation, in order to situate this specific discussion within the more general context of the role and function of law.

First, it is proposed that we need to take a very broad view of the nature and function of law; a narrow view does not reflect either its actual or proper function. Second, although it is a truism that law is a very important institution in our society, we need to recognize that this may be true in ways that are not always readily apparent. Together with medicine, law has become even more important than in the past, because of the decline in adherence to organized religion. Many of the values and functions that organized religion used to carry or perform, respectively, have had to be 'reallocated' or 'relocated.' In many instances, they have been relocated in law and in medicine. This shift is giving law and medicine, as institutions, burdens with which they are not necessarily designed to cope and is causing some problems and confusion for these institutions.

Third, law is one of the mirrors of our culture. As such, it reflects one aspect of 'truth,' or, possibly, one of many 'truths.' That is, there may be multiple truths concerning any given issue. I suggest that we can examine an issue through different prisms and that the 'answers' that we generate, even if they appear to be conflictual, can still be reflections of truths about that issue. It just depends on how we look at and deal with such conflict. If we insist that there can only be one truth, we must regard such conflict as intolerable. But if we allow that such conflict may reflect many 'truths' – including those beyond our present understanding – the multiplicity of our reflections will not be at odds with truth or unacceptable to those who seek to understand it as a whole, or to grasp even a part of it, in the welter of our apparently conflictual 'answers.'

Fourth, law not only reflects culture; it forms culture. There is an interactive dynamic between law and culture. It is particularly necessary to be aware of this characteristic of law in the context of AIDS.

Fifth, law not only reflects our society; it also reflects each of us as individuals. It also 'forms' both our society and each of us to greater or lesser extents. The doctrine of precedent in the law is a mechanism that both allows us to and requires that we reflect back into what we did and why. But it also allows and requires that we simultaneously project forward into what we see ourselves as risking and gaining in the future by the decision we are taking. In short, much of the operation of law, as a societal institution, is as a combined reflection and projection mechanism, where the reflection and projection are intimately linked.

I was particularly interested in one statement that Andy Fabo made at the 'Representing AIDS' conference in London, Ontario (11–13 November 1988). He said that art had moved to minimalist concepts, that is, that a work of art could be constituted by the barest line. He went on to say that perhaps one could even abandon image and form altogether, with the result that art could become pure concept. My free-association thoughts, as I listened to him, concerned the nature of law. Law, in one sense, is pure concept and, therefore, the question arises: Is law a form of art? It might be rather surprising to some persons to think about law as a form of art, especially those who see law as operating principally in, and as limited to, its punitive mode. It may even seem sacrilegious to or even denigrating of art to describe law as such. But, if law were a form of art, what questions would that cause us to ask?

They could include the following: What picture of our society does the law paint? What portrait does our use of law and our call for certain laws (for instance, in relation to AIDS) paint of us? One can also free-associate about who are the artists of the pictures that the law paints and consider whether there is any connection or similarity between lawmakers and artists. As I thought about this, the concept of authoritarianism came to mind. This is strong in the law, and traditionally very weak in the arts. (Persons involved in the arts are often regarded as anti-authoritarian, and the law and art differ with respect to imposition of penalties. One cannot realistically threaten, at least in a free society, that 'if you don't like my picture, I'll put you in jail'!) But I concluded that we should not let such differences, which may in some senses be superficial ones, get in the way of our seeing the similarities between the two disciplines. There are, I propose, many similarities between law and art and we might learn by exploring the notion not only, as we frequently do, of the artist as painting pictures of a society, but also of the lawmaker as an artist. That is, we could view the lawmaker as someone undertaking a creative function, where the 'end product,' law, is strongly influenced by the person and circumstances involved and by the person's aims, understanding, and talent.

Such is the approach taken in this paper. To explore the province and function of law in relation to AIDS, we need to look at the nature of law in general and of particular laws; the 'nature' of those who make law; the occasions on which it is made; and the reasons for which it is made. Moreover, we need to examine such questions at the conscious level (for example, the reasons we give for passing certain legislation); the unconscious level (the subliminal factors that cause us to enact certain laws); and the symbolic level (the wider effects of a given law, for instance, on societal values). Moreover, we need a global perspective, an integrated perspective, and a 'permeating' perspective (that is, more than a narrow, legalistic interpretation) of what law is and should be in our culture. With such considerations in mind and, as mentioned previously, in search of insights, I wish to address a series of issues that share the common theme of law, HIV infection, and AIDS. However, these issues by no means represent an exhaustive or comprehensive list of questions that can and must be asked in relation to 'law and AIDS.'

AIDS, Law, and the Need for 'Special' Law

A primary question in considering law in the context of AIDS is whether existing law suffices or whether new law, enacted to apply expressly to HIV infection and AIDS, is required and justifiable. Much existing general law can be applied, where appropriate and necessary, to AIDS situations. This incudes criminal law, labour law, constitutional law, family law, and many specialized areas of law, for instance, health-law doctrines. The latter include informed consent, 'living wills,' durable powers of attorney, confidentiality, autonomy, and inviolability (the basis for rights against compulsory testing), to name but a few. These doctrines reflect a wide range of issues that are addressed within contemporary health law and, importantly, in the context of HIV infection and AIDS, in particular, by law governing public health. The question raised here is whether we should enact 'new' law, specifically relating to HIV infection and AIDS. Such law is not necessarily invasive of the rights of persons affected by HIV. Indeed, it can be enacted to try to protect their rights. There have been some examples of this approach in the United States, where laws prohibiting discrimination in housing, insurance, schooling, and so on have been enacted specifically to protect persons with AIDS. However, some law suggested for enactment in this area would be highly invasive of rights: for instance, law that calls for isolation, quarantine, and mandatory testing in relation to HIV infection and AIDS, or for HIV-antibody negativity as a condition for crossing international borders.

In my view, we should work from a general presumption that we should not enact new or specific law in relation to HIV infection or AIDS. Only where current law is shown to be clearly inadequate, and proposed new AIDS-specific law is clearly justified (where those wishing to enact the law can show that it manifestly would do more good than harm) should such new law be promulgated. Such cases should be regarded as a justifiable exception to the general principle against enacting such law. At the same time, we (especially those of us who are involved in dealing with HIV infection and AIDS) must recognize that we should not argue for special exemptions from the general law in relation to HIV infection and AIDS. For instance, there are provisions in the Canadian *Criminal Code* that people who show wanton and reckless indifference to human life or safety commit criminal negligence and are guilty of an offence, if thereby they injure or kill another person. Just as one can be liable under these provisions for discharging a firearm in a crowded place, shouting 'fire' in a theatre, or driving under the influence of alcohol, so, likewise, persons ought to be liable if their conduct in relation to transmission of HIV shows wanton and reckless indifference to human life or safety.

Too often the 'two sides of the coin' are not considered. We should require that 'persons with AIDS' be treated in the same way as everybody else, including with respect to the use of law. But this approach means that there must be recognition that all people – persons with AIDS and persons without AIDS – carry the same responsibilities as well as rights, and that claims for special privileges or exemption must be avoided. There is both a reality and a message involved in this approach. All persons are entitled to fair and equal treatment, including before and under the law, whether they are persons with AIDS or persons without AIDS. That is, we must apply the principle that AIDS should not be 'treated in isolation,' including with respect to the use of law. This means that approaches consistent with those taken outside the area of HIV infection and AIDS must be taken with respect to HIV infection and AIDS and, to determine what these are, analogies must be drawn. For example, claims to treat persons differently, simply on the basis of their HIV/AIDS status and not of any conduct on their part, could be compared with treatment of persons who suffer from mental illness and have committed crimes in the past, or of persons who are alcoholics and could have very serious car accidents under the influence of alcohol. The law deals with such persons in the same general manner as everybody else and not simply on the basis of their status and what they might do in the future. They remain persons who live in the society under the general rules of the society. They are not incarcerated simply on the basis of their status, as is sometimes suggested for persons with HIV infection or AIDS.

Sometimes laws dealing with HIV infection and AIDS are suggested or enacted, not to treat persons with HIV infection or AIDS more harshly under the law than other persons, but in order to give them special protection. While such laws may, in some cases, be necessary, it has been well said that human rights can be most threatened when we act purporting to do good for others. Consequently, in this respect too some care needs to be taken, and the passage of specific law to deal with HIV infection or AIDS, even that which is intended to be protective of persons affected by HIV infection or AIDS, must be clearly justified in each instance.

In deciding whether to enact law or, if enacting it, what law to enact, or in applying the general law to situations involving HIV infection or AIDS, it is essential to ensure that any enactment or use of law fights HIV and its harmful effects on those affected, and not the *persons* affected by HIV infection or AIDS. Moreover, we must ensure that any enactment or use of law is likely to make irresponsible people responsible and will not make responsible people irresponsible. There is a danger that some laws could have the latter effect, because of the messages they carry of depersonalization, alienation, rejection, fear, and even hostility with respect to 'persons with AIDS.' Such messages, by reinforcing AIDS phobia, are likely to encourage further AIDS discrimination; moreover, they could hinder efforts to decrease the rate of HIV transmission by eliciting understandable hostile feelings from persons whose cooperation is needed in this effort and by reducing public awareness of the vulnerability of all communities to HIV infection.

AIDS, Law, and the Aims of Law

Law is not an end in itself; it is a means to an end. We must define and articulate what ends we hope to achieve by the use of law in relation to HIV infection and AIDS. One sometimes hears calls for the use of law 'to stop the spread of HIV.' These, I suggest, are often misguided in their perceptions of what the reality is and what it is possible to achieve with law. As a result, we are likely to pass inappropriate and even seriously harmful laws in response to such calls. We have to face the reality, and it is a sad reality, that probably, indeed almost certainly, we cannot totally stop the spread of HIV. What we can do, as mature people in a mature society, is to take those courses of action that will reduce the spread of HIV to the maximum extent. Therefore, the issue becomes, not how we can stop the spread of HIV but whether passing a certain law or not passing a certain law would give the best reduction in the spread of HIV. The laws that will achieve the latter may well be very different from those aimed at trying to achieve the former. In some circumstances, the laws indicated by each of these approaches will be in sharp contradiction.

We live in an open legal system, which means that everything is permitted unless it is prohibited. This reflects the value we place on our freedom, and, indeed, we have articulated this in the *Canadian Charter of Rights and Freedoms*. Applying these concepts, including in the context of HIV infection and AIDS, means that we should work from a principle that a law should not be enacted or used until, at least on the balance of probabilities, we have some evidence that it will do more good than harm. For example, mandatory testing laws have been shown to reduce, substantially, the willingness of people to be tested for HIV antibodies. This means that, in all probability, these laws would have the effect of increasing the spread of HIV – exactly the opposite result from the intention with which the law would be promulgated.

It is suggested that, if law is to be successful in reducing HIV transmission, three 'Rs' must be kept in mind. These are respect for persons and their rights; mutual responsibility; and mutual reassurance. The community, as a whole, needs to reassure people who are affected by HIV infection and AIDS that they are not 'out to get them.' But, likewise, persons and groups affected by HIV infection and AIDS need to reassure the communities of which they are a part that they are not going to harm them. This second form of reassurance is sometimes overlooked. It should not be, because it is important; even from a self-interested point of view, recognition of one's responsibilities and the provision of trustworthy reassurance of non-maleficence might well be more beneficial in eliciting responses that ensure protection of one's rights than some more direct demands for protection of these rights.

AIDS, Law, and Characteristics of Lawmakers

The laws that are proposed or enacted in relation to HIV infection and AIDS may sometimes reflect more the characteristics of the lawmakers who propose or enact them than the characteristics of the HIV infection and AIDS situations they are meant to address. A Montreal newspaper report (*The Gazette*, 5 April 1988, B5) is interesting in this respect. The headline states: 'Lawmakers tend to be authoritarian test results say.' This is not surprising. Robert Altemeyer, a professor of sociology at the University of Manitoba, found that of 100 Canadian politicians tested for authoritarian tendencies, several measured above 200 on a scale of 30 to 270. To put this in proper perspective, using the same scale, Altemeyer also did an assessment of Hitler. He was rated 205. That is, several Canadian politicians have overwhelmingly authoritarian tendencies. Those who scored high on the test tended to agree strongly with statements such as 'the way things are going in this country, it is going to take a lot of strong medicine to straighten out the troublemakers, criminals and perverts.' They tended to disagree with statements such as 'there is nothing immoral or sick in somebody being a homosexual.' In short, laws are made by men (and, to a large extent, men in the gender sense of this term, and not in its generic sense, have been the lawmakers). Lawmakers have their own values, attitudes, and beliefs, and a gender base from which they work. We must take this into account if we are to ensure that acceptable law is formulated in relation to HIV infection and AIDS.

This is not to say that persons who have strong beliefs cannot make valid and acceptable law. Everyone has his or her own set of values and those expressing strong beliefs may simply be more open and honest than some who say they are not sure what they believe. (One must be careful not to include within the latter group persons who are genuinely uncertain and have the courage and wisdom to admit this; even when such an admission may be detrimental to them, personally for instance, it is likely to be a politically nonviable response.) Those with strong beliefs may also be persons of greater integrity than those who change their beliefs to fit the prevailing fashion, especially in order to benefit themselves. Rather, we need to develop methodologies that will enable us to take factors such as lawmakers' 'tendencies' into account in formulating and analysing the law. We are relatively unsophisticated in such respects, possibly in part because of some residual influence of the traditional concept that law was divinely ordained and the lawmaker simply the spokesperson for the deity. Our consideration of the proper role and function of law in relation to HIV infection and AIDS may well make us more sophisticated and perceptive in these regards.

AIDS, Law, Risk, and Uncertainty

Western populations in the late twentieth century are very intolerant of identified risks. The word 'identified' should be noted. We live with great risk and are usually quite happy with this, as long as we do not know about it. People, in general, expect and even demand that 'identified' risk be reduced to a minimum. This is relevant to the current discussion because law can be used in an attempt to reduce actual or perceived, personal or societal risk, even when this use of law is seriously invasive of fundamental human rights. This is one way in which AIDS is going to test how real is our commitment to human rights. Will we act to respect human rights, as we have proclaimed we do, at a time when we did not feel personally threatened as a consequence of providing this respect? This is probably the first time that in a major way, in Canadian society as a whole, people who perceive themselves to be at some additional risk because of their support for human rights will have to choose either to oppose invasive measures being applied to people with AIDS that would breach their fundamental human rights, or to support such measures. Although, for example, our treatment of native peoples *should* have faced us with such questions, they have not done so in the same way that AIDS is now doing, probably because there has not been the same degree of personal identification with either the breaches of human rights involved or with the situations that give rise to these. Whatever the reasons, we have not previously had such an identified and widespread challenge, in practice, to our beliefs regarding human rights, at least in theory. In particular, we have not encountered such a challenge since our express articulation of human rights in legislative documents, of which the *Canadian Charter of Rights and Freedoms* is the most important example.

Express statements of human rights in official and authoritative form are also a late twentieth-century Western-democracy phenomenon. It is suggested that this phenomenon is another of our individual and societal responses to the decline in adherence to organized religion. When we no longer necessarily all recognize the authority of the Ten Commandments in a modern society, we turn to parliament. Pursuant to this reasoning, the Charter can be seen as a substitute for older forms of expressing, especially with respect to fundamental values, societal rules or societal consensus, which, it is important to note, are not necessarily the same. It is easy to say we abhor torture, we abhor apartheid, we abhor political imprisonment and similar appalling breaches of human rights that some other countries engage in, when we do not engage in such conduct, and are not faced with situations that could elicit such conduct. But, since we *are* faced with AIDS, we cannot avoid acting in relation to AIDS, which necessarily raises issues of human rights. Therefore, AIDS forces us to question ourselves, in terms of our real respect for human rights. Persons in Canada who have suggested, for instance, that law be enacted to allow compulsory testing of people for HIV infection must consider whether such a law would breach human rights. Happily, such approaches have been strongly rejected. In short, we cannot avoid being on 'home territory' in relation to respect for human rights in addressing issues raised by AIDS. Will our governments, and will we, act to respect human rights when there is strong evidence that they are being breached in our own community? I hope we will.

How we act will depend, in part, both on the reality and our perceptions of the risk and uncertainty with which we are faced. These are related, in that identified or perceived risk raises the level of uncertainty that is experienced. One solution is to try to reduce the risk. But, when this is too costly in terms of the harm that it would do to the delicate 'fabric' of our society (for instance, it would require breach of human rights), another solution is, I suggest, for us as individuals and as a society to learn to live more comfortably with uncertainty. This is not a common characteristic of our Western societies or of the people of whom they are composed. We will need to develop mechanisms to achieve this end.

AIDS, Law, and Impotence

By 'impotence,' I mean societal impotence: a feeling generated by the risk and uncertainty perceived to be faced in relation to AIDS and the fact that we are faced with an incurable, transmissible, fatal illness in relation to which there is not even a great deal we can do to prolong, substantially, people's lives. Inaction, in such circumstances, is intolerable for our societies, but action in the form, for example, of legal intervention, especially legislative intervention, may be contra-indicated. The danger is that, even where enacting law is contra-indicated, we might do this to simulate the taking of effective action in order to deal with the psychological discomfort caused by facing inaction and by uncertainty in the presence of perceived risk. Passage of law in such circumstances can be best described as a 'façade of action.' It can be compared with situations in which the government cannot afford to solve a problem and sets up a royal commission that costs 1 per cent of the cost of remedying the problem, in order to be seen to be 'doing something about it.' It is an example of what has been called the 'do something syndrome.' Very often this is what is happening with calls for the use of law in relation to AIDS. The passage of law would be a symbolic 'doing something,' while in reality it does nothing to reduce the spread of HIV or to help those affected by HIV. The danger is that this type of symbolic 'doing something' is not necessarily neutral; it can cause enormous harm. It can make people feel frightened, angry, hostile, and alienated. All of these feelings are counterproductive in reducing the spread of HIV.

AIDS, Law, and the Scientific Approach

The use of a so-called scientific approach is also related to needs for certainty. Politicians like to use a scientific approach as the basis for passing law. For example, they often prefer to rely heavily, and sometimes only, on statistical data regarding a certain issue, to the exclusion of considerations relating to values, symbolism, infliction of harm – all those rather soft considerations that can 'intrude' themselves in decision-making. The latter not only are more difficult to explain, and, as a consequence, more difficult to use as justifications, but also are more likely to elicit strong polarized responses. A 'scientific approach,' for instance one based on statistics, also seems to be founded on a more certain basis than many other approaches, and therefore is experienced as dealing better with the uncertainty element. Moreover, when it is used as the only basis justifying the passing of a certain law, it is easy for politicians to feel that they can back up that law. Consequently, adoption of a scientific approach is also related to political viability. To pass a law and not to be able to defend it is not politically viable, particularly because this causes a loss of politicians' credibility – an even more sensitive issue for politicians when their credibility is already low, as it seems to be at present. Political viability also often depends on adopting short-term solutions, even when long-term approaches are essential. A scientific approach (for example, medical or social-science research) is also relevant in this respect, but here it is more likely to 'harm' than to 'help' politicians, in that it can be used to identify the serious inadequacies and harms of short-term solutions. Difficulties of this kind that arise in relation to AIDS will be discussed a little later.

But there is yet another problem related to the adoption of a scientific approach (in the broad sense of this term) that is not of the politicians' making. This problem, which is inherent in the political system, is causing difficulties in relation to AIDS. The reality is that we have an enormously complex challenge to society with AIDS, and we are trying to deal with this challenge using institutions and instruments that were designed without any contemplation of issues of this complexity, including scientific complexity. Many 'AIDS issues' are showing up incapacities in the institutions and processes of our 'societal system' (for instance, our parliamentary, legal, and public-health institutions and processes) through their inability to deal with them satisfactorily. But this is not necessarily all bad. Dealing with 'AIDS issues' could well cause the whole 'system' to be revitalized. Tragic as the AIDS situation is, it offers opportunities for very major contributions to the change that is necessary in a society entering a new millennium.

AIDS, Law, and Symbolism

Susan Sontag, in *Illness as Metaphor*, proposes that each age uses an illness as the vehicle for carrying the symbolism of the evil in and disintegration of the society. Such illnesses are the 'scapegoat diseases.' The disease and the evil associated with it are 'driven out of the society into the desert,' by driving out, literally or metaphorically, those who have it. We need to recognize that, in a modern society, law can often be the driving-out mechanism. AIDS is a 'symbolic' disease; like AIDS, law carries symbolism. Therefore, law dealing expressly with

AIDS, or even as applied to AIDS, is doubly symbolic and, therefore, doubly powerful and important. It is powerful and important not just in relation to persons with AIDS, but especially in relation to what happens to and in our society as a whole.

AIDS, Law, and Infliction of Pain

Why are there such strong demands for the use of very invasive measures in relation to persons with HIV, including legal measures, when the data show that HIV is not transmitted by casual contact? Could this be for reasons of 'symbolic reassurance,' rather than as a practical measure to reduce HIV transmission? We may need symbolism that provides reassurance that there is something that can be done to protect us against AIDS. The use of invasive measures may also reflect a belief that there must be pain for a remedy to be effective. With this in mind, it is interesting to consider the history of pain control in medicine. Up to the beginning of the nineteenth century, it was frequently thought to be medically wrong to relieve pain, because of a belief that patients would not get better unless they suffered. The actions and reactions of societies and individual persons can reflect each other in many ways. Could our society be in some 'nineteenth-century state,' where people feel that there has to be pain for the society to 'get better'? Such a felt necessity for the presence of pain may be particularly likely to exist in relation to doubtfully effective or ineffective remedies, which I suggest the law often is in relation to issues raised by AIDS. If curative interventions are not possible (for instance, legal measures cannot stop transmission of HIV), and preventive interventions are of doubtful efficacy (for example, we do not know whether our AIDS education is effective), then pain-inflicting interventions may be more likely to be used. This might also occur, because, when cure is not possible, there is a desire or need to elicit some reaction or effect, and the only one available may be a pain response.

The infliction of pain may also be a disidentification mechanism. These mechanisms will be discussed shortly, but the possibility of infliction of pain functioning as such a mechanism merits consideration here. For instance, studies on child abuse show that parents who suffered abuse as children may be more likely than persons who have not suffered such abuse to abuse their own children. Inflicting pain on others that one could not bear having inflicted on oneself may be an attempt to show lack of fear where fear in fact exists, and, through this, to show that one is not identified with those others on whom the pain is inflicted or the situation in which they find themselves. Stated in another way, the person inflicting the pain is reassuring himself or herself that the reason for which, or the situation in which, the pain is being inflicted on the other person is not true of him or her, and will not become true. That is, the infliction of pain has disidentified the pain inflictor from the person who suffers the pain. Such a mechanism could operate not only in the context of child abuse, but also in that of AIDS.

AIDS, Law, and Political Viability

It has already been mentioned that what we need, in dealing with AIDS, are long-term 'hard' solutions. What we get from politicians (and let us be fair, what we request or usually demand from politicians) are short-term easy solutions. Usually, it is politically nonviable to do something that will only be beneficial ten years down the road. It is difficult to suggest how we are going to manage this problem.

An interesting example with respect to the use of law, in relation to AIDS, in order to maintain political viability, arises in the context of immigration and AIDS. The degree of interest in the issue of testing immigrants for HIV antibodies is quite out of proportion to any harm threatened. We have 135,000 immigrants to Canada each year. Most of them are families who come to set up a new life and to work to establish themselves. We have 40,000,000 visitors to Canada each year. If one considers one of the main modes of transmission of HIV, unsafe sex, this is much more likely to occur among persons on holidays or on business, and away from home, staying in hotels, than with immigrants. It would be illogical to test the 135,000 immigrants for HIV antibodies and not to worry at all about the 40,000,000 visitors, if the reason for testing were protection of public health.

It might be that immigrants are tested, and not visitors, because seropositive immigrants could prove to be too expensive (an 'excessive burden' in the words of the *Immigration Act 1976*) for our Canadian health-care system. We do not know the answer to this, and the arguments for and against will not be addressed here (M.A. Somerville 'The Case against HIV Antibody Testing of Refugees and Immigrants' *Canadian Medical Association Journal* 141 [1989]: 889–94). But there may be another reason, a more important one, for political interest in the subject of AIDS and immigration, in general, and the enactment of law in relation to HIV and immigration, in particular. Politicians may see themselves as 'damned if they do and damned if they don't' pass laws relating to AIDS. If they say there should be no law on AIDS because such law is invasive, wrong, and will do more harm than good, one segment of society expresses outrage at the failure of government to maintain standards of public health and morality. On the other hand, if they say there should be law on AIDS, another segment of society protests that civil liberties are infringed or individual human rights denied. In short, as can be true with law on abortion, politicians are at risk of losing 50 per cent of their voters whichever approach they take. What is the solution? Enact some 'tough' law, in order to demonstrate willingness to institute such measures, but have it apply only to persons who cannot vote for or against you. Who are these persons? The immigrants outside our borders who, if they are seropositive, will not be admitted to Canada. In short, by using such an approach, politicians can show that they are 'hard-line,' that is, willing to pass invasive law in relation to HIV, without having to impose such law on their home population, which in turn enables them to give a 'soft-line' message and retain the 'liberal' vote.

There might also be another reason why AIDS and immigration is an issue that attracts a disproportionate amount of attention. Testing potential immigrants and keeping out those who are HIV-positive may symbolize that AIDS is 'out there,' not 'in here,' and that we can take effective action to prevent its entry. This is yet one more form of disidentification from AIDS.

AIDS, Law, and Disidentification

A member of the WHO 'Global Program on AIDS' began an address with the statement that 'the one matter relevant to AIDS, about which there is consensus, is that it started in someone else's country.' We are all similar in identifying AIDS as coming from a 'foreign' source and blaming others for the AIDS epidemic, but we disidentify – 'unlink' from each other – in doing so. This tendency is strongly articulated when the unlinking takes the form of legislation, as for example if immigration legislation were to be passed, such as that referred to above, that prohibits entry to a country without an 'AIDS clearance.'

Infliction of pain as a disidentification mechanism has been mentioned already. This can be regarded as an active-aggressive form of disidentification, in comparison with other forms that are more passive-aggressive in nature. Labelling these forms of disidentification in this way may help us to distinguish the psychological roots of the process and to deal with its harmful social consequences. The importance of dealing with harmful disidentification becomes apparent when one realizes that it is a *primary* and *necessary* step in discrimination and stigmatization. Therefore, one way to address these problems would be at the level of cause (preventing disidentification) rather than of symptoms (punishing discrimination). An even deeper cause is the fear that gives rise to disidentification, and this must also be addressed, although it may be difficult to do so effectively.

The concept of 'rivers of disidentification' can provide important insights in relation to HIV infection and AIDS. There is a story that the prostitutes in Kinshasa were being interviewed about their role in the transmission of HIV infection. The prostitutes on one side of the river said: 'You shouldn't be interviewing us, we're the wrong people, we have no AIDS on this side of the river. It is the prostitutes on the other side of the river who've got AIDS.' So the researchers went over to the other side of the river to interview the prostitutes there. They said: 'You're on the wrong side, it's all the prostitutes over on the other side of the river who've got AIDS.' We need to ask what rivers of disidentification we are using in our communities, and, in particular, whether these include law.

Law can be used as a very strong river of disidentification. We can unlink from each other – disidentify from each other – through a use of law that has the effect of dividing a community into 'them' and 'us.' This might be done simply out of fear, but it might also be undertaken, whether consciously or unconsciously, to avoid responsibility. We mark off 'them' by saying the situation is their own fault, attributing guilt, and concluding that, therefore, we do not have to take responsibility for them. At the same time, and this is important, this conduct on our part does not excuse others from a duty to take responsibility for us, because we do not put ourselves into a 'them' category. The mechanism operative here, and one that is relevant to law, can be described as the concept of 'marker events' (M.A. Somerville 'Birth and Life: Establishing a Framework of Concepts' *Connecticut Law Review* 21 [1989] 667). A 'marker event' is a limitation device. It is an event with respect to which we make a rule that everybody on one side of the event is to be treated in one way, but everybody on the other side may be treated in a different way. We choose 'marker events' that will favour us. That is, we choose events that ensure that the precedents that we set in denying or doing to others what we would not want to have denied or done to us will not apply to us, and therefore will not harm us.

Finally, in relation to disidentification, we should consider whether we may be using or proposing to use law (for example, to isolate or quarantine persons with AIDS) not to deal reasonably with these people and the problems they are, or are perceived as, presenting, but in reality to conduct what has been called an 'isolation ritual' (D. Schulman 'Remembering Who We Are: AIDS and Law in a Time of Madness' *AIDS and Public Policy* 3 [1988] 75–6). It is important to recognize that the primary purpose of such a ritual is not so much to exclude the isolated persons as to bind together the persons concurring in and carrying out the isolation. It is pertinent to speculate, in this respect, whether the act necessary to achieve this type of bonding needs to inflict, or is more effective in achieving such bonding if it does inflict, pain on its victims. These rituals almost invariably cause severe suffering to those who are their targets, and guilt could well be generated by this infliction of pain. Indeed, one can speculate whether the bonding mechanism of those who do the isolation may be a shared sense of guilt and possibly communal denial of that guilt, which is often manifested, I would suggest, by vociferous justification of the laws that are employed in order to carry out the isolation rituals. It could also be that the use of law to impose such treatment allows denial, at the conscious level, that there is any guilt involved, on the basis that one cannot be guilty (at least, in the strict legal sense of that term) for doing what the law not only permits but directs to be done.

AIDS, Law, and Suffering

We tend to think of law (except for punitive provisions) as neutral in terms of inflicting suffering, or at best, as capable of relieving or preventing suffering, which some laws against wrongful discrimination in the AIDS context can be.

But if suffering is seen as occurring when there is a loss of control over what happens to oneself and perception of one's own physical or mental disintegration as a person, or a loss of self-esteem resulting from an actual or perceived denial of one's status as a person, then laws that result in such losses can be regarded as a direct cause of suffering. Laws allowing medical interventions without consent or breaches of confidentiality fall into this category. This is not to say that such laws are never justified; rather, we need to be conscious of the potential of law to inflict suffering when we are deciding whether there is justification for enacting and applying certain laws.

AIDS, Legal Precedents, and Wishful Thinking

Just as AIDS requires long-term, not short-term, approaches, AIDS will set far-reaching, long-lived human-rights precedents. We need to recognize that, in striking the balance with regard to both rights and responsibilities of both individuals and the community, the precedents set in the AIDS crisis will necessarily show the degree of our respect for each other and are likely to be the most powerful human-rights precedents that we set in many of our societies, at least for the next generation. Depending on their content, these precedents will support either respect for or breach of human rights. This realization is given particular force and importance when it is recognized that AIDS is not a short-term problem that can be 'fixed' by highly invasive and coercive measures. Unfortunately, it is a situation that will be with us for the foreseeable future, and, consequently, the ethics and law of our interventions are very likely to have a long 'half-life.' Therefore our interventions need even greater care than would measures that are likely to be temporary.

Wishful thinking may also influence legislative responses. There may be a psychological barrier that needs to be crossed in this regard. As we have already noted, placing 'rivers of disidentification' between different groups of people gives rise to a situation of 'us' and 'them' in the AIDS crisis, and serves to reduce the feeling that AIDS is a personal threat to us. Similarly, to reduce the threat that we perceive AIDS as posing to the existence of our society, we may allow ourselves to engage in another form of disidentification or denial: namely the promotion of false hopes and wishful thinking to the effect that AIDS is a temporary phenomenon. The danger of piercing this denial (which may for a society, just as for an individual, be a healthy coping mechanism in some circumstances) is that one can elicit serious, destructive depression or nihilism. In short, both as individuals and a society we need to learn how to live personally, ethically, legally, socially, and economically with the realization that 'AIDS is here to stay. It is like the day after Hiroshima – the world has changed and will never be the same' (J. Osborne 'AIDS: Politics and Science' *New England Journal of Medicine* 318 [1988] 444–7, 445).

Conclusion

Many key words have been used in this essay in examining the role of law in relation to AIDS. These include disidentification, symbolism, pain, suffering, politics, uncertainty, risk, and impotence. Many more could be added. AIDS challenges us to rethink our positions on many issues and not just the logical aspect of any given position, but also the emotional, moral, and symbolic aspects of it.

It seems almost unbelievable that a minute virus could elicit such an array of effects in so many fundamental aspects of our individual and societal lives. It is only in becoming aware of these multiple and complex effects that we will be able to use the 'AIDS crisis' as a source of linking to each other as humane and caring individuals and communities, and to avoid the unlinking that, although it may seem overdramatic to say so, could threaten to take us forward to a new 'dark age.' Dark is the absence of light. Although we have no light in the sense of a cure for AIDS, we should bear in mind that the light of our modern technology has enabled us to see the virus, and to recognize it for what it is, not some punishment or curse of a punitive god, but a part of nature to which we are still subject, devastating as this realization is in the context of the AIDS epidemic. We could also, to return to the subject of art, contemplate the relationship between art and light. Art needs light both to be created and to convey its message. Our challenge is to use the light of modern technology, the light of art, and, where necessary, the light of law, in the face of justified, imagined, or atavistic fears of AIDS, to fashion appropriate twenty-first-century responses to what is ultimately the fear of individual, societal, and even species death.

The State, Public Policy, and AIDS Discourse

BARRY D. ADAM

AIDS is something of a 'pure case' in the social construction of disease, having arrived as an unknown and unanticipated phenomenon at the site of some of the deepest anxieties of western civilization, namely sex and death. It was not long before this entirely novel entity was being encoded by highly charged rhetorics ready made by traditional debates over disease, sexual control, and homosexuality. Indeed, to make sense of the public debate over AIDS control policy in the 1980s requires a determined 'unpacking' of the AIDS languages that have formed since 1981 and a concerted probing into the deeper political forces which have generated conflicting discourses on the issue.

The Socio-historical Milieu

AIDS arrived into a highly developed political and ideological arena which gave it meaning and a 'place' on the historical stage. The late 1970s and 1980s, at least in the United States, the United Kingdom, and Canada, has been a period of conflict over the (dis)establishment of the nuclear family and the rights of people to take up new domestic and sexual arrangements outside the purview of patriarchal authority (Adam 1987). This might be understood in the broad historical sweep as an element in a larger process which has been underway for several

First appeared in *Contemporary Crises* 13 (1989). © Kluwer Academic Publishers (Dordrecht). Reprinted with the permission of the publishers.

centuries where the toleration of religious and political diversity has developed in opposition to church and state orthodoxies. Sexual debates are inheritors of older struggles which eventually disestablished state religions by redefining religious beliefs and practices as personal or private confessions. As well, they are the beneficiaries of the historical development of public and secular worlds supportive of norms of freedom of conscience, speech, and political pluralism. The erotic and intimate realms now seen to be the contested terrain of disputes between church- and state-sanctioned orthodoxies and the toleration or, even celebration, of single or multiple parenthood, gay and lesbian households, and fertility controlled by women. In this view, AIDS 'dropped into' the latest frontier of a profound historical change and so quickly came to bear a cosmological significance which other diseases escape.

Against any liberal, progressivist reading of these trends may be set the caveats presented by the work of Michel Foucault. A core theme in his work, not only in *The History of Sexuality*, but perhaps even more so in *The Birth of the Clinic* and *Discipline and Punish*, is how 'dark continents' of existence have been brought forward, massaged, shaped, and ultimately controlled by their articulation in discourse. In *The History of Sexuality*, Foucault (1978:11) wants 'to define the regime of power-knowledge-pleasure that sustains the discourse on human sexuality in our part of the world' and questions why sex is made to speak in the modern era and how it is carved into taxonomies of ostensibly discrete categories of perversity and normality. Talk about sexuality has always been much more than a simple contest between 'liberation' and 'control,' for the contest itself rises out of a deeper political play which constructs, produces, and disciplines the parameters of the debate and the use and meaning of sexuality. In *Discipline and Punish*, he notes how liberal reform movements participated in the larger disciplinary trends of the early nineteenth century where they ultimately 'set up a new "economy" of power to punish ... so that it should be distributed in homogeneous circuits capable of operating everywhere, in a continuous way, down to the finest grain of the social body' (Foucault 1979:80). The result has been the panoptic eye of the efficient jailer which both suppresses and 'produces domains of objects and rituals of truth' (Foucault 1979:194; 1980). It is probably fair to say that no one objects to the control and eradication of the causative agent(s) of AIDS, but AIDS control policy has always been much more and has inevitably raised the question of the supervision and regulation of sexuality. AIDS has ushered in a further development of sexual speech which cannot but partake of the larger twentieth-century 'obsession' with sexuality and its colonization by the professions, the media, and the state. Moving beyond Foucault's parameters, conflicts over the 'ownership' of the issue of AIDS raise again fundamental questions of feminism and gay liberation, in particular, who controls whose bodies?

Joseph Gusfield's classic study of Prohibition pointed out that social issues such as drinking are rarely fought out on their practical or intrinsic merits – whatever they may be – but as symbols of much larger and more difficult social changes. Gusfield showed that temperance debates were fueled by the much bigger concerns which the antagonists perceived to be at stake. 'Armed with the response of indignation at their declining social position, the adherents of Temperance sought a symbolic victory through legislation which, even if it failed to regulate drinking, did indicate whose morality was publicly dominant' (Gusfield 1963:111). In particular, Gusfield identifies the status anxiety of the small-town, American Protestants faced with increasing numbers of immigrants, Catholics, and minorities as the motor behind Prohibition.

The AIDS control debates, too, are indecipherable without recognition of their symbolic value for certain social constituencies. AIDS recapitulates aspects of other twentieth-century campaigns and debates around family, sex, and gender. Like earlier struggles over contraception, and more recent ones over abortion, the Equal Rights Amendment, and gay rights, many read AIDS control policy as a sign of the direction of larger historical forces.

As Dennis Altman (1986:28) points out, AIDS appeared at a particular moment in a particular society and these contingencies have shaped the career of the syndrome. It was first identified in the one western nation without universal health care during a government administration determined to cut spending on social programs. It appeared among homosexual men, Haitians, and drug users during an official retreat from the policy of protecting the rights of minorities. And AIDS appeared when the Christian right was ascendant with a program of traditional moralism and an ideological mold which had had a 'dry run' with herpes and was easily adaptable to the new affliction.

Adventures of the Discourse

To cite Gusfield (1981:53) again from an entirely different context, AIDS is very much the story of how 'uncertain, inconsistent, and inaccurate' knowledge is 'fashioned into a public system of certain and consistent knowledge in ways which heighten its believability and its dramatic impact.' AIDS has been made to fit the contours of the sexual politics of the 1980s and has been channelled into ready-made ideological ruts which have resulted in a 'public system of certain and consistent' categories impelling public policy. In the short history of the syndrome may be discerned three stages in the institutionalization of the 'strange virus of unknown origin.' From 1981 to 1983, AIDS was guarded in silence by taboos which forbade talk about sex, especially about the 'exotic' sex practices of gay men and about the stigmatized people it afflicted – again homosexuals, but also intravenous drug users and Haitians, who for the most part are poor black people. Only a few medical researchers and gay people, seeing their friends and neighbors rapidly waste away until death, anxiously discussed the new disease, but well outside the mainstream press. AIDS was made to speak from 1983 with the identification of higher status, more 'respectable' and 'innocent' victims of the disease, namely, children, people who had received blood transfusions, and in 1985, the popular Hollywood actor, Rock Hudson (Adam 1987). The breaking of the silence around AIDS punctured a logjam which led to an inundation of speculation, terror, 'facts,' and 'experts.' Still, there remained important repressions and silences around AIDS; the parameters of the spoken and the unspoken had shifted with new patterns of elision and separation encoding the new phenomenon. It is this AIDS discourse which occupies this section of the article. The 'third stage' emerging in the mid-1980s of state financial and legislative control of AIDS issues will take up the next section.

There is much to be learned from the history of contraception for understanding AIDS discourse. The most direct parallel involves conflicts over the implications of the use of condoms, but both issues raise again questions over the separation of sex from reproduction and of the right of people such as women, youth, and homosexuals to make their own sexual choices. As Linda Gordon points out, both suffragists and their opponents, and both the political left and the right, agreed on the immorality of condoms through much of the nineteenth century. But in the first decades of the twentieth century, the popular interest in contraception overcame the suffragist opposition to it, which rested on the 'fear of the other women – "fallen women" – who might undermine husbands' fidelity' (Gordon 1976:98). The women's movement, along with progressives of the day, swung around to the view that contraception was a fundamental right of women to control their bodies and their fertility. By the 1970s and 1980s, contraception had few effective opponents. The debate had relocated onto abortion. For traditionalists, abortion, like contraception before it, was yet another sign of the decline of the nuclear family because it allowed the escape of sex from family control, it released women from the obligations of motherhood and into the labor market, it permitted men to have sex while avoiding the responsibilities of family, and it let sex 'leak away' from the family to youth and to people who might stay unmarried, become 'loose' or 'bad' women, or prefer homosexual relationships. The conservative position, then, has typically resisted contraceptive technology and abortion in order to conscript sex for the family, naming abstinence as the only acceptable alternative.

This framework was employed during the 1910s and 1920s when public authorities in the United States became alarmed by the rising rates of sexually transmitted diseases (STDs) especially among soldiers (Brandt 1985). Public health authorities expended a great deal of energy and money attempting to counsel men to remain chaste and in closing down 'red light' districts across the United States. The results were ever-increasing rates of syphilis and gonorrhea. Infection rates were not brought down until the implementation of quite another policy by the federal government in the 1930s – and this was accomplished in the days before penicillin. The new policy abandoned the daunting task of trying to make sex unpopular in favor of a more practical approach of making condoms readily available and instructing men in their use. By separating the issue of infection (basically a question of placing a barrier between oneself and the infectious agent) from the question of sexuality, significant headway was made in controlling disease. It is noteworthy that in the United States and Canada, prophylactic means were given *only* to men and not to army women, that anti-STD campaigns were conceived solely from the male viewpoint complete with warning posters identifying women of bad morals as the source of disease, and that the 'clean-up' campaigns arrested women of 'bad character' such as prostitutes and not male soldiers who were apparently held blameless in the spread of STDs (Gordon 1976:358; Kinsman 1987:110). This 'democratization' of sexual information and technique from the educated classes to heterosexual men in general has yet to extend much farther and many of the sharpest debates today center around the distribution of information and technique to gay men and lesbians, youth, and to a lesser extent, women. Prohibitions against contraceptive information, which largely gave way in the postwar period, have been displaced by a censorship regime applied to safe sex (examined further below).

The upshot today is an AIDS discourse which recapitulates many of the themes and linkages of contraception, abortion, and STD policies. What has emerged is a closed rhetorical system which might be typified by the following suppositions:

- AIDS is an invariably fatal disease caused by the AIDS virus.
- AIDS can be contracted by having sex with an AIDS carrier.
- AIDS control, then, means finding out who the AIDS carriers are and stopping their irresponsible sexual behavior.
- Limiting sex to the traditional family is the most effective means of limiting the spread of AIDS.

From these articles of faith follow a number of moral and policy positions which Simon Watney (1987:124) has called the 'discourse of punitive fidelity.' The media and the state frequently repose the 'chastity-or-family' choice (sometimes qualified by 'if you must, use condoms') with obituaries on the putative 'sexual revolution' of the 1960s and claims of a 'return to family values.' In reviewing some very expensive television advertisements funded by the Canadian government and produced by the Canadian Public Health Association, Guy Poirier (1987:8) remarked that the ads presented

> straight white yuppies ... featuring a heterosexual couple and their children flaunting their supposed monogamy as the best protection against AIDS ... [The ads have] less to do with AIDS prevention than ... with the re-hegemonization of the monogamous heterosexual nuclear family as the only acceptable model for survival in the 1980s.

Educational materials have persistently advised first gay men and now the 'general public' to avoid 'promiscuity' and 'reduce the number of sex partners' as the first line of defense against AIDS.

From here, it is a short step to a 'wages of sin' argument, which has been articulated publicly primarily by the Reagan administration and fundamentalist preachers, where AIDS sufferers are held responsible for their own plight despite the fact that the greatest proportion of them were infected before AIDS was discovered and during the first 'silent' years of its history (Bayer 1985:589). Gordon's (1976:171) observations of medical attitudes to contraception in the 1920s ring eerily today:

> Injuries supposedly caused by contraception, such as venereal disease, were just punishments for sin ... condoms degraded love and produced lesions, ... 'God's little allies' in promoting chastity.

> It was almost as if doctors felt a subconscious satisfaction, a justification, when their patients developed infections.

Even when dealt with 'sympathetically' by the British media, people with AIDS have been presented as the victims of rejection by gay friends, lovers, and family (and not by governments, hospitals, and employers) and have been made to speak as guilty victims of past misdeeds (Watney 1987:124). James Jones' (1987:188) study of United States television drama notes how 'sympathetic' portrayals reinforce traditional scenarios:

> By placing the character within this largely heterosexual situation, the TV dramas create a discourse in which the character becomes the victim. The victim testifies as to the tragedy set upon him by forces beyond his control. He pleads for understanding and for acceptance ... hoping for a sympathetic ear. But the position of supplicant reinforces the status quo which maintains a separation between the heterosexual and the homosexual.

Jones (1987:196) observes that in stage plays, where gay writers have had some access, 'the gay person retains his individual humanity as well as his membership in the gay community, a realm which remains beyond the television screen.'

In addition to this sex-family complex, AIDS discourse is thoroughly riven by a fundamental structural opposition between guilt and innocence, a signification inextricably connected with self and other, and with power and powerlessness.[1] As Jonathan Elford (1987:545) writes, and has been widely noted elsewhere (Altman 1986:25; Watney 1987:33; Herdt 1987:1), 'disease transmission was often described as being from the culpable (gay men) to the blameless (women, haemophiliacs, recipients of blood transfusions) and ... scant attention was paid to the plight of those gay men with the disease.' Mapped over this deep structure is a moral/sexual hierarchy, identified by Gayle Rubin (1984:281), which ranges sexual activities and persons on a scale of virtue and vice. This symbolic system is further overlaid by a domino theory of contagion which postulates the disease progressing from the right-side categories to the left (table 1).

The 'risk groups' named by the United States Centers for Disease Control (CDC) have been inevitably interpreted against this semiologi-

TABLE 1. A domino theory of contagion

Theory	Categories		
Domino theory	Heterosexual men Good women Children	Bisexuals Prostitutes Loose women	Homosexuals Drug users Africans Haitians
Rubin's hierarchy	Heterosexual Married Monogamous Procreative Free Coupled In relationship Same generation At home No pornography Bodies only Vanilla	Homosexual In sin Promiscuous Nonprocreative For money Alone or in groups Casual Cross-generational In the park Pornography With manufactured objects SM	
Deep structure	Innocence Self Power	Guilt Other Powerlessness	

cal system. While the risk groups (homosexual men, IV drug users, Haitians, their sexual partners, recipients of blood products) came about as an initial orientation to the early data when the nature of AIDS was entirely unknown, the categories have lived on, even after the epidemiological evidence has provided a clear profile of a transmissible agent, probably Human Immunodeficiency Virus (HIV), which is semen- and blood-borne. By postulating types of persons instead of routes of transmission, the CDC has given rise to a set of popular ideas which have been purveyed in the media from time to time and repeated back to AIDS information workers. These ideas include: Only homosexuals get AIDS, or Anal sex causes AIDS. (This also has given rise to an odd set of writing on the 'strong vagina' and the 'weak anus.') The postulation of a Haitian risk group, in particular, masked a largely heterosexual transmission route, and the numbers of heterosexual people with AIDS jumped suddenly when the CDC abolished the Haitian category as a result of protests from Haiti and from Haitians in the United States.

This set of symbolic associations has also tended to anchor AIDS perceptions in the 'gay plague' complex, where the symbolic constructions of drugs and race have contributed little to the AIDS image and people with AIDS from the nongay risk groups have, in turn, tended to be rendered invisible to both their antagonists and to service agencies who would offer support. With the mid-1980s comparative decline of AIDS among gay men and rise among other groups which include disproportionate numbers of black and hispanic peoples both inside the United States and in the third world, it is an open question whether racial issues will shift the meaning of the syndrome in the future.

This discursive system controls and conceals a number of ambiguities, complexities, and alternative interpretations:

- Two conditions must be met for an AIDS diagnosis: (1) the patient must receive a positive result on an HIV-antibody test; and (2) the patient must suffer from one or more of the 'opportunistic infections' listed by the Centers for Disease Control in Atlanta. In other words, AIDS is the most serious manifestation of the spectrum of symptoms associated with HIV disease. After ten years of experience with this disease, the best medical findings point to about half of seropositive people going on to meet the AIDS definition after ten years. As of yet, it is not clear how many more will progress to AIDS or remain stable with more minor symptoms.
- Despite a clear pattern of transmission established from epidemiological research, there remains a possibility that HIV is not the 'cause' of AIDS, at least not the only cause, but is one of several factors (Duesberg 1987). This casts further doubt on the use of the HIV antibody test as an 'AIDS test.'
- AIDS control, then, is a question of avoiding contact between your bloodstream and the blood or semen of another person, and means providing people with the information and technical means of doing so.
- Various options remain open to people. Besides avoiding sex altogether, a range of 'safe' or 'safer' sex practices remain. Condoms properly used can make vaginal and anal sex 'safer sex.' Research into sexuality and public health suggests that the traditional 'family-or-chastity' choice is ineffective in disease control. Besides Brandt's study, rates of teenage and unwanted pregnancy, and rates of marital infidelity point to the ineffectiveness of a policy which has been

> promoted, after all, for centuries. The stress on monogamy is misleading in that an infected person entering a monogamous relationship will not reduce his or her risk and may endanger the other person. Conversely, safe sex practised with multiple partners should pose little or no risk of infection.

These propositions rupture the conflation of sex with STDs and deconstruct sex itself into a range of pleasurable practices thereby separating AIDS out from the grand moral schemes. Taboos against naming and thus acknowledging erotic variation enforce the chastity-or-family choice and guard against migration from sexual orthodoxy by installing a fear of the unknown at the site of the unspoken sensualities. The refusal to speak about safer sex establishes a secure terrain for blanket moralism. The dissemination of sexual how-to information risks disrupting the sex-STD elision by offering people the means to express their own particular sexualities.

To draw another analogy from the history of contraception, we might replace the 'refusal of motherhood' with the 'pursuit of homoeroticism' to see how prepackaged scripts about sex and gender can be revived to do new service for AIDS. In characterizing the position of the opponents to contraception, Gordon (1976:149) remarks:

> In refusal of motherhood, it seems personal and ideological feminism were joined: women's unnatural and false yearnings were threatening the entire race.

The State and Public Policy

AIDS thought then has flowed into pre-existing channels structured by a taken-for-granted symbolic universe. Increasingly the practical deconstructionists who would chip away or even upset the discursive edifice have found themselves at the peripheries of a world-view in the process of hegemonization by the state. The strength of AIDS language is not due to imminence, reason, or inevitability, but to concrete political forces. In the mid-1980s, legislative bodies in the United States, the United Kingdom, and Canada have been moving to guarantee a particular AIDS story through formal regimes of censorship and through funding the educational agencies which would promote the official story.

Most notable in this trend is the 14 October 1987 United States congressional ban on the 'use of federal funds for educational projects or materials that promote or encourage, directly or indirectly, homosexual sexual activity' (Bull 1987:1). That this law is intended to prevent safer-sex information which assesses the danger or safety of various sexual activities is clear from the debate where Republican congressmen brandished (privately funded) leaflets produced by community-based AIDS organizations and declared them 'obscene.' In February 1988, the British parliament moved to ban the 'promotion' or teaching of the 'acceptability of homosexuality as a pretended family relationship' and rescinded the right of municipalities to fund gay-related organizations or projects (Pincus 1988:1). Its own public service announcements stressed AIDS fear and the 'just-so' story where family life is the antidote to disease (Watney 1987: epilogue). A Canadian government bill, which died on the order paper in 1989, would have prevented health educators from:

- counseling the use of condoms during anal intercourse since all 'encouragement' of anal sex is forbidden, whether safe or unsafe;
- mentioning that masturbation or ejaculation upon a person are safe-sex practices as both are forbidden;
- pointing out that the use of erotica/pornography is itself a no-risk expression of sexuality as it is banned altogether.

The bill forces the accused to establish that any 'matter' has 'an educational, scientific or medical purpose' thereby potentially subjecting AIDS education organizations to have to justify every publication, communication, and seminar while the courts strike a 'balance of probabilities' among the 'erotic,' 'pornographic,' 'artistic,' 'educational,' and 'scientific' aspects of each item. The bill also denies absolutely the educational/scientific/medical defense to sex education material directed to those under the age of eighteen. At the same time, school curricula have been prepared which decry 'promiscuity' while remaining mute on safer-sex and which stress the safety of monogamy and the fallibility of condoms (Kinsman 1987:4).

British and Canadian Customs have also been inclusive in their interpretation of obscenity:

> Safe sex guidelines and letters about safe sex experiences are routinely censored from magazines aimed at gay men. Even advertisements for condoms are somehow construed to be

> depictions of anal intercourse and are therefore blanked out of Canadian editions of some magazines. (Armstrong 1986: 1–2)

While censors have consistently suppressed popular and explicit talk about sex in favor of clinical descriptions, AIDS educators strongly suspect that the former literature is far more widely distributed, more easily understood, and influential. They have sought to use it to popularize the safer-sex message. Research done by Michael Quadlund and associates (1987) has shown that men shown erotic films featuring safer-sex activities made the greatest changes in their sexual behavior compared to men exposed to other educational techniques. The state, at the same time, suppresses popular forms and texts which disrupt the official story.

With traditionalist script in place, the HIV-antibody test presents an almost irresistibly attractive technological fix to the AIDS problem. By reconstructing the procedure as an 'AIDS test,' mandatory HIV-antibody testing and quarantine arise as central tools in AIDS control. The United States president, in his only public address on AIDS, called in 1987 for 'mandatory HIV testing for federal prisoners, potential immigrants and possibly for patients in Veterans Administration hospitals.' Reagan also suggested that states consider routine testing for marriage license applicants and state and local prisoners (Westheimer 1987:1). The United States military was by then already testing all of its members. Colorado authorized quarantine for those who fail to '"cease and desist" [in] behavior believed to be "dangerous" by public health officials' (Poggi 1987:1). Illinois mandated quarantine of HIV+ people through a court order, as well as marriage testing, required testing of those convicted of sex and drug offenses, mandatory reporting of HIV+ children to school superintendents, and safe-sex education limited to 'preaching abstinence until marriage' (Botkin 1987:3). Minnesota required 'forcible testing and quarantine of people who show a "careless disregard" for the transmission of AIDS' (Halfhill 1987:1) and an HIV+ prisoner in that state was convicted of 'assault with a deadly weapon' for biting a guard. British Columbia authorized quarantine by order of a medical officer of health (Kinsman 1988:4). In Ottawa, Halifax, and Calgary, people with HIV disease have been jailed on the grounds that others have been or may have been exposed through their blood donations or having sex.[2] The trend among public health authorities in the late 1980s has been to demand the right to detain forcibly and without trial those seropositive people whom they regard a 'irresponsible' (see *American Journal of Public Health* 79 [1989] n.7).

On Democracy and Social Control

The major constituency for alternative discourses on AIDS is the community-based organizations devoted to offering personal and practical support to people with AIDS and to disseminating safer-sex information and techniques. Most of the community groups in North America and the United Kingdom originated in the periods of silence and hysteria about AIDS, and have evolved into alliances of gay and nongay members as increasing numbers of women, blacks, and hispanics have joined, as well as people with backgrounds in volunteer, medical, and social service work. The community organizations have generally involved a great many people lacking the luxury of believing themselves beyond infection and who, therefore, have found no place for themselves in the traditional discourse which assigns AIDS to the guilty Other. Though by no means unitary in their approaches, the community groups have been central in generating practical and emancipatory understandings of empowering themselves to resist AIDS.

Governments have displayed considerable ambivalence when faced with the community groups. Especially conservative governments, such as British Columbia and Queensland, have denied any public money to community work. Texas preferred having the Houston Institute for Immunological Disorders close, rather than offer it support once its AIDS patients ran out of money for medical care. In other cases, community groups have received 'soft money' through government grants, though the sums pale in comparison to funding granted specifically for AIDS to the established public health and social welfare sector which became interested in AIDS with the appearance of government money.

Government funding poses new problems for community groups. Safer-sex information must be typically financed from local fundraising and apart from government money. Like the contraception movement, AIDS groups experience a 'pull' toward the official version of AIDS and face the possibility of redirection. While many early contraception activists went to jail in the early part of the century for distributing how-to information, the movement eventually made a transformation to respectability by shifting focus from 'birth control' to 'family planning' and by withdrawing information to unmarried people (Gordon 1976:365). Like other community groups before them when faced with the prospect of state funding, AIDS organizations are subject to internal dissension and problems of patronage and cronyism in allocating money. There is no lack of precedent for social and health reformers being displaced or converted into social control agents doing the work of the state. In several major cities, new activist groups in 1987 and 1988 have sprung up to confront public officials on slow drug testing and quarantine legislation.

The fundamental issue underlying the AIDS debates of the 1980s is: who has the right to make sexual choices? Traditional conservative forces, whether based in the church, state, or 'patriarchy,' seem more than a little reluctant to cede the power to be sexual (including homosexual) to the masses, but would rather have it done surreptitiously and have its practitioners 'suffer the consequences.' The psycho-scenario is familiar to analysts of unwanted pregnancy. Contraception is not used when 'it is easier to deal with guilt about sex by viewing one's adventures as one-time-only slips, promptly repented – over and over' (Gordon 1976:407). The issue has been run through once in the closing of bathhouses in major cities. While community AIDS groups often (but not always) saw bathhouses as vehicles for offering safer-sex information and condoms, empowering gay men to make sexual decisions which avoid AIDS transmission, local authorities saw bathhouses as sites of uncontrollable sex and contagion (see Collier 1985).

Much of the educational issue has been not just one of talking about sex but also of providing the means for individuals to take control of their sexuality by being able to separate it from reproduction and disease. Framing it in ethical terms, Ronald Bayer, Carol Levine, and Susan Wolf (1986:1769) postulate that 'individuals be treated as autonomous agents who have the right to control their own destinies.' For community organizations, whose participants are closest to the affliction itself, AIDS control is a question of the most pragmatic and effective means of preserving themselves, their friends, and their community from rapid death without sacrificing erotic bonding. It is, says Jonathan Silin (1987:34), 'an emancipatory vision focusing on the ability of *each* to choose and fulfill his / her ambitions rather than a managerial one, concerned with the control of behaviour.'

Acknowledgment

The paper was first presented to the Workshop on Feminism, Critical Theory, and the Canadian Legal System and the Canadian Sociology and Anthropology Association meeting with the Learned Societies of Canada, Windsor, Ontario, and then revised for the 'Representing AIDS' conference at the University of Western Ontario in London, Canada.

NOTES

1 For further discussion of these associations, see 'The Politics of Guilt and Guilt Expiation Rituals' in Adam (1978).

2 To date, only Cuba has been reported to have instituted mandatory quarantine for all HIV+ people, a move consistent with the concentration camps it set up for homosexuals in the 1960s. On legal aspects of quarantine, see Parmet (1985:53). Collier (1985:301), Nichols (1984:315). All agree that quarantine is illegitimate.

REFERENCES

Adam, B. 1978. *The Survivial of Domination*, New York: Elsevier / Greenwood

– 1987. *The Rise of a Gay and Lesbian Movement*. Boston: G.K. Hall / Twayne

Altman, D. 1986. *AIDS in the Mind of America.* Garden City, NY: Anchor

Armstrong, R. 1986. 'Customs Bans AIDS Information.' *Censorship Bulletin* 5 (Winter) 1–2

Bayer, R. 1985. 'AIDS and the Gay Community.' *Social Research* 52 (3) 581

Bayer, R., C. Levine, and S. Wolf. 1986. 'HIV Antibody Screening.' *Journal of the American Medical Association* 236 (13) 1769

Botkin, M. 1987. 'Thompson Signs Quarantine Bill.' *Gay Community News* 15 (12) 3

Brandt, A. 1985. *No Magic Bullet.* New York: Oxford University Press

Bull, Ch. 1987. 'Congress Guts AIDS Education.' *Gay Community News* 15 (15) 1

Collier, S. 1985. 'Preventing the Spread of AIDS by Restricting Sexual Conduct in Gay Bathhouses.' *Golden Gate University Law Review* 15: 301

'The Constitutional Rights of AIDS Carriers.' *Harvard Law Review* 99 (1986, 6) 1274

Duesberg, P. 1987. 'Retroviruses as Carcinogens and Pathogens.' *Cancer Research* 47 (March 1) 1188

Elford, J. 1987. 'Moral and Social Aspects of AIDS.' *Social Science and Medicine* 24 (6) 543

Foucault, M. 1978. *The History of Sexuality.* Vol 1. New York: Pantheon

– 1979. *Discipline and Punish.* New York: Vintage

– 1980. *Power / Knowledge.* New York: Pantheon

Gordon, L. 1976. *Woman's Body, Woman's Right.* New York: Grossman

Gusfield, J. 1963. *Symbolic Crusade.* Urbana: University of Illinois

– 1981. *The Culture of Public Problems.* University of Chicago Press

Halfhill, R. 1987. 'Minn. Opts for Quarantine.' *Gay Community News* 14 (46) 1

Herdt, G. 1987. 'AIDS and Anthropology.' *Anthropology Today* 3 (2) 1
Jones, J. 1987. 'The Sick Homosexual.' In *Current Issues.* Proceedings of the International Scientific Conference on Gay and Lesbian Studies, Amsterdam
Kinsman, G. 1988. 'Quarantine Legislation Passed in B.C.' *Rites* 4 (8) 4
– 1987. *The Regulation of Desire.* Montreal: Black Rose
– 1987. 'Ontario Misinformation About AIDS.' *Rites* 4 (7) 4
Nichols, Ch. 1984. 'AIDS – A New Reason to Regulate Homosexuality?' *Journal of Contemporary Law* 11 (1) 315
Parmet, W. 1985. 'AIDS and Quarantine.' *Hofstra Law Review* 14 (1) 53
Patton, C. 1985. *Sex and Germs.* Boston: South End
Pincus, E. 1988. 'God Save the Queers.' *Gay Community News* 15 (32) 1
Poggi, S. 1987. 'Colo. Mandates AIDS Reporting.' *Gay Community News* 14 (43) 1
Poirier, G. 1987. 'Public Forum Votes Canadian Ads the Worst.' *Rites* 4 (1) 8
Quadlund, M. et al. 1987. *The 800 Men Study.* New York
Rubin, G. 1984. 'Thinking Sex.' In C. Vance, ed, *Pleasure and Danger.* Boston: Routledge & Kegan Paul
Silin, J. 1987. 'Dangerous Knowledge.' *Christopher Street* 113: 34
Watney, S. 1987. *Policing Desire.* London: Comedia.
Westheimer, K. 1987. 'Reagan to Force HIV Testing.' *Gay Community News* 14 (45) 1

Sacrificial Sex

ARTHUR KROKER

So, that is what we have then. Two orders of sexuality at the end of the world: cynical sex and sacrificial sex as indifferent signs of the body in ruins (see plates 59, 60, following p 239).

Cynical sex is sex without secretions. The dark dreamworld of all the California technicists who, in flight from the retroviruses of body invaders and under the impact of the neo-fascistic politics of Body McCarthyism, speak longingly now of a telematic body, a cyber-body, technified to such a degree of abstraction and intensity that it becomes a virtual body. And sacrificial sex? That is the emblematic sign of the postmodern panic body at the fin-de-millénium – just that point where sex re-enters the dark domain of mythology and is spoken of now in the ritualistic language of surrogate sacrifice and victimization.

In an earlier meditation on panic sex in America, I talked of the existence of a cynical sex, a sex without secretions, which had about it the empty quality of Foucault's cynical power. One of the conditions of its acceptability was precisely the limits it placed on human freedom, a power made all the more seductive because it occluded consciousness of its own cynicism.

And a cynical sex, too, which had as one of its conditions of acceptability that sex now would have no existence other than an empty sign onto which could be inscribed all of the seductions and vampiric imaging associated with designer representations of sex. In fact, a virtual sex in the age of cyber-punk where computer-imaging technology did for the sex organs what it had previously done for the eyes and hands and even personalities. You know, like those new cyber-beings generated in the laboratories of California or Boston, where when you wear a simu-skull (a designer helmet that substitutes virtual vision for normal ocular vision) and simu-hands (cyber-fingers for moving around in the irreal world of virtual space), you acquire the possibility of projecting multiple schizoid personalities outwards simultaneously, and, why not, multiple sex organs for the age when sex comes under the sign of virtual satisfaction and virtual desire. Not waterworks as much as simu-works: a virtual penis, virtual vagina, and even now an exteriorized glass womb for the body telematic. Sex without secretions, therefore, as the dreamworld of the body cybernetic: the body where William Gibson's *Neuromancer* comes alive as an actual model of a cybernetic culture in which the body drifts away from itself into the matrix of cyberspace. Here, the mind is on its way to being exteriorized, the dominant mode of exchange is proscribed biologicals for the body half-flesh/half-metal, the real world is data, and the old male cock has one last half-life jacking off into cyberspace. The body in cyberspace, then, is meat after the fall, a kind of outlaw zone, a deliberately unsupervised playground for technological experimentation, where technology as virus subordinates the body as servomechanism to the threefold biological logic of viral invasion, replication of its genetic code, and cloning.

Or is it just the opposite? Not so much the invasion of the body by technology as virus, but the contamination of technology by the human virus. The whole psychopathic intensity of predatory-like behaviour at the fin-de-millénium blown into technology, and from there blowing out across the mediascape. Sacrificial technology, therefore, where it is no longer technology as domination of a passive human species, but the domination of technology to the point of its victimization by predator / parasites living on the dark mythic side of the postmodern condition. A virtual world, therefore, where we live on the edge of a postmodern subjectivity that is colonized by telematic images of the cyborg body and that takes its vengeance by reducing technology to a sacrificial scapegoat.

A virtual sexuality, then, which works to place limits on our knowledge of bodily fluids as a viral contaminant, a kind of parasite/predator, racing/tracing across the postmodern field of our bodies. Here, cynical sex for the body telematic has one last function as the transgression that confirms the disappearance of natural sexuality into the discourse of sexuality, and then the vanishing of seduction as the key sign of discursive sexuality into simulation, and finally, at the end of the millennium, the appearance of a fourth order of sexuality for the postmodern condition: sacrificial sex.

Sacrificial sex? That is the flip side of cynical sex. Not sex without secretions as the simulated sign of the death of seduction at the end of the world, but the regression of sexuality itself now into a final spasmodic phase of originary violence and the desperate search for sacrificial victims, what Bruce Jackson calls the 'killable other.' The existence of sacrificial victims depends on two preconditions: first, their subjectivity, their bodily existence, must be ethically exterminated so that they are 'disappeared' (as South Americans would say) as a site of communal moral responsibility; and second, they must be translated into the privileged and fantasized object of the revenge-seeking will as surrogate victims whose 'disappeared' moral subjectivity makes their bodies a free-fire zone for all the revenge-seeking displacements of the ruined social order. Sacrificial victims, like persons living with AIDS, whose bodies can be targeted as privileged repositors of individual responsibility for all of the public anxieties of the social – its intense fear of viral contamination reflected by the panic search now for the drug-free body, the virus-free body; and who can simultaneously serve as sacrificial displacements, actually mythical expiations, for all of the violence and vicissitudes of the revenge-seeking will.

Anyway it was predictable. In *Violence and the Sacred*, René Girard talked about the formation of sacrificial culture as the founding, generative act of violence, the serial act of violence, in Western culture. For Girard, sacrifice can be the genetic code of Western culture because it fuses a desperate fear of nature and social nature with a primitive displacement of this fear onto chosen scapegoats, sacrificial victims, who serve simultaneously as sublimated communal representatives tracing on their bodies all of the contradictions, anxieties, and guilt of the social, and as privileged sacrificial sites to allay the furies of mythic recurrence. These killable others are in the mythic sense monstrous doubles: part victim, part symbolic representative, part sacrificial host, part fantasized threat, part objects of metaphoric language to excess, part real bodily suffering.

With this difference, however. In just the same way that Pietr Sloterdij has remarked in the *Critique of Cynical Reason* that cynicism in the postmodern condition exists now only in its reversed and opposite form (not any longer the original 'kynicism' as philosophy, rebellion, from below, but cynicism now as truth-telling by the ruling élites who deny they can act otherwise); so too classical sacrifice now also has been reversed. No longer sacrifice in the classical sense of ritualized victimization to appease the gods, but postmodern sacrifice as a whole panic scene of an empty ritualized displacement of ressentiment over our own botched and bungled instincts onto a mean-spirited search for the 'killable other': the sacrificial victim, like the AIDS sufferer, who can be so immediately scapegoated because the virally contaminated body now is the privileged site of a threefold displacement on ideological, political, and psychological grounds.

1. Ideologically, for example, people with AIDS can be chosen sacrificial victims because AIDS is now an inscribed political siting for a twofold crisis tendency of the middle class, the class that typically defines public policy in the short term. In a superb essay, 'Anxiety and Politics,' written in German after he had fled the Nazis, the theorist Franz Neumann prophesied that intense bourgeois anxiety would soon give rise to an ideology of salvation. A frantic need to save (that is, to 'justify' in a religious sense) the authoritarian personality would result in a neo-fascistic search for a strong political leader, while a no less urgent drive to satisfy the revenge-seeking will would lead to the victimization of the weak, the poor, and the sick. For Neumann, the bourgeoisie exists today under the intense pressure of two moments of anxiety: an outer anxiety, marked economically by fears of loss of disposable income and thus their privileged class position (marked biologically now by panic fear of the contamination of the body by viral invaders); and an inner anxiety distinguished by the classic syndrome that when the bourgeois self retreats into its interiority to find refuge from a threatening external situation, it finds only a vacated ego, a sense of identity that has long ago been exteriorized, actually ablated, in the ideological constitution of the bourgeois self. In times of acute public and personal crisis, when history and autobiography co-mingle, when the outer anxiety meets the inner anxiety, the political outcome is the re-emergence of the neo-fascistic authoritarian personality to the tune of 'Don't worry, be happy': a grisly politics of psychological discharge into the public situation marked by a ruthless search for sacrificial scapegoats onto whose bodies can be displaced anxieties over the threatening external and internal situations; the recuperation of sadism towards the weak and the marginal; the election of political leaders who mirror the revenge-seeking will of the masses by assuming the position of predator-parasite (like Ronald Reagan first, followed by the weak force of George Bush); and the

creation of a whole frenzied public scene where ruined America, with its population leaking contaminated bodily fluids, re-energizes itself by constantly reversing field and seeking out new sacrificial scapegoats.

2. Politically, the ultimate result of the reappearance of Neumann's ideology in waiting is the resurfacing in North America of Body McCarthyism: which is not like McCarthyism of the 1950s where political discourse was reduced to the fundamentalism of loyalty oaths, but is a new kind of fundamentalism where political discourse is reduced to the purity of your bodily fluids.

A urinal politics, therefore, which this time on the terrain of bodily fluids rather than loyalty oaths insists on the (unattainable) ideal of absolute purity of the body's circulatory exchanges as the new gold standard of an immunological discourse. Less a traditional style of McCarthyism, with its refusal of political pluralism and its insistence on absolute commitments to America as the new Holy Community, than a hyper-McCarthyism of the fin-de-millénium, with its biological vision of the fundamentalist body: a hyperdeflation of the body to the quality of its internal fluids.

A urinal politics would be one that privileges the body anew as the target of the power of the panopticon, sublimates anxieties about the catastrophe without onto the body as a text for an immunological discourse, and speaks the discourse of clean bodily fluids with such evangelical zeal because, like the radiating waves from a long past explosion of a gigantic supernova, it has only now reached the telematic sensors of Planet One. The rhetoric of clean bodily fluids is really about the disappearance of the body into the detritus of toxic bodies. It reflects the fractal subjectivity, cultural dyslexia, drug-induced terror, and simulation-is-all mentality of the postmodern condition. The intense fascination with sanitizing the bodily fluids is also a *trompe l'œil* deflecting the gaze from the actual existence of the contaminated body towards the ludicrous ideal of clean urination for the nation. Yet the existence of the contaminated body depends, ironically, on the polluting conditions of the high-intensity market society – a telematic society in which bodily fluids become obsolete in so far as they are treated as surplus matter.

As the insurgent basis of urinal politics in contemporary America, the desperate rhetoric of clean bodily fluids signals the existence of the postmodern body as missing matter in the cyberspace of a society dominated by its own violent implosion in loss, cancellation, and parasitism. Body McCarthyism is, then, a biologically driven politics in which the strategies and powers of society come to be invested in the question of the transmission of bodily fluids and which, if inspired by the conservative and deflationary vision of the fundamentalist body, also feeds parasitically on generalized panic about the breakdown of the immunological systems of contemporary society. It is a hygienic politics that can be immediately powerful because it is deeply mythological, and it *is* powerful because, as the body is recycled in the language of medieval mythology, political control over it becomes intensely localized and subjective. In the Middle Ages sin was the sign of the body in ruins. Now, however, the fallen body is mythologized by a whole panic scene of secreting, leaking bodies exposed on (and for) the hysteria-inducing media.

Ultimately, the politics of Body McCarthyism, which is motivated by panic fear of viral contamination, is steered by a eugenic ideology: William F. Buckley, in a further outbreak of the fascist mind, demands the tattooing of AIDS victims. Body McCarthyism, moreover, responds to a double crisis moment: the crisis without as the breakdown of the immunological order in economy (panic finance), culture (panic media), and the body (panic genetics); and the crisis within as the existential breakdown of the postmodern mind into a panic scene when the realization grows that Lacanian misrecognition is the basis of the bourgeois ego (the substitution, that is, in the postmodern bourgeois mind at its mirror stage of an illusory, fictive, panic identity for a principle of concrete identity). Body McCarthyism focuses on the illusory search for the perfect immune system and inscribes on the body of the PWA a whole scene of panic medicine. The body of the PWA becomes like Foucault's illusory but ideologically fantasized individual before it: a silent sign of the body in ruins – interpellated by warring medical languages; colonized by revenge-seeking ideologies; inscribed by a thousand metaphors; policed by the disciplinary therapeutics of a cynical state. What emerges is a whole cynical scene of media hystericizations and political scapegoating where the sacrificial victim, the AIDS sufferer, is ethically suppressed into silence in order to be offered up in sacrifice repeatedly to the revenge-seeking will.

3. If Body McCarthyism is the ideological sign of sacrificial sex, then psychologically the age of sacrificial sex is driven onwards by Nietzsche's slave morality as the dominant form of public consciousness

at the fin-de-millénium. For Nietzsche, majoritarian opinion in the last triumphant days of history in ruins would be a doubled sense of slave morality, typified by passive deference to authority, and contempt to the point of oppressing the weak and powerless as a kind of cruel sport. In a culture marked by a 'strong sense of self, but a weak ego,' slave morality is the psychological fuel feeding a grisly recurrence of gay bashing, and an ethical indifference to the point of 'viciousness for fun' against the victims of AIDS. Here, we see once more that a sexual politics based on the 'pleasure of sadism' directed against the gay-community specifically, and against AIDS victims more generally, has finally made its way across the Atlantic from Europe in ruins to be the distinguishing force of the politics of ressentiment. In the politics of ressentiment, therefore, we can detect a double complicity between the active nihilists and the passive nihilists. The active nihilists are our 'creative leaders,' who, knowing that there is no longer any substantive purpose to their willing, would prefer to go on acting – whether sacrificially or suicidally – rather than not to act at all. They are the perfect emblems of Nietzsche's 'will to will to will.' Their accomplices, the passive nihilists, are the growing majority of slave moralists, who used to want no more than entertainment and would blink at anything remotely serious. But now, if shows like Morton Downey's recently cancelled TV celebration of nihilism in LA is to be believed, they are beginning to seek revenge for their own botched and bungled instincts by engaging in simulated orgies of collective fury against sacrificial scapegoats.

How, then, does our society deal with the threat of mythic recurrence? Not by sacrificial renunciation, as in the Middle Ages, but by sacrificial excess. The fetishistic act of selecting a surrogate victim of the day serves to appease the bad conscience of slave morality. In slave morality the monstrous double goes inside. No longer is Marx's priest the inner calculative spirit of bourgeois society: now it is grisly ressentiment fuelled by our own knowledge of ourselves as predator-parasites in the postmodern scene. And that is why our society *must* have surrogate victims onto whose bodies can be inscribed all the suppressed violence of the retrashed fascism that passes for advanced capitalist culture.

Greetings then to the survivors of sacrificial culture from shamanistic theory! A shamanistic theory that seeks to provoke once again rituals of mourning as a way of meditating upon the intimations of deprivation in the post-catastrophe that is sacrificial culture.

Sacrificial sex
Sacrificial art
Sacrificial commodification
Sacrificial fashion
Sacrificial death

That's the subjectivity of the sacrificial body: the body in ruins as it re-enters the domain of panic mythology, and is reinscribed by the whole dark, but retrashed, mythical languages of exclusion, victimization, sacralization, fantasization, scapegoatism, and ritualistic displacement at the end of the world. The second recovery of mythology, then, is as panic mythology for the panicked body that alternates between the victim positions of predator and scapegoat.

The Possibilities of Permutation: Pleasure, Proliferation, and the Politics of Gay Identity in the Age of AIDS

SIMON WATNEY

for George Cant and Tony Whitehead

> Safer sex was above all a form of resistance developed by gay men acting in micro-networks linked by their own newspapers in an imagined national and international community.
>
> Cindy Patton[1]

> There's a battle for and around history going on at this very moment which is extremely interesting. The intention is to stifle what I've called the 'popular memory,' and also to propose and impose on people a framework in which to interpret the present.
>
> Michel Foucault[2]

Introduction

In his preface to the 1957 edition of *The Book of Imaginary Beings*, Jorge Luis Borges distinguishes between 'the zoo of reality' populated by named, discrete species, and 'the zoo of mythologies ... whose denizens are not lions but sphinxes and griffons and centaurs. The population of this second zoo should exceed by far the population of the first since a monster is no more than a combination of parts of real beings, and the possibilities of permutation border on the infinite.'[3] From its origins, sexology has offered a similar potential for the proliferation of sexual identities, grounded in the specialized pleasures of the body. For example, as is well known, Krafft-Ebing's *Psycho-*

pathia Sexualis grew 'from 45 case histories and 110 pages in 1886 to 238 histories and 437 pages by the 12th edition of 1903.'[4] Weeks, Foucault, and many others have charted the emergence of the modern categories of sexuality, defined in relation to what Freud termed 'object-choice,' that is, 'the act of selecting a person or type of person as love-object.'[5] Choice, in this context, is not to be understood as conscious or deliberate, but an irrevocable and determining aspect or potential of an individual's unconscious being.

How object-choice enters consciousness is contingent upon a multitude of social, cultural, and psychic factors. Sexual object-choice thus furnishes the grounds for identity, but is not a natural or inevitable identity in or of itself. Moreover, as Laplanche and Pontalis have pointed out, there is a significant difference between the notion of object-choice in relation to *individuals* (eg one's father, one's wife), and object-choice in relation to *types* of people (eg homosexual, heterosexual).[6] It is in this latter sense that object-choice has been narrowed into the categories of sexuality, as a system of knowledge, which should not be confused with actual sexual behaviour. Sexual anthropology demonstrates the extraordinary diversity of ways in which different societies estimate what is 'correct' sexual behaviour for women and men. Yet it seems that it is only in the West, and in comparatively recent times, that object-choice has been so rigidly socially codified, and has taken on such a central role in relation to fundamental notions of the Self, and of collective social identity.

For almost two millennia, Christian metaphysics offered a picture of the soul and its place in Creation that was not, in this modern sense, an identity at all. Yet as Christianity lost its grip on the institutions that possess the power to define 'human nature,' other systems of knowledge emerged with alternative but no less universalizing claims to provide the base for our sense of Self. Class, science, race, gender, sexuality, and nationality have all competed to provide 'totalizing' identities in the past hundred years, though in practice most people will identify with several, or all, of these available categories of self-knowing in ways that are frequently conflicting. Thus a black British lesbian may experience sexual prejudice in the black community, racial prejudice amongst other lesbians, and xenophobia elsewhere in her life. However, sexuality has increasingly dominated Western notions of identity, though as Carole S. Vance has noted, 'in traditional sexual science, heterosexuality remains an unexamined and naturalized category, and little in popular culture causes heterosexuals to consider their sexual identity or its origins and history.'[7] It is in this context that we should consider the vagaries of the categories available to women and men whose object-choice is homosexual. In all of this it remains helpful to distinguish between homosexual *desire* and the many ways in which it has been lived in the modern period. The late nineteenth century offered a proliferation of 'explanations' and identities, from the 'third sex' hypothesis of Karl Ulrichs, with its biologistic base, to the more strictly 'scientific' theories of Krafft-Ebing and Karoly Benkert, who invented the category of 'the homosexual.'[8] This was not however intended as a medical category – though its formulation accords with the wider contemporary discursive framework of sexology – but was 'placed in a political/juridical context that had nothing to do with medicine or psychiatry.'[9]

The invention of sexuality, with its binary distinction homosexual/heterosexual, was thus a tactical strategy on the part of the homosexual' theorists. Their strategy was subsequently appropriated by the institutions of medicine, psychiatry, and the law, which pathologized 'homosexuality' and naturalized and de-historicized 'heterosexuality' in order to undermine the original, pluralist, social implications of these terms. None the less, the homosexual/heterosexual distinction has never been uniformly accepted without resistance, and subcultural groupings organized around the shared experience of homosexual desire continue to provide local nomenclatures and identities. Furthermore, it is far from clear that 'heterosexuality' should properly be regarded as an *identity*: rather it is an ideology, characterized precisely by its taken-for-grantedness, save in exceptional circumstances. As I have observed elsewhere: 'Taking itself for granted, "heterosexuality" remains largely oblivious to its own object-choice, and is inhabited in a variety of ways, from the identities of parenting, of domesticity, of sexual fantasy, gender, and so on. It is only when the coherence of the ensemble of roles and relations that constitute "heterosexuality" are perceived to be at risk, that object-choice emerges as a primary term for individual identification – an identification moreover that is overwhelmingly negative, and defined by exclusions, repudiations, displacements and denials.'[10] Indeed, the psychology of sexuality is characterized by an overwhelming negativity. It is at this point that the emergence of gay identity reveals its full significance as a distinct refusal of the categories of sexuality. Again, as I have written elsewhere:

> Historically, 'the homosexual' has been incited to think of his core essence as a perverse negative of heterosexuality, which is

> taken as the norm right across the major discursive fields of sociology, anthropology, psychiatry, jurisprudence, politics, education, and psychoanalysis. The gay man, on the contrary, affirms his sexuality in a category which is fundamentally socio-political, and implies no intrinsic common factor with other gay men beyond the workings of power on the entire range of homosexual desire in all its variant forms, which are unified only in their collective affirmations of value and validity. This is quite different from the identity of 'the heterosexual,' for whom heterosexuality does not designate desire for the opposite sex, so much as a rejection and denial of homosexuality. Thus, homosexual identity involves a primary and self-abasing awareness of *not* being heterosexual, whilst heterosexual self-awareness involves an equally primary sense of *not* being homosexual.[11]

Gay identity thus offers a positive term for collective and individual experience that 'escapes the entire frame of reference, and the power relations invested within the epistemology ... of sexuality as such, which is simultaneously produced and policed in the negative persons of "the homosexual" and "the heterosexual."'[12]

Gay politics thus aims to recruit identities away from 'homosexuality,' whilst simultaneously promoting a theory of sexual diversity that can also challenge discrimination against particular sexual identities and practices. Hence the significance of gay identity: it presupposes a sexual politics that rejects 'the morality of [sexual] "acts" which has dominated sexual theorizing for hundreds of years ... in the direction of a new relational perspective which takes into account context and meanings.'[13] Gay politics aims to cut off object-choice from the ideological and political forces that have been so massively invested in it, via differential age-of-consent laws and other legislations founded on the institution of marriage considered as the only sacrosanct focus for adult sexual activity. Gay identity stands for the recognition and acknowledgment of *all* forms of consensual erotic and sexual behaviour. In place of a simple 'majority / minorities' model of sexuality, it offers a dynamic picture of affective and sexual relations that is highly sceptical concerning the monolithic categories of 'homosexuality' and 'heterosexuality' alike.

Hence the tension between this pluralistic, embrasive approach to sexual politics, and the more limited identities associated with particular sexual practices that have flourished under its permissive umbrella, threatening a return to the anomic proliferation of Krafft-Ebbing's late-nineteenth-century inventory of individual sexual 'perversions.' It was this danger that Foucault repeatedly addressed in his insistence that whilst we have to affirm human rights concerning sexuality: 'What we must work on ... is not so much to liberate our desires but to make ourselves infinitely susceptible to pleasure. We must escape and help others escape the two ready-made formulas of the pure sexual encounter and the lovers' fusion of identity.'[14] Foucault's sexual politics was consistently opposed to any notion that there exists an 'essence' of hidden or repressed sexual identity that might be 'liberated'; rather, he proposed a dynamic model that aspires to a far more open-ended and, as he emphasized, 'creative' relation between sexuality and the rest of one's being.[15] In this way the rigid moralism that is attached to the binary construction 'homosexual / heterosexual' might give way to a wholly new sexual ethics, together with an erotics that could effectively challenge what he saw as the miserably impoverished values and institutions that dominate Western notions of sexual satisfaction and affective relations.[16] In spite of its name, Gay Liberation seemed admirable and radical to Foucault precisely in its challenge to the authority of heterosexual models in same-sex relations, and its demand for relational rights that exceed sexuality as it is known, instituted, and fleshed out in individual lives.

At this point it is also necessary to consider HIV infection and disease in relation to the ways in which their emergence among gay men in the West has been widely interpreted as something intrinsic to gay identity. At the very moment at which gay politics seemed poised to strike a major challenge to the power relations of sexuality as a structure of knowledge and identities, HIV has been massively exploited to provide the pretext for an aggressive restatement of the authority of the ancient discourse of sexual 'acts.' HIV has also been used to justify the project of a would-be universal moralism that cunningly appropriates the crudest form of sexual naturalism to notions of 'public health,' which 'homosexuality' is held to threaten. This process aspires to nothing less than the wholesale reclassification of gay men as the voluntary, culpable inhabitants of a 'depraved' sexual underworld that cannot be sufficiently policed. In this manner epidemiology, virology, and immunology are harnessed to still potent premodern notions of contagion and sin, which in sexually puritanical societies such as Britain, Canada, and the United States provide the grounds for juridical initiatives that far exceed the worst nightmares of Ulrichs or Benkert concerning the criminalization of same-sex relations a hundred years ago.

For example, who could have imagined in the early 1980s that the British parliament would enthusiastically endorse new legislation in 1989, across party political lines, that forbids 'the promotion of homosexuality' by local government authorities, or that the U.S. Senate would in 1989 support similar new legislation that prevents all federal funding in the field of the arts for the production, distribution, and 'promotion' of 'obscene and indecent materials, including but not limited to depictions of sadomasochism, homoeroticism, the exploitation of children, or individuals engaged in sex acts'?[17] Such laws only serve to reveal the full extent to which sexual identity has now entered the foreground of ideological and political contestation in the West, and cannot be casually dismissed as 'marginal.' For what is ultimately at stake here is not only 'sexual freedom,' but the aggressive contemporary re-assertion of the categories of sexuality as the exclusive legitimate means by which women and men are to be officially permitted to identify their erotic needs, individually or collectively.

HIV Disease and Gay Identity

The distinguished American writer Robert Glück has described how 'AIDS creates such magnitudes of *loss* that now death is where gay men experience life most keenly as a group. It's where we learn about love, where we discover new values and qualities in ourselves.'[18] Writing in 1988, in the context of some 60,000 cases of AIDS in the United States, Glück noted how the increasing scale of the epidemic increases the fears of those most closely affected, whilst at the same time he personally felt 'less afraid, because of treatment and the "companionship" of so many normalizing factors, articulations, groups and institutions.' Since diagnosis means 'work and struggle,' AIDS 'has become a kind of career.'[19]

In societies where HIV was most widely transmitted among gay men before its existence was known or suspected, it is only from within the gay community, and the AIDS service organizations that it established, that we hear such powerful statements of the complex and conflicting day-to-day realities of HIV disease, as it is experienced by those who continue to be the most directly affected. This *collective* experience remains significantly absent in accounts of those same constituencies, viewed from the outside. For example, a recent full-page article in the *New York Times* describes how 'Gay men find sadness colors life as they make the most of their days.'[20] Journalist Dena Kleiman sets the picture: 'Nationwide the disease has been diagnosed in more than 57,000 men since it was first recognised in 1981. A majority of them have died and no one has been cured. But the worst is yet to come: studies indicate that hundreds of thousands of gay men, including a majority of gay men in some cities, including New York and San Francisco are infected with the AIDS virus. Medical experts predict that most of those infected will eventually develop severe illness. Over the years, the original shock has evolved into a kind of sad stoicism and dogged, even hopeful, determination.'[21] Kleiman interviewed a number of gay men living with HIV disease, with a resulting montage of gruelling personal accounts: 'You would think it would get easier. It doesn't'; 'Everything is tinged with a certain sadness'; 'My biggest fear is that what happened to David is going to happen to me'; and so on. The key term here is 'sadness,' announced in the article's headline, and repeated as its leitmotif: 'some gay men are ill, fighting an invisible invader and against time, frustrated by the pace of medical progress. Many more, still healthy, know they carry the AIDS virus, or might. Others have discovered that they are probably free of the virus. But all share the sadness.'[22] Unaccustomed to the rather more civilized 'humanist' values of much American journalism, British and other readers may initially find such commentary almost unimaginably sympathetic, in comparison to the routinely insensitive output of the British and other national print industries.

None the less, it is important to note the way in which the established conventional image of the supposedly powerless 'AIDS victim' survives within this new ideological framework of humanist pathos. For example, we learn nothing of the 'work and struggle' described by Robert Glück from *within* the gay community. Nor do we learn anything of the huge scale of national and international information exchange and political organizing associated with groups such as the AIDS Coalition To Unleash Power (ACT UP) that has played such a vital role in making new treatment drugs available to those in need, and in challenging bigotry at all levels of society. Instead, we find isolated individuals, and one couple, all presented as doomed and more or less hopeless, whilst biomedicine stands by, doing its limited best. Yet nobody interviewed seems to exist in a wider social context than that of their double diagnosis: gay and HIV-antibody positive. The epidemic is thus represented in a strangely paradoxical manner.

On the one hand we are told that literally hundreds of thousands of gay men are directly affected, whilst at the same time we are only permitted to 'meet' them singly, or at most in pairs. Thus the entire structure of urban (and rural) gay culture is conveniently erased *as if it had never existed.* There is thus no way that readers could ever appreciate that *all along,* lesbians and gay men have constituted the leading force in Western HIV education, even and especially where national governments have abdicated all responsibility for their citizens in relation to the right to effective health education.

When Robert Glück described AIDS as 'a kind of career,' he was speaking from the direct experience of someone caught up in the complex structure of formal and informal organizations that have been created in response to the officially neglected and changing needs of communities living with the multiple consequences of HIV infection. An article describing the common experience of doctors being educated about biomedical aspects of HIV by their patients briefly draws attention to the vast international network of treatment-related information concerning experimental drugs and clinical trials that is rarely available to people living with HIV from within the field of professional medicine.[23] Purportedly written by a doctor, though subsequently exposed as the work of a consultant anaesthetist, the article none the less offered a fascinating insight into professional attitudes towards sexuality. 'There really is a gay community, isn't there Clive?' asks the 'doctor.' 'You look after each other in a very practical way.'[24] It is rather as if the writer had discovered a national network of curiously philanthropic Martians, helping one another out. Furthermore, it would seem that these Martians are everywhere and, worst of all, are virtually undetectable – undetectable that is until they give themselves away, through strange 'sexual acts' or previously unknown (and incurable) diseases. Moreover, the medical disguise donned by the author tells its own story concerning the relative authority of different voices speaking about HIV in the public domain.

Journalists almost invariably turn to the medical establishment in relation to all aspects of the epidemic, from treatment issues to housing and welfare benefits. Whilst this medical establishment is, of course, as divided and unstable as any other branch of professional science, its attitudes to sexuality are generally homogeneous and consistent, not least because sexuality has, since its inception, been widely understood to belong under the wider aegis of biomedical science. By a cruel paradox, this has meant that few doctors receive any specialized education in the sociology of sex, and that heterosexuality is thus deeply inscribed within biomedical discourse and professional medical identities. In its institutional and theoretical understanding of health, Western medicine can only acknowledge the existence of gay men from the limited perspective of genito-urinary medicine, which in turn has traditionally been an undervalued branch of professional medicine by reason of its 'unsavoury' associations with sex and sexuality.

From the first identification of a syndrome, hypothetically derived from acquired immunological impairment, HIV has been written about as a disease of 'homosexuals.' This is hardly surprising, given the shocking ignorance of sex and sexuality displayed throughout the epidemiological literature of AIDS[25]. Indeed, it was frequently unclear whether a new disease or a new social constituency, 'homosexuals,' had been discovered. Gay men's bodies continue to be enrolled into clinical trials as if our very physiology were distinct from that of 'heterosexuals,' and, by extension, as if 'findings' in such studies would not be predictive for other men. As a result of ignorance and prejudice, journalists effortlessly translated the homophobia of professional medicine and epidemiology into the dominant 'public' picture of AIDS.[26] Indeed, HIV continues to be widely considered as a disease that results from specific so-called 'homosexual acts,' though of course there is nothing that gay men do sexually that is not also done by 'heterosexuals.' If, as seems increasingly likely, the cells lining the rectum are biologically susceptible to retroviral infection, this would say nothing about the 'rights' or 'wrongs' of anal intercourse. The extreme unlikelihood of arguments against *vaginal* intercourse, on the grounds of the vagina's vulnerability to yeast conditions, minor abrasions, and known sexually transmitted diseases, reveals much about the underlying tendency to dress up prejudice and phobia in the 'respectable' mantle of biomedical discourse.

The figure of 'the homosexual' that has been widely established as the focal figure of AIDS commentary is thus constituted primarily in relation to an imagined repertoire of 'sexual acts,' from which both disease *and* identity are imagined to derive. In countries such as Britain, where gay identity has never been officially accepted as a political position, HIV has afforded a widespread opportunity for 'heterosexuality' to further its authority by treating the terms 'homosexual' and 'gay' as if they were synonymous. Thus the strategic refusal of gay men to root an identity within the historically pre-given power relations of sexuality has little or no public acknowledgment, and the gap that gay men feel between their perceptions of themselves and the constructions made of them in the mass media and popular culture continues to widen. This is largely a function of the specific nature of British parliamentary politics, and of the general absence of a discourse of diversity in British political life. Furthermore, it should be noted that the *ideological* figure of 'the homosexual' has come to play an increasingly significant role in the production and marketing of the concept of 'the family,' which is so central to the consolidation of Thatcherism as a *national* cause and identity.[27] In Britain, as in North America and parts of Western Europe, the epidemic has thus engaged an especially complex set of conflicting currents of opinion and belief concerning gay men. The vast publicity given to AIDS throughout the media, in health-education campaigns, and elsewhere has undoubtedly established the straightforward *fact* of sexual diversity as never before. Yet the range of interpretations derived from the acknowledgment of sexual diversity remains volatile in the extreme.

This new visibility is frequently expressed in opinion polls, which demonstrate the contradictory nature of the situation. For example, 74 per cent of those questioned in one major British survey in 1988 believed that 'homosexual relationships' are 'wrong.' This compares with a mere 62 per cent in 1983.[28] An astonishing 88 per cent of people believed that 'extra-marital relationships' are 'wrong,' whilst only 25 per cent are opposed to premarital sex. There is also a growing belief that more money needs to be spent on medical research relating to AIDS, though 'fewer than one in 10 wants more spending on care for people dying of the disease.'[29] Whilst the great majority think that people with AIDS 'have only themselves to blame,' there is also a belief that 'AIDS patients receive less sympathy than they deserve.'[30] In other words, it seems clear that the wider context of social and cultural change is reflected in attitudes towards AIDS. It would certainly seem that the increasing gulf between cultural ideals concerning sex and marriage and actual experience results in something of a retrenchment around 'safe' conventional moral values. Indeed, it may well be that moralistic condemnations of 'AIDS victims' are connected to other forms of fantasized magical self-protection.

Yet the same voices that speak confidently and aggressively against 'pornography' or 'promiscuity' are equally unlikely to be overjoyed by the prospect of their own sons and daughters marrying the first person they ever go out with. The cultural ideal of falling in love with the girl or boy next door and settling down for a life of monogamous joy remains very powerful, but it is increasingly challenged by the inevitable acknowledgment of the high proportion of teenage marriages that break down, and the growing recognition that most adults in the

West will in fact be involved in a series of sexual relationships in the course of a lifetime. In this respect, it would appear that the sexual morality of gay men, with its emphasis on honesty within relationships, its recognition of 'serial monogamy' as the dominant cultural norm, and its ability to transform broken love affairs into lasting friendships, has much to offer the rest of society. Perhaps this is one reason for the resurgence of anti-gay prejudice. In this way, doubts about available models of child-raising and 'family life' can simply be projected away onto lesbians and gay men, and painful conflicts thus resolved, however temporarily. Certainly the new cultural permission to be frankly anti-gay meshes with a far larger situation in which anti-gay prejudice has never been considered bizarre or in any way problematic or extraordinary.

Activists and Assimilationists

Gay men thus face a virtually unprecedented situation. We have had to organize and campaign at every stage in the history of the epidemic for adequate local and national funding for medical and social services, health education, and so on, whilst living through an ever-increasingly terrible and tragic reality in our midst. At the same time, the rest of the population frequently appears only too glad to stand back as onlookers, variously indifferent, hostile, or openly contemptuous as our friends and loved ones sicken and die. In this respect, the cultural response to HIV disease invariably follows the patterns of gay-community politics as they existed *before* the start of the epidemic, regionally, nationally, and locally. Wherever gay men have congregated in the past thirty years and become involved in local community politics, their situation is likely to be far better than in cities or localities where there has been no such concentration of gay men, and no subsequent cultural or political representation of gay issues.

This is very clear in Europe, where for example France had lacked a strong gay movement in the early 1980s, or a campaigning gay press, and consequently lacked an institutional base from which effective community-based AIDS service organizations might have emerged. Britain, on the contrary, in spite and to some extent because of the high levels of national anti-gay prejudice, was able from very early on to develop support services and health education for gay men, in spite of government hostility and a chronic shortage of funds. It has only been in very unusual circumstances, as in Australia and California, that gay men have from the outset been consulted by state authorities, and their first-hand experience recognized and respected.[31] The different experience of HIV disease, according to local epidemiological factors in this wide variety of national gay cultures, has had profound effects on gay identity itself. Initially one can detect the emergence of a reinvigorated 'assimilationist' tendency within the gay movement alongside a new confidence around the organizing concept of 'AIDS activism.'

Whilst not wishing to read too much into a single publication, I regard the appearance of Marshall Kirk and Hunter Madsen's *After the Ball: How America Will Conquer Its Fear and Hatred of Gays in the '90s* from a major publishing house as one indication of the 'assimilationist' position, on which I have written elsewhere.[32] As Michael Bronski has pointed out: 'Deriding what they see as the excesses of the past – gay pride parades, angry protests, equal-rights demands, celebrating gay sexuality through drag or leather, even attempting to explain why "gay is good" to heterosexuals – as counterproductive to making straights accept us, the authors have come up with a revolutionary idea for social change: advertising.'[33] Mass-media campaigns should present lesbians and gay men as ultra-respectable, according to Kirk and Madsen, in order to persuade the rest of the world to change its attitudes (and laws). Yet, as Bronski argues, 'their simplistic advertising strategy ignores the incredible complexity of how social change occurs: a process that works on myriad levels – psychological, economic, political – and not by some clever marketing trick that makes people switch from Diet Pepsi to Diet Coke.'[34] Indeed, the very title of their book immediately and succinctly summarizes their thesis in little: gay sex is dirty, we had too much of it, we got HIV as a result, and now we need to work doubly hard to take the sex out of homosexuality. Yet it is *homosexuality* that is their key term, and it is a pre-gay-liberation social world that they would wish to restore: a world of 'discretion' and of exemplary citizenship to 'compensate' for an inevitable deviance which is the cross that 'homosexuals' must apparently bear.

It is surely significant that such attitudes last flourished in the 1950s and 1960s amongst law-reform groups such as Britain's Albany Trust.[35] At heart, 'assimilationism' always defers to the authority of dominant ideology and institutional politics. It aims at 'tolerance' for what is accepted as an intrinsically dislikeable and possibly contemptible form of sexuality. At most it can only aspire to an 'equality in difference' with straight society, and regards sexuality as a primarily personal, individual issue that is best kept private. Any notion of a gay politics that reaches out to challenge the entire governmental rationality of sexuality is thus out of the question. This conclusion certainly accords with Mark Gevisser's shrewd observation that 'lesbian and gay students, like most students in the late 1980's, are at college to gain a place in society, not to relinquish the place they already have. Far from rejecting mainstream society, they seem intent on achieving that essentially American goal of cultural assimilation. They want to be upright solid citizens. Openly gay upright solid citizens.'[36] Similar attitudes may be encountered on the American Left, as in Gregory Kolovakos' 1989 review in *The Nation* of Larry Kramer's *Report from the Holocaust*.[37] Whatever else might be said about Kramer's writings, it is vital to recognize that he was actively involved in the struggle to communicate information about AIDS from the beginning of the epidemic, and that any discussion of his strategies should rest on that acknowledgment. For Kolovakos, Kramer is simply 'biased and repetitive.' He is accused (horror of horrors!) of equating 'sexual freedom with promiscuity' in a manner that would not be unworthy of the editor of the *New York Post*. Worst of all, according to Kolovakis: 'Caught up in his personal drama, Kramer is immoral in representing the presence of the virus in a segment of the gay population as a death sentence for all homosexuals.'[38] Yet Kramer has never said more than that AIDS was, and remains, a perpetual threat to everyone not having safer sex, and especially to gay men, whom it has so terribly affected. Moreover, Kolovakos' picture of HIV as a discrete presence within 'a segment of the gay population' strongly suggests that he understands nothing of the need to establish the threat of HIV infection to all gay men, regardless of their known or perceived HIV-antibody status.[39]

AIDS can thus be presented as a problem for a minority within a minority. Where Kramer sees genocide-by-neglect, Kolovakos sees only the success of the gay movement in 'placing AIDS on the national agenda, in developing hospice care, in demystifying the disease.'[40] This is all very well, but entirely overlooks the fact that such state funding as is available to AIDS service organizations is entirely dependent upon the recognition, as is so often stated, that HIV is not 'just' a gay disease. It also overlooks the inconvenient fact that in many U.S. cities, and in countries such as Britain, gay men continue to make up over 90 per cent of AIDS cases cumulatively. AIDS is a crisis for *all* gay men, regardless of our HIV-antibody status, and effective HIV education is entirely dependent upon sustaining a strong confident sense of gay identity in such a way that the word 'gay' comes to *mean* 'safer sex.'[41] It is precisely this vision of community development that seems to appal commentators such as Kolovakos, who seems to care very little about the ongoing catastrophe and scandal surrounding so many aspects of medical treatment and clinical research.

Elsewhere in his review, Kolovakos agrees with Gore Vidal that the categories of sexuality 'make no sense.'[42] As far as he is concerned, 'the vast majority of gay men and lesbians simply want to go to work, to shop in the local malls, to watch sitcoms, to lead lives in which sexual preference is not the lightning rod Kramer would have it be.' Yet it is not Larry Kramer who is responsible for American homophobia, but a dense, complex mosaic of cultural, psychological, and ideological factors. Kolovakos' position exemplifies the way in which many gay men continue to imagine the project of a gay politics *as if AIDS had never happened*, or as if AIDS were simply *an inconvenient distraction* from the inexorable progress of civil rights in the field of sexuality. Kolovakos seems quite content to abandon the entire project of post-gay-liberation gay politics in grateful exchange for an identity that is virtually indistinguishable from that of the 'equality'-seeking liberal 'homosexual' of the 1950s. He even notes, in an archly 'surprised' aside concerning the use of the term 'sissy,' 'How gay men hate that word!', as if he finds such fundamental questions of language, power, and identity entirely trivial and beneath him.

This then is the new 'gay realism' of the Reagan/Bush era, bravely lining up behind Randy Shilts and Gore Vidal in a vision of comfortable, easily realizable sexual pluralism that might emerge if only gay men and lesbians would give up their unfortunate and regrettably 'shrill' style of politics and embrace more 'traditional' civil-rights strategies. This of course conveniently overlooks the fact that the modern civil-rights movement was constituted in civil disobedience. It also ends up protecting the overall structure and *savoir-pouvoir* of sexuality. For it is profoundly naïve to imagine that the categories of sexuality 'make no sense.' On the contrary, they remain indispensible to the current workings of state power and the hegemony of 'heterosexuality,' forged in compliant sexual identities.

This type of *de haut en bas* rejection of the activist tradition of gay politics is still more marked in the writings of Darrell Yates Rist. In July 1988, the *New York Native* published a letter signed by Rist and Kolovakos, together with Kathleen Conkey and Rosemary Kuropat, strongly criticizing a demonstration by the AIDS Coalition To Unleash Power (ACT UP) against the presence of New York's Mayor Ed Koch at the official opening of a Gay Pride and History Month.[43] AIDS, they wrote, 'is undoubtedly the major health issue facing the gay community, and indeed, the nation, today (though we note that it is not the one issue that ought to concern us). Activism is part of a long tradition for our community, but we distinguish between well-placed and well-timed activism and fascistic tactics that are no more acceptable when we implement them than when they are used against us. We are eight years into an epidemic that is killing many thousands of gay men ... We have a right to heal, and events like the kick-off of Gay History Month offer us a meaningful respite.' According to Rist and his colleagues, the priority of gay politics should be the task of teaching society 'to respect us.' Hence their polemic against 'a band of screaming activists who seem bent on working against the causes of their own community.' Instead, they recommend 'a well-orchestrated campaign to increase funding levels for AIDS services at appropriate forums.' For 'if AIDS is not a gay disease, as we so regularly protest, why does ACT UP choose to ruin a Gay Pride event?' As Vito Russo commented in the same edition of the *New York Native*:

> All those good and polite little boys and girls who have been whining about how ACT UP trashed its own party and how this wasn't the time or the place to zap the mayor are not activists, they're a bunch of politically naive asswipes. For such people the right time and place never seems to come because they're too busy begging for a pat on the head or a position in local government. These people are like the Jews who said, 'Don't throw rocks at the Nazis. You'll make them mad at us.' How much worse can this administration possibly be? It seems like anybody who's willing to be publicly identified as gay these days is termed an activist. I would like to remind all of these so-called 'activists' what activism means. Activists do things that you're not supposed to do. Activists are not respectable ... Activists are not dazzled by the crumbs off a table from a mayor who is allowing their friends to die. Activists are not grateful for some rinky-dink exhibit which 'allows' us to celebrate our history while our history is being systematically wiped out.[44]

The position that Russo described as that of the 'polite little boys and girls' was succinctly put in another letter to the *New York Native* signed by Julia Friedlander and another fourteen signatories. They accused ACT UP of censorship, and argued that 'forbidding the mayor from speaking about gay and lesbian people is not likely to improve his policies on AIDS.'[45] They repeat the Darrel Yates Rist assertion that although 'AIDS is obviously an extremely important issue ... It is not the only issue for our community in this decade.' The letter ended with a rallying cry: 'We need each other. If our community is ever to build unity around a particular agenda or strategy, we must develop debate and dialogue from a base of mutual respect. We cannot turn contempt against one another.' Yet, as Larry Kramer pointed out in the same issue of the *Native*, 'There is no way in the world there is ever going to be "unity" in any population as large as ours. It's a waste of breath even wishing for it. It's totally unrealistic. There are too many constituencies, which is as it should be.'[46]

Through all of this, a number of factors should be noted. Firstly, there was never any question of ACT UP's trying to prevent anyone visiting the gay-history exhibition. Their target was the mayor of New York, who, as ACT UP explained, 'has whipped the gay leadership of New York into submission, convincing them to accept an unacceptable record on AIDS, and then expecting the rest of us to honor him for all he has done. That's hypocrisy, and if we made people uncomfortable, if we embarrassed them in front of the mayor, if we refused to allow them to ignore the reality of the mayor's record on AIDS, that's good ... We are not going to let the mayor feel welcome at any gay or AIDS-related event in this city until he proves that his words have the force of action behind them.'[47]

Secondly, there is evidently a growing division between those for whom HIV disease is 'just' another issue and those for whom the epidemic is the central key issue, to which all other aspects of gay politics are related for the foreseeable future. The former will regard ACT UP demonstrations as 'censorship,' oddly failing to recognize that politicians rarely lack opportunities to reach large audiences, whilst the AIDS movement has limited access to media representation. The latter will insist, and I believe correctly, that the principle of freedom of speech in such circumstances gives precedence to the weak and the marginalized rather than to professional politicians. It is hardly consistent to call for 'debate and dialogue' when one side is literally fighting for its life, whilst the other is holding a scented handkerchief to its offended nostrils and turning away.

Thirdly, a distinction between a politics of civil rights, founded in lobbying, is increasingly being opposed to a politics of direct confrontation. Yet this is a naïve and ultimately harmful approach, since it both falsifies the history of civil-rights politics and poses lobbying and activism as if they were alternatives. Activism only becomes a necessity when other forms of negotiation are refused, or break down. However, it is transparently clear that only direct action has guaranteed the provision of such vital innovations as the fast-tracking of experimental new drugs and effectively challenged unethical protocols for clinical trials, as well as raising collective community consciousness about such issues.

Fourthly, one may detect a conflict between an older model of gay culture and politics, based in the idea of a 'natural' and inevitable unity of lesbians and gay men, founded in our sexuality, and more recent strategies that proceed from the premise that gay identity is always contingent on specific and constantly changing circumstances and priorities. From the former perspective, any criticism of this mystical (and misty) vision of gay harmony is regarded as treacherous, whilst from the latter perspective the concept of 'gay community' is an ideal that must acknowledge the actual complexity of issues and objective situations that confront lesbians and gay men in terms of their class, gender, race, age, and specific sexual preferences.

As Jeffrey Weeks has pointed out, sexual object-choice can only provide at most an unstable base for political identities. He distinguishes helpfully between the *tactical* aim of the gay movement, which is to defend and assert gay rights, and its *strategic* aim, which 'must be not simply the validation of the rights of a minority within a heterosexual majority, but the challenge to all the rigid categorisations of sexuality, categorisations which exist not to delineate scientifically one type of person from another but which act to control people's behaviour in very rigid ways.'[48] This entire debate resurfaced nearly a year later when Darrell Yates Rist published a highly contentious article in *The Nation* claiming that 'even the homosexual heart for AIDS beats false; it beats only for men of a certain age, a certain color – in fact, a certain social class.'[49] According to Rist, 'the battle against anti-gay violence languishes, while assaults have soared specifically as a backlash to the disease.' Rist's total inability to comprehend the specific, unique, personal experience of AIDS among hundreds of thousands of gay men and lesbians in cities such as London and New York is reflected in the absurdly rhetorical questions that he poses: 'Can no threat but AIDS ignite our indignation? Why do we care so little, in fact, even for the sanctity of our relationships? Why is there no ACT UP specifically to protest laws forbidding same-sex marriage, banned in every state? Why no marathon protests at marriage licence bureaus, no sit-ins at state legislatures, no class action suits?'[50] And in a statement of almost unparalleled vulgarity and plain stupidity, he writes that gay men wearing ACT UP or GMHC (Gay Men's Health Crisis) T-shirts to his local gym are not sufficiently courageous to 'boldly advertise a more identifiably gay and therefore riskier issue.' It seems to have escaped his notice that for most Americans, gay now *means* AIDS, and vice versa. His assertion that 'a certain interest in AIDS has become the trendy code for suggesting one's homosexuality without declaring it, what being a bachelor and an artiste used to suggest,' is as profoundly insulting to the courage and achievements of American AIDS activists as it is revealing of Rist's own values, which betray a strange mixture of gay-liberationist ideas about the supposed intrinsic value of public disclosure, and a contemptuous dread of organized civil disobedience.

It is almost as if the check that HIV has posed to the cosy assimilationist fantasy of tolerance just around the corner is being displaced back onto AIDS activists, and especially onto people living with HIV and AIDS. How else can one possibly interpret Rist's extraordinary criticism of anti-discrimination legislation for people living with AIDS on the grounds that such laws won't help lesbians or 'the average homosexual or bisexual man who, whatever our hysteria, would not test positive for HIV either.' The sheer callousness of such a response all but beggars belief.

Ultimately, Rist's brand of self-proclaimed 'gay liberation' amounts to little more than the demand for the right to same-sex marriages, a strategy he curiously shares with Larry Kramer. That 'gay marriage' is advanced as an alternative and higher priority to HIV-related issues denotes the full measure of the ethical bankruptcy of the 'equality'-seeking, assimilationist 'homosexual' tradition of gay politics, as it survives in the Age of AIDS. It is not gay men who have to learn the sovereign joys of marriage from heterosexuals; on the contrary, the gay movement needs to sustain its critique of sexuality, embodied *most precisely* in the institution of marriage, which should be our target, not our goal.

However, Rist's unforgiveable error has been his constant and unrelenting hostility to AIDS activism. He clings, almost lovingly, to his own identity as a 'true' gay 'radical,' presenting himself as the spokesman of a gay-rights movement that has supposedly been 'shouted down by the politics of this epidemic.'[51] He has consistently and single-mindedly contrasted the political struggle against homophobia and on behalf of gay rights to the AIDS situation, as if the entire history of the epidemic had not exemplified the most murderously homophobic social policies and attitudes, at all levels, seen anywhere on earth since the fall of the Nazis. This leads him inexorably to attack AIDS activists, whom he caricatures as mere social careerists 'chumming with the Liz Taylors.' It is as if his main anger about AIDS is the way in which the epidemic has derailed his own career prospects as an erstwhile gay Savonarola for the fin-de-millénium. Hence his breathtakingly astonishing conclusion that really, gay men are making a lot of fuss over nothing when it comes to AIDS. After all, as he points out: 'Even if 1.5 million died off ... a minimum of 9.7 [million] homosexually active men ... would remain uninfected and sentenced to life.'[52] But by this point it should be clear that Darrell Yates Rist has become the gay equivalent to the Holocaust-never-happened school of historians.

We may thus identify profound disunity amongst many gay men at the very point at which a very high level of established consensus might have been expected. For I believe that the single, central factor of greatest significance for all gay men should be the recognition that the current HIV-antibody status of everyone who had unprotected sex in the long years before the virus was discovered is a matter of *sheer coincidence*. We need to think very seriously indeed about our personal relations to an epidemic that affected millions around the world long before anyone even dreamed it was taking place. This is why most analogies with other diseases such as herpes and hepatitis B are so dreadfully misleading and misplaced. Every gay man who had the good fortune to remain uninfected in the decade or so before the emergence of safer sex should meditate most profoundly on the whim of fate that spared him, but not others. This is why HIV disease is, and will always remain, an issue for *all* gay men, regardless of our known or perceived antibody status. Those of us who chance to be sero-negative have *an absolute and unconditional responsibility* for the welfare of sero-positive gay men. Would they have written us off if we had been infected, in the way that Darrell Yates Rist and his comrades seem so callously prepared to write off those living with HIV today, together with all those who have died? This is the question we must ask ourselves, and the future of gay identity hangs on the answer that we find. Those who continue to interpret HIV as an issue for a minority within a minority only reveal the crippling poverty of their own moral, political, and spiritual resources.

That it was the left-wing *Nation* that eventually published Rist's diatribe only serves to underscore the problems that lesbians and gay men face from mainstream political culture in the Age of AIDS. As Larry Kramer has pointed out, 'it is "perversely sad" that *The Nation* ran the story when they have virtually ignored the AIDS issue, only running a handful of stories over the last eight years. The left wing and all the major left wing intellectuals haven't talked about AIDS ... because the left wing has a terrible history of homophobia.'[53] Yet it is not that history that concerns Rist, or the criminal neglect of the Reagan, Bush, Thatcher, and Mulroney administrations. Rather, in the tradition of liberal 'tolerance' that he so eloquently represents, he prefers to blame gay men themselves, very much in the moralizing manner of Randy Shilts: 'It wasn't a virus that for centuries has deprived us gay men and lesbians of our freedom, nor is it the epidemic that now most destroys our lives. Nor is it bigotry. It's our own shame, a morbid failure of self-respect and sane, self-righteous anger. If we care about nothing but AIDS now, it is because identifying with sexually transmitted death plays to some dark belief that we deserve it.' Yet among the tens and hundreds of thousands of women and men who have given so much of their time and energy and passion in the fight against AIDS throughout the 1980s, who is there who cares 'about nothing but AIDS'? I have yet to meet such a person.

What Rist so tragically fails to comprehend is why so many gay men who had not previously been actively involved in gay politics became involved in AIDS service organizations. The American gay movement is especially vulnerable to a leadership model that has assumed the existence of a coherent minority behind it – a minority often held in more or less open contempt for not 'coming out.' One of the many things that AIDS teaches is the profound inadequacy of this top-down, mandarin model of sexual politics. It is therefore especially distressing, if not entirely unpredictable, to find a number of gay intellectuals rushing to openly champion Rist's 'cause.' Thus Gore Vidal reveals only his own Olympian distance from the harsh realities of U.S. health-care provision in his arrogant and intolerably callous 'suggestion' that there should be 'less fretting over an "epidemic" that is nothing but a familiar pretext to exert more and more controls over everyone through mandatory blood, urine and lie-detector tests.'[54] Whilst the point about biomedical control over the body is undoubtedly important, it is staggering that a gay man, in 1989, can literally not see an 'epidemic' beyond the question of testing.

Nor could Rist's loyal disciple, black lesbian Jewelle L. Gomez, resist the opportunity to rush into print to defend him. Whilst it is undoubtedly true, as she states, that 'racism and sexism have hampered the movement for gay rights,' it should also be pointed out that the racism and sexism that are most dangerous to the movement are not so much within it as outside it, and campaigning against its very existence.

Indeed, one of the most distasteful aspects of Rist's pontificating style is his tendency to hide behind the sturdy skirts of anti-sexist and anti-racist rhetoric. At the 1988 National Lesbian and Gay Health Conference in Boston, he even went so far as to claim that books on AIDS are directly preventing the publication of writings by women of colour!

Yet it is the entirely misleading comparison between HIV disease and breast cancer made by both Rist and his old friend Rosemary Kuropat that is most revealing. If it could be demonstrated that breast cancer is caused by an infectious agent, and if treatments were routinely withheld from women with breast cancer, and if health education was denied, and the known evidence that the cancer could be transmitted to men was used as a pretext to impose massive legal curbs on female sexuality – then, and only then, would the analogy hold. As things stand, such spurious comparisons only serve to distract attention from the larger question of how alliances can be forged and sustained between different groups of the disabled and chronically sick, who share so many unnecessary problems concerning housing and finance and medical treatment.

Rist presents a picture of wealthy white AIDS service organizations, systematically starving out resources from other communities of need. For anyone remotely involved in the *real* world of fund-raising, the truth is very different. This is not to ignore the regrettable disparity of funds available to different communities, but such an observation should not be allowed to eclipse the wider point concerning the total abdication of the state's responsibility *throughout this crisis* for the health and welfare of *all* citizens, black and white, gay and straight. Hence the significance of Robert Massa's thoughtful and carefully weighed comments:

> It may be sentimental to argue that AIDS has brought maturity to the gay movement, but surely it has brought increased political activism. Rather than narrow our focus, AIDS has raised consciousness about gut issues like access to health care and the rights of surviving lovers. Why complain that the community donates to Gay Men's Health Crisis when even Reagan's own task force conceded that support services are woefully underfunded? Why sow discord by claiming lesbian issues have suffered when examples abound that the epidemic has deepened the bonds between gay women and men? Why argue that we've neglected gay youth – what greater legacy than that we stood up firmly against calamity? And even if AIDS had distracted from other

> battles, so what? Infectious disease *is* a more urgent issue than gay rights. What do civil rights mean in the grave?[55]

On the basis of her many years' experience of AIDS service organizations around the world, Cindy Patton has described her sense 'that there is a strong commitment to pursuing a broad, leftist, gay liberation agenda within AIDS work ... It may be difficult to see the multiplicity of issues that progressives are working on under the rubric of "AIDS" ... This politics is rather more transversal and post-Marxist than dialectical. It attempts to speak into an ideological battle against repression parading as public health ... The really political work going on ... is to wrest HIV and the bodies of those we care about and serve from the icy grip not of death, but of a science that can only consider humans to be giant agar plates.'[56] It is this cultural politics of language, and images, and identities, that Darrell Yates Rist seems unable or unwilling to recognize in the field of AIDS activism. Rather than trying to establish absolute distinctions between 'gay rights' and 'AIDS activism,' we should be working to develop effective interventions in relation to *all* the institutions that frame and determine the experience of *all* people living with HIV disease, and our communities.

Effective AIDS activism begins by establishing clear issues that have been thoroughly researched. Subsequent lobbying targets the institutions that exercise power and authority, and direct action follows if they refuse to respond or negotiate. AIDS activism is also concerned with the symbols by which such institutions, from the press and TV to the medical profession and pharmaceutical industry, assume and maintain their power, including the words and images by which they attempt to define the world in the likeness of their own prejudice and vested interests. AIDS activism has taught us much about the nature of institutional politics and ideology that the gay-rights movement had little or no opportunity to explore or discover before the epidemic. Far from displacing the issue of gay pride, AIDS activism has developed strategies and techniques that make earlier forms of lesbian and gay lobbying look wildly outdated. There is no point in standing at the barricades if 'the enemy' is a multinational corporation that can transfer funds and information to the other side of the globe in a microsecond.

From his experience working with the National Gay Rights Advocates, and the AIDS Civil Rights Project, Ben Schatz has also eloquently challenged any idea of a watertight distinction between 'gay politics' and the epidemic. Speaking at the fifth annual International AIDS Conference in Montreal in June 1989, he forcefully argued that in the early days of the epidemic 'we didn't emphasize that gay people play an important part in everyone's life, that we are not beamed down to earth from another planet. We are instead part of everyone's family and friendship circles ... instead we say things like: "AIDS is not a gay problem – it's a human problem." Aren't we human too?'[57] He also noted how funding for gay men's health education has always been grossly inadequate: 'A northern Californian funder donated $650,000 to the AIDS battle provided not one cent went to the gay community. In the *America Responds to AIDS* campaign, not one poster or television commercial is aimed at gays.' Exactly the same situation obtains in Britain and most other Western nations. Schatz continued: 'A common response to my complaint is that there is now little transmission in the gay community or that AIDS is moving out of the homosexual population. I say that AIDS is not moving out of the gay community; it is simply moving into other communities. Furthermore, don't believe there is little transmission among gay men. Thousands of gays continue to seroconvert annually. If it were the same number of white heterosexual doctors, there would be an uproar.' It should also be noted that much AIDS education has been aimed at gay men as part of a much wider population, frequently referred to as 'men who have sex with men.' Such campaigns are targeted at men who may not think that they are at risk, because they don't have a gay identity, whether for reasons of age, or class, or culture. Sometimes such campaigns have resulted from the pressures of censorship on explicitly gay-affirmative materials.

Yet in this way forms of community development have emerged that other forms of gay-rights politics could never have envisaged. For example, the recognition of the full extent of sexual transmission between Hispanic men, and other men of colour, has led to the emergence of a new and long-overdue dimension of anti-racism within the overall field of AIDS education. Such work has almost invariably derived from gay and other non-government AIDS service organizations, since state AIDS education cannot imagine the existence of such groups, let alone try to reach them. Furthermore, the similar official denial of lesbians as a constituency in need of specific health-promotion campaigns has likewise brought home the full extent of straight society's indifference to the rights of lesbians. This in turn has tended to make the gay movement stronger, by leading us back to shared aspects of lesbian and gay oppression. As Ben Schatz insisted at the end of his Montreal speech: 'We must never, never apologize for being lesbians or gay men.'

The forms of gay identity that AIDS activism has produced are, of course, specific to the complex varying local circumstances of the epidemic, but they none the less continue patterns that had been broadly established before the epidemic. Whilst some gay men have settled into monogamous relationships out of fear – 'cocooning' as it has been described – others have developed safer sex as a way of sustaining their commitment to erotic pleasure and freedom of choice. The widespread formal and informal institution of 'jack-off' groups and parties, in the United States and Amsterdam for example, evidently sustains a cultural identity that confidently refuses the crude anti-sex messages that make up so much official government-sponsored AIDS 'education.'[58] The message from voluntary-sector AIDS service organizations, however, has consistently aimed to build on pre-AIDS sexual practices and identities, in order not to make safer sex seem like a set of negative, and entirely proscriptive, new rules.[59] Such safer-sex education has maintained that safer sex is an issue for *all* men having sex with men, that we are *all* responsible to and for one another in relation to HIV transmission, and that we are *all* safer-sex educators.[60]

This multilateral resistance to official AIDS discourse has brought gay men together as never before and affirmed gay identity in relation to the collective achievement of drastically lowering rates of HIV incidence, and helping and supporting one another through the rigours of this seemingly endless health crisis. Most gay men have had their moments of heroism in the course of the epidemic, and most of these stories will never be told for the simple reason that they involve acts of private, quiet heroism that are rarely talked about. We can all think of such examples. It is this level of AIDS activism, together with the extraordinary collective empowerment that groups such as ACT UP have sustained over time that Darrell Yates Rist and his friends seem so stubbornly unable or unwilling to acknowledge. In the final analysis, this is their great loss.

Gay Culture and the Counterdiscourse of Gay Identity

Prior to the emergence of HIV among gay men, seven structures 'rationalizing' anti-gay prejudice were widely prevalent in Western societies. First, a theory of 'arrested development,' founded in neo-Freudianism, that presents homosexual desire as 'infantile' and 'regressive.' Second, there is the more ancient concept of 'the unnatural,' which has also been given a pseudo-scientific gloss as 'perversion,' in spite of the wide cultural and historical frequency of behaviour and identities founded in homosexual desire. Third, there is the argument that homosexuality is non-procreative and barren, which roots morality in sexual reproduction. For this argument an infertile marriage would be as 'sterile' as a lesbian or gay relationship. In this way the frequency of lesbian and gay parenthood is also conveniently erased, and the heterosexuality of 'the family' is thus protected. Fourth, there is the theological concept of sin, commonly expressed in terms of 'abomination' in codes of sexual conduct that are imagined as divinely ordained. Fifth, there is a widespread cultural critique of supposed unmanliness, which singles out 'effeminate' men and 'masculine' women, as if gendering were a simple system of opposed yet complementary characteristics. Sixth, there is the accusation that homosexual desire stems from a hatred of the opposite sex, that gay men deliberately 'reject' women as their sexual partners. Homosexuality is thus an extreme version of misogyny from this point of view, which is sadly shared by some feminists, especially if they theorize lesbianism as a deliberate 'rejection' of men.[61] Finally, there is the common equation of homosexuality with paedophilia, which reads gay relationships as an age-based surrogate for heterosexual gender difference.

The first three of these structures are overwhelmingly naturalistic, offering heterosexual desire as a biological imperative that can brook no variations or expansions. The fourth category is frankly metaphysical, whilst the last three are based on various complex assumptions and attitudes concerning gender. AIDS has been widely used to amplify and reinforce all these categories, whilst a new and potent fatalism has been added to gay identity, at least as it is perceived and conceived by non-gays. From this latter perspective, homosexual desire is often regarded as not only deadly for gay men, but an active threat to the rest of the population. This perspective is typified by talk of the supposed threat that gay men now pose to our very species.

Yet homosexual object-choice has provided the grounds for cultural groupings and aspects of identity in many societies, and never more so than when aggressively stigmatized. However, the 'mollies' and 'margeries' and 'poofs' of earlier generations all seem to share a common tendency to accept derogatory classifications and to socialize in relation to them, even if, as seems likely, these terms of abuse took on ironic or counterdiscursive meanings for those whose identities were formed and lived out under the stigmatizing influence of such nomenclature. The emergence of gay identity in the course of the twentieth century provides an alternative structure of identity that proceeds from a collective refusal of such strategies, although it co-exists with 'homosexual' and 'queer' identities that continue to be produced, especially away from the social and geographical bases of gay culture in the major urban conurbations of the West. Official AIDS commentary constantly fails to recognize the significance of the distinction between gay and homosexual identity. Thus, a major British quality newspaper will typically announce in a headline 'AIDS epidemic among gays "near peak,"' whilst the first line of the story informs readers that 'the current AIDS epidemic among male homosexuals may be reaching its peak, according to a new report.'[62] Whether gay culture and identity will prove sufficiently resilient to resist such pressure remains to be seen. AIDS has stimulated a contradictory set of cultural pressures on gay identity. While gay men are united as never before in the collective struggles around the epidemic, the larger popular culture works at all levels to re-homosexualize gay identities.

In a moving article written in 1988, the American gay writer John Preston considered the situation of young men coming out as gay in the age of AIDS:

> I'm struck by the fact that they are still coming out. Is there some smaller number of young men arriving into our community than there would have been before? I can hardly discern it. I can only see the numbers growing ... What is most striking to me is that this new generation has learned the new forms of sexuality and is still able to use sex and celebrating sex as a way to find community ... I believe that the salvation of our sexual history and our erotic imaginations is one of the greatest challenges we have ever faced. The transformation of our movement into a multi-generational community is another ... We who are older and more experienced need to look at the *obligations* of gay men to our youth. We need to resurrect and honor the concept of role models that was so important to the early gay movement ... We claimed our erotic imagination for ourselves and our community and we need to affirm it as a valued part of our history.[63]

It would certainly appear that the fear of death that has been culturally associated with homosexuality per se is not shared by most gay men, and this in itself is an eloquent testimonial to the effects of safer-sex education instituted by and for gay men. Yet 'official' HIV/AIDS education continues to be based on strategies that misguidedly attempt to frighten the rest of the population away from *all* sexual activity outside marriage, and it is the inevitable long-term resentment that such campaigns foster that offers a major threat to the larger project of gay rights. This again is why the issues of AIDS and gay politics are, for the foreseeable future, inseparable.

Gay political resistance to official AIDS commentary is nowhere more apparent than in the immediate experience of shared losses and mourning. Most gay men and lesbians will by now be familiar with the relentless routine of farewells and funerals for dearly loved friends and colleagues. Given the close bonding of gay culture, this means that large networks of ex-lovers and families are often involved, and there can be no aspect of the epidemic that is more at variance with 'official' accounts of the supposed 'meaning' of AIDS than such funerals and memorial gatherings. Indeed, AIDS has generated a wholly new type of funeral that frequently blends elements of religious ceremony with secular gay culture. To take but one personal example, the recent funeral of a friend of mine, George Cant, who had played a very active and important role in the British AIDS movement (see 'Our Lady of AIDS,' pp 108–9 in this volume), brought together at his request Sid Vicious's recording of *My Way*, together with a passage from the Verdi *Requiem*, one of Strauss's *Four Last Songs*, and Paul Simon's *Bridge over Troubled Water.* It is difficult to put into words the complex associations that such a sequence of music produces in such circumstances. Suffice to say that the music at George's funeral spoke for a life of great richness and emotional range, which was also movingly representative of the richness and range of gay culture as a whole.

Nothing exemplifies this cultural response to the profound personal dimensions of the epidemic more eloquently and successfully than the NAMES Project, better known simply as 'the Quilt.' Memorializing many of the thousands who have died as a result of HIV disease, the Quilt embodies precisely that relation of the individual to the collective that underpins all aspects of gay identity. As Cleve Jones, the project's executive director, has pointed out, the Quilt 'was created in homes across America by the families, friends and lovers of people lost to AIDS. While they represent a great diversity of people and backgrounds, they are united by their shared experience of a devastating epidemic.'[64] Only the meanest of spirits could object to this extraordinary testimony to the actual complexity of AIDS, witnessing to the range not only of tragedy, but also of achievement. From the stark 'RICK DIXON AGE: 31,' to the appropriately Warholian spray-paint repetition of 'MICHEL FOUCAULT 1926–1984,' or simply 'Love You Dad' with a homely montage of embroidered hearts and ribbons, and the many, many extraordinarily inventive images commemorating different lives, the Quilt effortlessly gives the lie to any notion of HIV as a disease of 'outsiders,' or 'the family' as a simple uniform institution, or sexual identity as a direct biological entity.

As early as 1985, a major survey revealed that the average gay man in New York City had already known 'four men who either had died of AIDS or were ill with AIDS ... These numbers have increased dramatically since then, resulting in a secondary epidemic of bereavement growing at a logarithmic rate in the gay population.'[65] When I visited San Francisco in 1987 I was at first surprised to find that the gay scene seemed to be carrying on very much in a business-as-usual fashion, save for the leather bars, whose clientele had already largely perished. As a foreigner, I failed to comprehend or take in the ways in which gay men in that city had responded to the enormity of loss in their lives precisely by celebrating dead friends and loved ones *on their own cultural terms*, in bars and clubs, with disco music and a quiet determination that the gay life of San Francisco would survive as a testimonial to the values of pluralism that are so central to gay identity. As the epidemic has worsened in other cities, I have seen the same process repeated throughout western Europe, from London to Stockholm. Whilst there is a growing literature on individual bereavement patterns in relation to AIDS, there has been little time to look beyond the urgent requirements of the present to the long-term mourning process that will follow the epidemic for the entire lifetimes of many millions of lesbians and gay men. Just as John Preston has described the 'obligations' of older gay men to younger gay men, so in the decades ahead those of us who survive the epidemic will undoubtedly need the long-term support of all those who 'come out' after the peak of the epidemic in the 1990s.

Writing at a time when HIV was already being more and more widely transmitted amongst gay men since nobody knew of its existence, Michel Foucault qualified the modern period in relation to death: 'Wars are no longer waged in the name of a sovereign who must be defended; they are waged on behalf of the existence of everyone ... If genocide is indeed the dream of modern powers, this is not because of a recent return of the ancient right to kill; it is because power is situated and exercised at the level of life, the species, the race, and the large-scale phenomenon of population ... One might say that the ancient right to *take* life or *let* live was replaced by a power to *foster* life or to *disallow* it to the point of death.'[66] In Foucault's terms we may productively analyse *all* the various cultural and political practices generated in response to the epidemic in relation to two sets of historically given procedures of power, or *disciplines.* The first of these involves 'an anatomo-politics of the human body' that centres on the body as if it were a machine, concerned with its productivity, its obedience, its recalcitrance, its *utility.* The second involves 'a biopolitics of the population' that is effected through a multitude of regulatory controls, centred on the body understood primarily as a participant in the life of the *species*: 'the body imbued with the mechanics of life and serving as the basis of the biological processes: propagation, births and mortality, the level of health, life expectancy and longevity, with all the conditions that can cause these to vary.'[67] If, as Foucault argues, in the modern period, the 'old power of death that symbolized sovereign power was now carefully supplanted by the administration of bodies and the calculated management of life,'[68] we may apply his analysis of corporeal power to the types of disciplinary control exercised throughout 'official' AIDS and safer-sex education campaigns.

The meaning of the body that informs such campaigns may in turn be traced in other practices, from journalism and television coverage, to the protocols of clinical trials, the statements and policies of politicians, medical practice, and so on. These all accrete around the compliant identity of the 'AIDS victim,' who must totally and willingly aquiesce to the meanings that the coincidence of disease and sexuality have made his body speak. As Foucault emphasizes, it is precisely this proliferation of disciplinary technologies, targeting the body and legitimated in consenting identities, 'that enables us to understand the importance assumed by sex as a political issue.'[69] As he has famously observed: 'Sex was a means of access both to the life of the body and the life of the species'[70] – both terms being central to the dominant practices and discourses surrounding and defining the course of the epidemic.

Yet this ensemble of practices and discourses is not, of course, uncontested. Since 1983, the identity of the 'person with AIDS' or 'person living with AIDS' has effectively refused the entire logic of the epidemic that is condensed in the concept and carefully policed image of the 'AIDS victim.'[71] Furthermore, it is increasingly clear that the practices and values developed by gay men in the name of safer sex have not merely rejected these official messages, but have *expanded* many of the central tenets of pre-AIDS gay politics. For example, non-government AIDS service organizations have repeatedly drawn attention to the risks of HIV infection to social and sexual constituencies whose very existence the dominant AIDS discourse and commentary cannot admit, such as gay teenagers, gay people with disabilities, and so on, all of whom are also recognized to be fully sexual. Amongst gay men, safer sex has constituted a range of sexual practices that not only take over pre-AIDS sexual pleasures, but also defend these in the face of official contempt.

One need only consider the language of the U.S. Helms amendment of 1987 to grasp the significance of the terrain on which the meaning of AIDS is contested. For example, Helms described a Gay Men's Health Crisis workshop for participants to learn how to 'feel comfortable practicing safer sex.' Such a fundamental aspect of safer-sex education among gay men is simply dismissed by Helms as a 'revolting project,' since his aim is to prevent gay sex *in its entirety.* This is congruent with the tendency seen throughout the history of the epidemic to argue that gay men should give up sex altogether. It is equally evident in the assertion that gay sex somehow 'caused' HIV in the first place. Gay Men's Health Crisis had submitted a grant proposal for funding based on the assumption that 'as gay men have reaffirmed their gay identity through sexual expression, recommendations to change sexual behaviour may be seen as oppressive. For many, safer sex has been equated with boring, unsatisfying sex. Meaningful alternatives are often not realized. These perceived barriers must be considered and alternatives to high-risk practices promoted in the implementation of AIDS risk-reduction education.'[72] Such a statement derives from the mainstream of non-government AIDS education, which Helms described as 'so obscene, so revolting, that I am embarrassed to try to discuss it.'[73] Yet he was compelled to discuss it, and at great length, in order to persuade his fellow senators to effectively dis-fund GMHC at the very height of an unparalleled health crisis. It *amazes* me that heterosexual commentators have so completely failed to recognize the plainly genocidal purpose behind the Helms amendment, and other such legal manoeuvres. Liberals piously denounce the genocidal policies of the Pol Pot regime in Cambodia and all are agreed in their condemnation of murderous terrorist assaults on civilians. Yet the Helms amendment has attracted almost no commentary whatsoever, despite its almost naked aspiration to prevent gay men from defending themselves and one another from HIV.

Such experiences teach us the full extent to which AIDS issues and 'gay rights' are now related. For whilst the Dannemeyers and Helmses of this world are relatively easily identified, it is the wider climate of barely conscious consent to their policies that is far more seriously alarming. We should not attribute such consent simply to a supposedly unified and pathological condition of homophobia, because by so doing we lose sight of the more important point that such aggressive indifference to the lives of gay men is profoundly structured in the roles and relations that make up 'heterosexuality.'

The direct, long-term experience of HIV disease has taught large numbers of lesbians and gay men a series of brutal lessons concerning the differential power relations of sexuality. Such lessons make a mockery of the linear, juridical model of gay politics espoused by figures such as Darrell Yates Rist. Yet the situation surrounding HIV disease is never predictable, and it is important to recognize the full extent to which gay people have been able to determine many aspects of social policy determining the course of the epidemic from *inside* the state. At the same time, organizations such as ACT UP and AIDS ACTION NOW! (Toronto) demonstrate the ability of AIDS activists to successfully challenge the power of a wide range of institutions that oversee and control the position of people living with HIV disease and their communities, from local and national government to the multinational pharmaceutical industry. It is in this context that we must not neglect the intellectual and political critique of sexuality that has been directly responsible for so much unnecessary suffering. This task is greatly encouraged by the insights of psychoanalysis, with its understanding that sexuality 'does not mean only the activities and pleasure which depend on the functioning of the genital apparatus: it also embraces a whole range of excitations and activities which may be observed from infancy onwards and which procure a pleasure that cannot be adequately explained in terms of the satisfaction of a basic physiological need (respiration, hunger, excretory function, etc.); these re-emerge as component factors in the so-called normal form of sexual love.'[74] It is this deep scepticism concerning the supposed 'normality' of heterosexuality that makes psychoanalysis so useful to the development of gay politics and gay identity.

Conclusion: Gay Identity and Popular Memory

In a major article on British cultural responses to the loss of life during the First World War, David Cannadine described a situation in which, 'where traditional ceremony and traditional religion seemed inadequate in the face of so much death and bereavement, alternative attempts were made to render such losses bearable ... Two responses in particular merit attention: the one official, public and ceremonial; the other private, spontaneous and individualistic. The first was the construction throughout the country of war memorials, and the gradual evolution of the ritual of Armistice Day. The second was the massive proliferation of interest in spiritualism.'[75] The NAMES Project stands as a form of public, commemorative response to the epidemic, albeit constructed in terms of what amounts to an alternative cultural nationalism in the United States. Ironically, the Quilt promotes a nationalism that can value drug users and gay men as *citizens* in the context of a catastrophe that the state has yet to register in any meaningful symbolic sense. Hence the grim significance of the poster produced by Gran Fury (the graphic artists' collective associated with ACT UP), which asks directly: 'When a Government Turns Its Back on Its People, Is It Civil War?' Gran Fury were also responsible for a major installation in the Broadway window of New York's New Museum of Contemporary Art, in 1987. This included a series of pictures of figures such as Jerry Falwell, together with grossly offending quotes, against enlarged photographic stills from the Nuremberg trials of Nazi war criminals, beneath a hugh neon sign proclaiming: 'Silence = Death.'

The 'Silence = Death' motif, with its pink triangle summoning memories of the treatment of gay men in the Nazi concentration camps, has provided a dramatic rallying symbol around the world, recruiting lesbians and gay men to an identity that is centrally informed by our awareness of the scale of social injustice in the AIDS crisis. It has now effectively joined the concept of 'gay pride' as a fundamental symbol and slogan defining both the new gay politics and gay identity. Like the Quilt, it offers a radically innovative strategy for raising gay-community AIDS awareness, without resorting to more traditional forms of political rhetoric. Yet the 'Silence = Death' logo emerged in New York, where the epidemic has been so especially severe, and neither it nor the Quilt can necessarily be understood in other parts of the world that currently remain less badly affected. For example, I recently heard of a gay cultural worker in the Scottish city of Glasgow, whose only comment concerning the Quilt was that it appeared to be 'badly made.' This is similar to criticism by a British gay critic of an exhibition of photographs questioning the dominant visual imagery of isolated 'AIDS victims,' on the grounds that the show did not include enough KS lesions. He concluded: 'We must have portraits from the camera to rival Velasquez's paintings of dwarfs and fools or Géricault's of the insane.'[76] This High Art approach is deeply embedded in gay culture, especially in the assimilationist notion of a supposedly timeless 'gay sensibility,' and is clearly incompatible with the emergent gay AIDS-activist identity. Such observations strongly suggest that a profound struggle over the gay 'popular memory' of AIDS is already under way. The result of that struggle will be decisive for gay identity and community strength in the immediate and foreseeable future.[77]

If projects such as the Quilt and Gran Fury's 'Let the Record Show ...' installation represent gay cultural interventions against the grain of the mass-media construction of the 'meaning' of AIDS, a more private response is also becoming apparent, especially in the United States. For example, *The Advocate*, which describes itself as 'The National Gay Newsmagazine,' has contained a full-page advertisement from the Pride Institute of Minneapolis in every issue for the past few years. The ad announces: 'More Gay Men and Lesbians Have Died from Chemical Dependency than from AIDS,' a claim that it follows up with the assertion that seven million lesbians and gay men 'are struggling with the disease of chemical dependency.' The Pride Institute offers what it describes as a chance 'to recover a healthy personality, without the distractions of your everyday routine ... based on a proven combination of 12-step experience and clinical expertise ... We also offer you a chance to explore the history and heritage of being gay in a straight world. Our goal is to send you back into the world full of the enthusiasm, talent and energy that makes you who you are: proud, clean, sober and ready to go ... *Recover with pride.*' As Ellen Herman has observed, such 12-step 'recovery' programs 'have become so popular within the gay and feminist communities that they virtually constitute a 12-step "movement."'[78] Certainly gay and feminist bookshops in the United States contain shelves of books on the subject of Addiction and Dependency that are virtually unknown in Europe. Moreover, the 12-step 'movement' was the largest single grouping at the 1988 and 1989 gay-pride marches in San Francisco. Recovery programs of this sort all share the common metaphysical strategy of appealing to a Higher Power, which is invoked as a healing force in relation to addictions that are understood as purely individual matters. One thus comes across 12-step programs to 'cure' lesbians who are 'addicted' to love, gay men who are 'addicted' to sex, and so on and so forth. All this is announced in the cheery New Age tones of the American therapy industry, which seems totally unable to even begin to address the complex social and economic determinations of sexual behaviour, alcohol consumption, and drug use. It is this metaphysical individualism that makes the 12-step movement so worrying – the equivalent to a new Mystery Religion. It is only possible to understand why readers of *The Advocate* are not incensed and appalled by the grotesque insensitivity of the Pride Institute's publicity in the context of the cultural disorientation caused by the epidemic, a disorientation that makes many people very vulnerable to this kind of pseudo-spiritual snake oil.

How else can one explain the emergence of a popular discourse concerning supposedly 'healthy' personalities and the lure of a 'new sobriety'? Such messages tap deeply into the notion that AIDS resulted from sexual excess, and that sexual abstention will somehow make us all 'clean.' It is highly significant that this type of violently anti-political analysis can also tap into the concept of gay pride, and even recruit 'the history and heritage of being gay' to its cause. It is of course equally significant that the aim here is to lead to an acceptance of 'being gay in a straight world,' with no question of any analysis or challenge to 'straight' power. The 12-step movement offers a chimerical *personal* solution to the direct consequences of the organization of sexuality, class, and race in modern America. As such it partakes in the wider 'cultism' of the U.S. therapy industry, associated with such mass-media gurus as Louise Hay and Shirley MacLaine. In a moving and eloquent survey of such attitudes, Allan Bérubé concludes that 'AIDS is a profound tragedy, not a golden opportunity. It is neither an exterminating angel who came into our lives to punish us nor a guardian angel come to offer us the chance to be born again. If we have anyone to thank for the changes we have made, it is ourselves and each other, not AIDS ... The caricature of our past doesn't do justice to the depth and maturity of our lives before AIDS, including the sexual creativity that has enabled us to protect ourselves and each other by eroticizing safer sex.'[79] Just as the gay-liberation movement grew out of the disparate, conflicting experience of 'homosexuals' in the 1950s and 1960s, so a new gay identity is emerging from the harrowing experience of AIDS. This is everywhere uneven, and responses are unpredictable and often understandably extreme.

The work of Foucault, Weeks, and others demonstrates that the Victorians were every bit as interested in sex as we are, and as David Cannadine has forcibly argued, 'it is no solution to our very real contemporary problems to try to put the clock back to some idealized, mythical and non-existent nineteenth century golden age, where it is erroneously believed that these matters [of death and dying] were coped with more effectively than they are by us today.'[80] It may therefore 'be necessary to re-think that beguiling and nostalgic progression from obsessive death and forbidden sex in the nineteenth century to obsessive sex and forbidden death in the twentieth. For even if that model is of some relevance in the realm of public attitudes, it says little of value about the world of private experience.'[81] This is especially true for lesbians and gay men, who have come to live cheek by jowl with death throughout the 1980s in ways that our contemporaries cannot begin to imagine. Whilst martyrology is distasteful, especially if it lends a posthumous sense of purpose to the accidents of epidemic disease, it is none the less salutary to record and recall the political history of the HIV epidemic as it enters its second decade. For if we accept that gay identity is not fixed or given, but a complex historical result, it becomes apparent that it is at the level of popular understanding and memory of the epidemic that gay identity will be re-shaped and re-directed. In spite of all the dangers of an overly juridical model of history, we must strive *as if* we might achieve a verdict.[82]

Yet we should never expect the future of gay identity to involve the constant reproduction of people like ourselves. Indeed, the entire project of gay liberation aimed to undermine the processes by which homosexual desire was previously shaped into the self-abasing likeness of 'the homosexual.' At one extreme it seems that we are currently threatened with a widespread cultural return to just that likeness, and it is the very *possibility* of the ongoing project of gay identity that is now at stake. The jury that will eventually decide the 'truth' of AIDS has yet to be called, and in the meantime hundreds of thousands of the leading witnesses are already dead or dying. Right now it is at the level of the public 'meaning' of AIDS that the future of gay identity is being fought over. As Walter Benjamin observed in an earlier moment of twentieth-century cultural crisis: 'Only that historian will have the gift of fanning the spark of hope in the past who is firmly convinced that *even the dead* will not be safe from the enemy if he wins. And this enemy has not ceased to be victorious.'[83]

NOTES

1 Cindy Patton 'What Science Knows: Formations of AIDS Knowledges' in *AIDS: Individual, Cultural and Policy Dimensions* ed P. Aggleton et al (London, New York: Falmer Press 1990) 5

2 Michel Foucault 'Film and Popular Memory' *Foucault Live* ed S. Lotringer (New York: Semiotext(e) 1989) 102
3 Jorge Luis Borges 'Preface to the 1957 Edition' *The Book of Imaginary Beings* (Harmondsworth, Eng.: Penguin 1974) 13–14
4 Jeffrey Weeks *Sexuality and Its Discontents* (London: RKP 1985) 67
5 J. Laplanche and J.-B. Pontalis *The Language of Psycho-Analysis* (London: Hogarth Press 1983) 277
6 Ibid
7 Carole S. Vance 'Social Construction Theory: Problems in the History of Sexuality' in *Homosexuality, Which Homosexuality?* ed Dennis Altman et al (London: Gay Men's Press 1989) 29
8 Frederic Silverstolpe 'Benkert was not a doctor: On the nonmedical origin of the homosexual category in the nineteenth century,' paper delivered at *Homosexuality, Which Homosexuality?: International Conference on Gay and Lesbian Studies* (Amsterdam 1987), ed Altman et al
9 Ibid 209
10 Simon Watney 'The Homosexual Body: Resources and "A Note On Theory"' *Public* issue 3 (Toronto 1989)
11 Watney *Policing Desire: Pornography, AIDS, and the Media* (Minneapolis: University of Minnesota Press 1987) 27
12 Ibid
13 Jeffrey Weeks *Sexuality* (London: Tavistock 1986) 81
14 Michel Foucault 'Friendship as a Way of Life' in *Foucault Live* ed S. Lotringer (New York: Semiotext(e) 1989) 206
15 Ibid
16 Foucault 'The Social Triumph of the Sexual Will' *Christopher Street* 64 (New York 1982)
17 'U.S. Senate Moves to Censor' *Capital Gay* 405 (London) 11 August 1989, 8
18 Robert Glück 'HIV 1986–1988' *City Lights Review* 2 (San Francisco 1988) 42
19 Ibid
20 Dena Kleiman 'Gay Men Find Sadness Colors Life as They Make the Most of Their Days' *New York Times* 7 February 1989, B6
21 Ibid
22 Ibid
23 Jon Williams 'AIDS in a Time of Ignorance' *The Independent* (London) 21 March 1989
24 Ibid
25 For example, see Jan P. Vandenbrouke and Veronique P.A.M. Pardoel 'An Autopsy of Epidemiological Methods: The Case of "Poppers" in the Early Epidemic of the Acquired Immunodeficiency Syndrome (AIDS)' *American Journal of Epidemiology* 129, no 3 (March 1989)

26 See Meyrick Horton and Peter Aggleton 'Perverts, Inverts and Experts: The Cultural Production of an AIDS Research Paradigm' in *AIDS: Social Representations, Social Practices* ed P. Aggleton et al (New York, London: Falmer Press 1989).
27 See Simon Watney 'Introduction' in *Taking Liberties: AIDS and Cultural Politics* ed E. Carter and S. Watney (London: Serpent's Tail Press 1989).
28 Lucy Hodges 'Snapshot of Changing Views on Life and Love' *Daily Telegraph* (London) 3 November 1988
29 Ibid
30 Ibid
31 For example, see Dennis Altman and Kim Humphrey 'Breaking Boundaries: AIDS and Social Justice in Australia' *Social Justice*, forthcoming
32 Watney *Policing Desire* chap 1. See also Marshall Kirk and Hunter Madsen, *After the Ball: How America Will Conquer Its Fear and Hatred of Gays in the '90s* (New York, Toronto: Doubleday 1989).
33 Michael Bronski 'Dirty Dancing' *The Advocate* 528 (Los Angeles), 4 July 1989, 60
34 Ibid
35 See Jeffrey Weeks *Coming Out* (London: Quartet 1977).
36 Mark Gevisser 'Lesbian and Gay Students Choose' *The Nation* 26 March 1988, 413
37 Gregory Kolovakos 'AIDS Words' *The Nation* 1 May 1989. I would like to thank Paula Treichler for drawing my attention to this article.
38 Ibid 600
39 See Watney 'Safer Sex as Community Practice' in *AIDS: Individual, Cultural and Policy Dimensions*.
40 Kolovakos 'AIDS Words' 601
41 See Watney 'Safer Sex as Community Practice.'
42 Kolovakos 'AIDS Words' 600
43 Kathleen Conkey et al 'Zapping the Mayor or Zapping Gays?' *New York Native* 4 July 1988, 6
44 Vito Russo 'Why ACT UP Zapped Koch' *New York Native* 4 July 1988, 6
45 Julia Friedlander et al 'An Open Letter to the Members of ACT UP' *New York Native* 4 July 1988, 8–9
46 Larry Kramer 'A Word from Larry Kramer' *New York Native* 4 July 1989, 8
47 David Kirschenbaum 'Why ACT UP Zapped Mayor Koch' *New York Native* 4 July 1988, 6
48 Jeffrey Weeks 'Capitalism and the Organization of Sex' in *Homosexuality: Power and Politics* ed Gay Left Collective (London: Allison & Busby 1980) 19

49 Darrell Yates Rist 'The Deadly Cost of an Obsession' *The Nation* 13 February 1989, 198
50 Ibid 199
51 Ibid 200
52 Ibid 198
53 David Anger 'Author, Activist Larry Kramer in Town' *Equal Time* 183 (Minneapolis), 12 April 1989
54 Gore Vidal 'Gay Politics and AIDS' *The Nation* 20 March 1989, 362. I would like to thank Michael Bronski for drawing my attention to this letter.
55 Robert Massa, letter to *The Nation* 1 May 1989, 607. I would like to thank Craig Carnahan for drawing my attention to this letter.
56 Cindy Patton, unpublished letter to *The Nation* 1989, personal communication
57 Neil Smith 'The De-Gaying of AIDS' *Info* (Ottawa) July/August 1989, B7
58 See Cindy Patton 'What Science Knows.'
59 See Cindy Patton 'Thinking on Your Feet: A CMM Approach to Training Peer Educators' publication forthcoming.
60 See Watney 'Safer Sex as Community Practice.'
61 For example, see Celia Kitzinger *The Social Construction of Lesbianism* (London: Sage 1978). This work exemplifies the type of revolutionary feminist 'theory' that gives social constructionism a bad name. See Vance 'Social Construction Theory.'
62 Liz Hunt 'AIDS Epidemic among Gays "near peak"' *The Independent* (London) 4 September 1989, 1
63 John Preston 'Gay Men and Sex in the Eighties' *Mandate* (New York) 14, no 4 (April 1988) 87
64 Cleve Jones 'Afterword,' in C. Ruskin *The Quilt: Stories from the NAMES Project* (Pocket Books 1988) 157
65 John L. Martin 'The Impact of AIDS-Related Deaths and Illnesses on Gay Men in New York City' *Focus* (San Francisco) 3, no 7 (June 1988) 2
66 Michel Foucault *The History of Sexuality, Volume 1: An Introduction* (New York: Vintage Books 1980) 137
67 Ibid 139
68 Ibid 138
69 Ibid 145
70 Ibid 146
71 See Simon Watney 'AIDS and Photography (1987)' in *The Critical Image* ed Carol Squiers (Boston: Bay Press 1990).
72 *U.S. Congressional Record – Senate* 14 October 1987
73 Ibid
74 Laplanche and Pontalis *Language of Psycho-Analysis* 418

75 David Cannadine 'Death and Grief in Modern Britain' in *Mirrors of Mortality: Studies in the Social History of Death* ed J. Whaley (London: Europa Books 1981) 219
76 Philip Core 'Unseen Enemy' *The Independent* (London) 14 April 1989
77 A conference on the subject of HIV disease and gay identity took place at the Landsforeningen for bøsser og lesbiske, in Copenhagen, in February 1990, papers forthcoming.
78 Ellen Herman 'Getting to Serenity: Do Addiction Programs Sap Our Political Vitality?' *Outlook* (San Francisco) Summer 1988, 10
79 Allan Bérubé 'Caught in the Storm: AIDS and the Meaning of Natural Disaster' *Outlook* (San Francisco) Fall 1988, 18
80 Cannadine 'Death and Grief in Modern Britain' 240
81 Ibid 241
82 See Mark Cousins 'The Practice of Historical Investigation' in *Post-Structuralism and the Question of History* ed D. Attridge et al (Cambridge: Cambridge University Press 1987) 135.
83 Walter Benjamin 'Theses on the Philosophy of History' in *Illuminations* (London: Cape 1970) 257

Notes on Contributors

BARRY D. ADAM is professor of sociology at the University of Windsor and author of *The Survival of Domination* and *The Rise of a Gay and Lesbian Movement*. He is past president of the AIDS Committee of Windsor and is currently working on a project concerning the impact of HIV on personal, family, and work relationships.

BART BEATY is a student in the undergraduate film program at Carleton University and intends to pursue his interest in film criticism and cultural theory at the graduate level in the United States. In 1991 he was a student in the Western Literature and Humanities seminar on AIDS and the Arts at the University of Western Ontario. In the summer of 1991 he worked with Greenpeace in Toronto.

MONIQUE BRUNET-WEINMANN completed her graduate work in art history at the Université de Montréal with a thesis on the figural painting of Louise Gadbois. She has published extensively on the art scene in Quebec, and has contributed to numerous arts programs on Radio-Canada. In 1990, as director of CRITIQ (Complexe de réalisations indépendant transculturel et interartiel du Québec), she organized a conference on apocalyptic themes in contemporary art at the Centre Saidye Bronfman in Montreal.

CLARENCE CROSSMAN has been the education coordinator of the AIDS Committee of London since 1987, and a leader in London's gay and lesbian community since 1981. A founding member of the Visual AIDS Committee and a clergyperson in the Metropolitan Community Church, he has initiated many AIDS education projects including the 1991 video *Going Home*, which examines a rural family's response to the epidemic.

MONIKA GAGNON is a Toronto-based writer and critic who has published in numerous magazines and journals, including *Parachute, C, Vanguard, border/lines, Third Text*, and *Cinéaction*. She has also contributed essays to several anthologies, notably *Work in Progress: Building Feminist Culture, Yellow Peril: Reconsidered*, and *Thirteen Essays on Photography*. She participated in SIDART at the Fifth International AIDS Conference in Montreal in 1989. She is co-editor of *Parallelogramme*, published by the Association of National Non-Profit Artist-Run Centres (ANNPAC/RACA).

JOHN GORDON graduated from King's College (London, Ontario) in 1989 with a degree in social work. From 1988 to 1990 he worked as a counsellor with the AIDS Committee of London and as an activist for persons living with AIDS in Southwestern Ontario. He continues to be active in the New Democratic Party at a federal level.

JOHN GREYSON is a video/film artist whose titles include *Moscow Does Not Believe in Queers* (1986), *The ADS Epidemic* (1987), *Urinal* (1988), and *The Making of Monsters* (1991). He produced the Deep Dish TV compilation of AIDS tapes entitled *Angry Initiatives, Defiant Strategies* (1988), and was co-founder of the Toronto Living With AIDS project (1990), a series of thirteen half-hour tapes addressing the AIDS crisis from various community perspectives. His tapes about AIDS include *The Pink Pimpernel* and *The World is Sick (sic)*. His current project, *Zero Patience*, is a feature musical about the Air Canada flight attendant accused of bringing AIDS to North America.

JAN ZITA GROVER edits *Artpaper* in St Paul, Minnesota, and is a member of the editorial collective of *PWAlive!*, a newsletter written by and for people living with AIDS. She has written about cultural struggles around AIDS since 1986. In Minnesota, she can do that and canoe, too – a healthy compromise.

DANIEL HARRIS has been writing for gay newspapers and magazines since the early 1980s, and is currently a columnist for *The Quarterly*. His essays and reviews have appeared in *Harper's*, the *Washington Post*, *The Nation*, and the *Los Angeles Times*.

DAVID KINAHAN is a doctoral student at the University of Western Ontario. His dissertation explores issues of contemporary cultural theory in relation to sixteenth-century English poetry. In 1988 he helped to found the 'Visual AIDS' exhibition and was an original member of Western's interdisciplinary graduate seminar on AIDS and the Arts.

ARTHUR KROKER is professor of political science at Concordia University in Montreal. He is the author of numerous books on postmodern culture, including *The Postmodern Scene* (1988), *The Panic Encyclopedia* (1991), and *The Possessed Individual* (1992). He has also edited with Marilouise Kroker *Body Invaders* (1988) and *The Hysterical Male* (1991).

JAMES MILLER, Faculty of Arts professor at the University of Western Ontario in London, is the author of *Measures of Wisdom: The Cosmic Dance in Classical and Christian Antiquity* (1986). In 1988 he initiated an interdisciplinary seminar on AIDS and the Arts at Western – the first such course at a Canadian university. He is the curator of 'Visual AIDS,' an international exhibition of AIDS posters that has been touring Canada, the United States, and Western Europe since October 1988. In 1989 he joined the order of the Gay Fathers and marched behind their banner, with his eldest daughter, during the 1991 Pride Day celebrations in Toronto.

JEFF O'MALLEY has worked with a variety of non-government organizations concerned with cross-cultural education, human rights, cultural activism, and the Developing World. In 1989 he helped to organize a conference of such organizations during the Fifth International AIDS Conference in Montreal. From 1990 to 1991 he was an officer in the Global Program on AIDS at the World Health Organization in Geneva.

BRIAN PATTON is completing a doctoral dissertation on Andrew Marvell and seventeenth-century political writers for the English Department at the University of Western Ontario. In 1988 he attended the first 'AIDS and the Arts' seminar at Western and worked on the commentaries for the original 'Visual AIDS' exhibition at the London Regional Art Gallery.

DAHLIA REICH covered the medical beat at the *London Free Press* from 1988 to 1990, winning numerous awards from the Western Ontario Newspaper Association, the Ontario Reporters' Association, and other organizations during that period. Besides the local impact of the AIDS epidemic, her assignments have included the Ethiopian famine in 1985 and the return of adopted children to their native Bangladesh. In 1991 she wrote on European affairs while staying in France on an eight-month journalism scholarship.

DR MARGARET A. SOMERVILLE has published widely in medicine, ethics, and law, and is very active in 'presenting' these fields in all forms of media. Her current appointments at McGill University are as Gale Professor of Law, professor in the Faculty of Medicine, and director of the McGill Centre for Medicine, Ethics, and Law. She has served as a consultant to the Global Programme on AIDS at the World Health Organization, and in 1991 became a Fellow of the Royal Society of Canada.

SIMON WATNEY is the director of the National AIDS Manual (NAM UK), and the author of *English Post-Impressionism* (1980), *Policing Desire: Pornography, AIDS, and the Media* (1987), and *The Art of Duncan Grant* (1990). He has written on the politics of AIDS representation for such journals as *Radical America, October*, and *Impulse*, and has contributed essays on sexuality, racism, and cultural activism to several anthologies, notably *Taking Liberties, Coming On Strong*, and *Out There*. Forthcoming is a collection of his essays entitled *Practices of Freedom*.

THOMAS WAUGH has been associate professor of film studies at Concordia University since 1976, and is currently chairing Concordia's HIV/AIDS advisory committee. He is the editor of *'Show Us life': Towards a History and Aesthetics of the Committed Documentary* (1984), and the author of a forthcoming history of gay male erotic film and photography to 1969.

DAVID WHITE, a doctoral candidate at the University of Western Ontario, is writing a dissertation on the representation of AIDS in gay literature under the supervision of Professors James Miller and Alice Mansell. In June 1989, along with Andy Fabo and other AIDS activists, he participated in the demonstration at the opening of the Fifth International AIDS Conference in Montreal. In the fall of that year he taught Western's first undergraduate course on AIDS and the Arts.

Photo Credits

Plates

1 John Tamblyn, for Visual AIDS
3 Lennart Nilsson
4 Art Services (UWO)
5 Taro Yamasaki
7 Peter Sterling
9 Ethan Hoffman
10 Max Winter, Tim Dillon
11 James D. Wilson
12 Glenn Mansfield
13–15 Gay Men's Health Crisis
16 Gypsy Ray
17–18 Jane Rosett
19 Duane Michals
20 Nicholas Nixon
21–4 Courtesy of Monika Gagnon
25–37 Nick Wells
38 Art Services (UWO)
39 Courtesy of André Durand
40 Courtesy of Gallery John A. Schweitzer
41–2 John Tamblyn, for Visual AIDS
43 Courtesy of Galerie Christiane Chassay
44–5 John Tamblyn, for Visual AIDS
46 Philip Hannan
47–9 John Tamblyn, for Visual AIDS
50 Philip Hannan

51–4 John Tamblyn, for Visual AIDS
55–6 Susan Bradnam (photos in feature); John Tamblyn (photos of layout)
57 Art Services (UWO)
58 Art Services (UWO)
59–60 John Tamblyn, for Visual AIDS

Portfolio One

1–12 John Tamblyn, for Visual AIDS

	Portfolio Two	*Art information*
1	Courtesy of Mary Scott	mixed media, n.d.
2	Wyn Geleynse	acrylic on canvas, 1987
3	Wyn Geleynse	mixed media on paper, n.d.
4	William Kuryluk	T-pins on copper, 1988
5	Carmen Lamanna	oil, tempera, wax on plywood, 1987–8
6	John Tamblyn	ceramic installation, 1988
7	Diana Church	oil on canvas, 1981
8	David Reynolds	typewriter photo collage, 1989
9	Isaac Applebaum	mixed media on parchment, 1988
10	Ian McCausland	oil on canvas, 1988
11	Ian Murray	urine, Indian Yellow, on Harumi paper, 1987
12	Tony Wilson	mixed media on antique engraving, 1987

Index

abstinence (chastity) 116, 131, 149, 173, 194, 201, 309, 311, 313, 358, 362

academics: and activists 4, 7, 12, 15, 22, 56, 138, 147, 177, 185–214, 350; and artists 7, 12, 15, 17, 20, 22, 138, 201, 216, 360–1

Acquired Immanent Divinity Syndrome 110, 259, 268

activism. *See* AIDS activism; cultural activism

ACT UP (AIDS Coalition To Unleash Power) 5, 8, 18, 21, 29, 37, 39–40, 71, 77, 108, 118–19, 136, 158, 163, 183, 186–7, 204, 207, 211, 221, 235, 241, 266, 335, 342–6, 352, 359, 360; *plates* 20, 50

Adam, Barry 14

A Day without Art 158

A Death in the Family 112, 123, 124, 126, 128–9, 130, 134

Advertising Age 43–4

Advisory Committee of People with AIDS 28

aestheticism: and/as activism 10, 11, 16, 66, 79, 96, 98, 108, 129, 136–45, 203, 206, 217–21; versus activism 15, 17, 22, 39–42, 62, 68–9, 82, 108, 119, 131, 135, 157–9, 168, 196, 265–6, 360; *plates* 1, 19, 39, 44

A Fake Video Script 139–45

Africa 169, 178–80, 182, 183, 190, 217, 312; as origin of disease 74, 76, 101, 142–3, 170–1, 280, 301; *plates* 46, 48; Portfolio One 1, 2, 7; Portfolio Two 1

Against Nature 136; exhibition 136–7

Agathon 20

Age of AIDS 11, 18, 66, 91, 120, 149,178, 189, 203, 216, 219, 226, 262, 264, 267, 329, 347, 354; criticized 19, 199, 201, 209, 257, 270, 281; paradoxes of 10, 86–7, 102, 202, 335–6, 346

Ahasuerus 95

AID (Acquired Immune Deficiency) 27, 47

AIDS (Acquired Immunodeficiency Syndrome)
- as 'invariably fatal' sexually transmitted disease 72, 74, 83, 92, 108, 153, 179–80, 183, 228, 231, 241, 310
- casual transmission of 28, 33, 171, 179–80, 279
- diagnosis of 24, 27, 34, 91, 131, 156, 190–2, 223, 227, 232, 251, 255, 259, 313, 334, 335
- economic impact of 15, 154, 171, 179, 213, 349
- epidemiological history of 3, 15, 25, 26, 27–31, 36, 43, 47, 84, 101, 142, 154, 156, 169, 171, 180, 188, 190, 198–9, 278, 308, 310, 312–13, 333, 334–5, 341, 347, 351, 356
- etiology of 26, 28, 31, 48, 152, 264, 265, 306, 312–13, 358
- in Third World 47, 101, 151, 169–76, 213, 301
- living with 36–9, 40, 87, 118, 138, 151–3, 155, 175, 187, 192, 211–13, 222–7, 232, 234, 238, 256, 282, 303, 323, 334–9, 346–7
- naming of 4, 27, 46–7, 128, 152, 181, 209, 241
- symptoms of 23, 30, 61, 62, 84, 180, 182, 188–92, 223, 232, 237, 255, 261–2, 266, 269, 313
- treatment of 24, 29, 40, 102, 103, 104, 109, 129, 153, 155, 212–13, 225, 226–7, 255, 296, 303, 336, 338, 349
- virology of 15, 102, 114, 276–80, 333

See also HIV

AIDS ACTION NOW! 5, 141, 144–5, 186, 204, 207, 211, 359; *plate* 50

AIDS activism: and civil disobedience 342–6; and lobbying 350; and mourning 163–8, 266, 334–5, 355–6; concept of 16, 36–7, 40, 66, 87, 108, 141, 178, 211–13, 250, 266–7, 340, 343, 345, 350–2; history of 3–6, 25–9, 34, 37–40, 42, 48, 54–6, 112, 117–19, 155, 163, 185–6, 191, 249, 318, 339, 341–3, 345; in Africa 9, 175–6, 179; in Britain 3, 5, 104, 105, 108, 210, 339, 355; in Canada 3, 5, 87, 135–45, 147, 154, 157–8, 185–8, 206–11, 213, 241–53; in Europe 9, 132, 150, 155, 210, 339; in Latin America 175, 183; in United States 3, 5, 9, 25–53, 117–19, 135–45, 155, 163, 210, 249, 334–6, 340–6, 359–60; representation of 66, 70, 77, 117–18, 221; success of 359; versus assimilationism 339–52, 361; *plates* 17, 50; Portfolio One 9. *See also* ACT UP; AIDS ACTION NOW!; cultural activism

AIDS advocacy, 246–9

AIDS allegory 92–4, 149, 151, 180–1, 192, 197, 200, 219, 266, 275; of Flesh and Spirit 99, 101, 104, 107, 148, 181, 258–64; *plates* 41–3. *See also* Christian; death; moralism

AIDS and the Arts (seminar) 11, 12, 53, 177, 194, 206–7, 208, 216; *plates* 52–3

AIDS apocalypse 131, 151, 180, 184, 199–200, 202, 209, 321, 328

AIDS archives, 44–5

AIDS awareness 19, 22, 114, 177, 202, 232; as activist aesthetic project 4, 9, 21, 202; as defence 178, 182–3; as defiance 178, 180–1; as desire 178, 183–4; as fear of death 178, 179–80; as social cause 3, 114, 120, 202, 216

AIDS carrier 35, 154, 179; myth criticized 310; *plate* 9

AIDS Civil Rights Project 350

AIDS Coalition To Unleash Power. *See* ACT UP

AIDS comedy 141; satiric 131–2, 164, 227, 241, 244, 248
AIDS commentary. *See* AIDS discourse
AIDS Committee of London (ACOL) 208, 242, 243, 244, 246–9, 253, 256
AIDS Committee of Toronto (ACT) 141, 224
AIDS conferences: as site for activism 3, 185–8, 351; Atlanta (First) 28, 36; Boston 349; international 87; London, Ontario 15–19, 21, 53, 54, 68, 83, 134, 138, 207, 242, 288, 318; Montreal (Fifth) 12, 153, 154, 156, 159, 185–92, 194, 200, 210, 351; San Francisco (Sixth) 210; Stockholm (Fourth) 51; *plates* 1, 50
AIDS control policy 305–6, 308, 310, 313, 316, 324, 344. *See also* AIDS politics; AIDS prevention
AIDS crisis, 3–6, 9, 10, 11, 14, 15, 17, 55, 68, 74, 78, 84, 90, 102, 108, 112, 114, 117, 119, 120, 124, 127, 130, 135–6, 138–9, 154, 177, 186, 188, 194, 196–201, 205, 216, 221, 262, 265, 266, 268, 292, 303, 324, 341, 349, 352, 358, 360
AIDS: *Cultural Analysis / Cultural Activism. See* Crimp
AIDS discourse (commentary) 4, 6, 8, 12, 14, 17, 19, 29–30, 42, 56, 62–3, 74, 124, 125, 169–76, 188, 191–3, 216, 218, 234, 261, 273, 307–14, 335, 337, 352, 354–5, 357–8
AIDS discrimination 3–6, 14, 19, 25, 31, 95, 119, 177, 193, 209, 222, 227, 232, 238, 247–54, 256, 281, 290, 292, 300, 302, 305, 335, 346
AIDS education 27–39, 155, 173, 174–5, 177–84, 194, 203–4, 206, 213, 223, 239, 242, 244, 247, 252, 298, 313, 314–15, 317–18, 336, 339, 341, 351–2, 354–5, 357–8
AIDS facts 12, 19, 22, 24, 175, 209, 239, 257, 273, 274, 278–9, 282, 283, 308
AIDS-Hilfe Schweiz 150; *plate* 59
AIDS Info-Docu Schweiz 177, 210
AIDS legislation 14–16, 19, 39, 212, 242, 289–92, 296, 300, 318, 346
AIDS literature 21, 138, 159; chronicle history 8, 257–65; fiction 8, 13, 257, 264–5, 283; medical 14, 27–30, 276–82, 337; non-medical 6; novels 257–70; plays 133, 311; poetry 8, 11, 164, 191; testimonial 8, 14, 282–3; video script 139–45; women's 269–70; *plate* 45
AIDS phobia (panic) 28, 31, 35, 37, 69, 84, 92, 102, 103, 117, 122, 132, 143, 148, 153, 178, 179–80, 182, 186, 191, 192–3, 197, 209, 211, 222–4, 226–7, 233–4, 238, 241, 249, 250–1, 264, 266, 291–2, 300, 304, 308, 315, 317, 324–8, 334; *plates* 42, 57; Portfolio One 1–4
AIDS politics, 7–8, 14–16, 116–17, 137, 155, 163, 175, 186–8, 197–8, 206, 209, 211–13, 266, 273, 297, 299–300, 305, 307–14
AIDS prevention campaigns 16, 19, 22, 36, 43, 156–7, 169–84, 193, 228–9, 244, 310, 315, 351, 352, 355, 358; *plates* 40–2, 46–9, 51–3, 59–60; Portfolio One 1–12
AIDS-Related Complex. *See* ARC
AIDS representation: diversity of 8, 30–3, 135, 176, 192, 205, 209, 355–6; ethics of 6, 39–40, 230–1, 236–9, 241–53, 281; isolating effect of mainstream 35, 39–41, 42, 50–1, 61, 72–3, 84, 90–2, 115, 126, 169, 175, 224, 226, 228, 234,

241, 261, 282, 291, 297, 335–7, 344, 351, 360; medical 15, 17, 24, 31, 61, 182; politics of 6, 12, 14, 16, 31–2, 39–41, 54–5, 61–2, 69, 78, 84, 93, 102, 104, 195, 108, 112–13, 118–19, 121, 124, 131–2, 165, 181–4, 194, 203, 209, 216, 275–6, 317–18; private 163–8, 226; problematics of 7, 16, 24–5, 29, 40–2, 61, 63, 68, 70, 113, 124, 128, 133, 137, 152, 163, 169–76, 179–84, 208, 272–84, 297; rupturing strategies of 11, 63, 66, 84, 86, 136, 145–6, 146–60, 185–8, 314, 316; verbal 8, 10, 14, 24, 33, 95, 117, 139–45, 241, 257–84; visual 8, 10, 12, 17–18, 24, 30–53, 61–3, 68, 72–4, 84, 89–90, 96, 102, 115, 117, 135–45, 234

AIDS service organizations 141, 150, 155, 157–8, 175, 179–84, 203, 208, 210, 224–5, 242–3, 246, 247–53, 315, 334, 339, 341, 343, 348–9, 350, 351, 352, 358

AIDSpeak 19. *See also* AIDS discourse

AIDS-Staat 9, 18

AIDS-Timmy 228, 231–2, 234–5

AIDS tragedy 19, 92, 94, 96, 115, 117, 118, 196, 199–201, 234, 278, 297, 311, 355, 362

AIDS 'victim' 4, 8, 10, 11, 13, 17, 19, 23, 25, 32, 33, 34, 35, 37, 41, 48, 50, 62, 93, 101, 108, 126, 144, 154, 187, 191, 202, 228, 232, 233–5, 236–9, 247, 255, 266, 267, 268, 281, 311, 326, 327, 335, 338, 357, 360

AIDS virus 48, 198, 226, 281, 335; myth criticized 200, 209, 277–80, 284, 310; *plates* 3, 4, 47. *See also* HIV

Albany Trust 340

Alberta College of Art 65

Alice Doesn't Live Here Anymore 111

Altemeyer, Robert 293

Altman, Dennis 307, 311

Altman, Lawrence K. 153

American Foundation for AIDS Research 267

America Responds to AIDS (campaign) 19, 351

Amsterdam 352

amyl nitrate 57, 165

anal sex. *See* sex

Andrews, Stephen 215, 219; Portfolio Two 9

androgyny 89, 101, 144

And the Band Played On. *See* Shilts

An Early Frost 35–6, 122, 133

Ansel Adams Center 210

Apocalypticism. *See* AIDS Apocalypse

Apollinaire, Guillaume 76, 79

ARC (AIDS-Related Complex) 55, 222, 223, 224, 225, 232, 237, 253–4

art: activist 4–10, 62, 66, 69, 77, 119, 135–45, 192, 194, 203–5, 266; apotropaic 103, 104, 110; as advertisement 265–6, 340; as agitprop 138, 141, 163, 204; as commodity 62, 72, 135, 143, 157–8, 265–6; as enlightenment 304; conceptual 288; elegiac 8, 10, 66, 132, 136, 138, 159, 164, 355–6; epitropaic 104, 108; figural 10, 66, 86, 96, 205, 217–21; graphic 17, 21, 211, 284; high 361; homoerotic 9, 79, 136, 219; medieval 72, 85, 150–1, 180; memorial 8, 11, 16, 71, 80, 159, 265–6, 267, 355–6; minimalist 288; modern 70, 96; performing 16, 118, 158, 229; political 69, 217–21; postmodern 4; public 11–12, 16,

179–84; religious 8, 10, 12, 93–109, 159, 264; sacrificial 327; theurgic 97–9; transcendent 12, 42, 62, 68–9, 82, 98, 105, 119, 128, 140, 143, 204, 206, 218; vain 189, 192. *See also* aestheticism; AIDS representation; artist
Art Against AIDS (auction): Montreal 157–9; New York 157; *plate* 44
Artemis 99, 100
Artforum 141
artist: allied with critics 3–8, 12, 15–19, 22, 53, 55, 97–100, 201–11, 216, 266, 288; at odds with critics 39–40, 108, 123, 135–7; dismembered 83–4; role of 41, 62, 81–2, 86, 105, 110, 129, 155–60, 205, 215, 221, 266; with AIDS, 211; *plates* 25, 33, 35, 37. *See also* Fabo; Durand
Arts Action Now (agenda) 12, 202, 203, 204–6
Art SupporT 157, 159
Aschenbach 140–1, 143–5
Asians 218
As Is 123, 124, 125, 127–9, 130
A Space (gallery) 65
assimilationism 14, 339, 361; fantasy of tolerance 346; reinvigorated by AIDS crisis 340–4, 361–2
Athens, plague of 20, 192
Atlanta 28, 30, 36, 313
Augustine, St 80, 109
Australia 149, 150, 182–3, 205, 339; Queensland 317; *plate* 41; Portfolio One 8
authoritarianism 289, 293, 324
authority: crisis of 138, 272, 305, 333; of dominant ideology 340–1, 350; of medical establishment 61, 117, 138, 155, 182, 282–3, 336; of representations 25–6, 289; *plate* 2
A Virus Has No Morals 112, 131–2
AZT 29, 37, 234

Barracks, The 65, 76
Baryshnikov, Mikhail 267–8
bathhouses 131, 318; as gay underworld 65, 165, 198, 257, 258
Baudrillard, Jean 151–2
Bay Area Reporter 163–8; *plate* 45
Bayer, Ronald 318
Beardsley, Aubrey 79
Beaty, Bart 11
Beijo da rua 175; *plate* 49
Benjamin, Walter 363
Benkert, Karoly 331, 334
Benner, Dick 127
Bentham, Jeremy 81
Berlin 9, 14, 66, 210
Berliner AIDS-Hilfe 210
Bersani, Leo 74, 88
Bérubé, Allan 362
bestiality 142, 171, 268, 279–80
Bible 182, 230, 262, 267, 295; Genesis 114, 119, 179, 191, 264; Ecclesiasticus 260; Esther 95; Job 263; Revelation 107
billboards 43, 229
bisexuals and bisexuality 57, 91, 92, 226, 269, 279, 280, 281, 312
Black Death. *See* plague
blacks 101, 317; as 'high-risk' group 16, 25, 29, 40, 89–90, 308, 313, 351; discrimination against 4, 114, 142, 177, 179; gay, 78, 137; Marxist 169; men 180, 217; women 179, 217, 330, 348, 349; *plates* 38–9
Blake, William 81, 230
blindness, AIDS-related 263
blood 92, 171, 313, 316; banks 28, 35, 156, 213; screening 281; supply 'poisoned' 33, 35, 209, 258, 312
body: abject 10, 56, 63, 129, 218; Christian 216; contaminated

323–6; cybernetic 321–2; disappeared 323; emprisoned 71, 73, 83, 92, 219, 220; erotic 12, 16, 36, 89–90, 101, 129, 216, 217, 221, 266, 267, 312, 329; exotic 217; female 54, 56, 60–1, 63, 76, 89–92, 179, 213, 216, 217, 219, 220, 261–2, 308; fundamentalist, 325–6; gay/homosexual 55–6, 61–3, 67–8, 74, 82, 87, 219, 221, 337; geometric 81–2; male 36, 89–90, 101, 217, 219; Marxist 216; mechanical 357; militarized 276–84; of hysterics 56–63; of PWAs 62–3, 89–92, 102, 129, 179, 216, 219, 221, 255, 326, 350; opposed to soul 75, 80, 83, 109, 144, 218, 220, 258–60; panic 321–4, 328; pathetic 71, 86, 218; postmodern 325–6; purified 259, 261–2, 275, 323, 325–6; ruined 61, 63, 85, 100, 132, 148, 179, 218, 219, 255, 258–9, 261–2, 326, 328; social constructions of 53–63, 81, 90, 165, 172, 179–84, 203, 207, 209, 215–21, 229, 275–7, 280, 282, 307, 323, 357; spiritualized 80, 82–3, 102, 181, 258–61; telematic 321–2; tortured 219, 220, 261–3, 268, 328; under duress 17–18, 216, 218–19; *plates* 25–37, 52–3, 59–60; Portfolio One 1–2, 5–8, 10–11; Portfolio Two 1–12

Body & Society. *See* The Body & Society

Borchelt, Frances 260–4

Borges, Jorge Luis 329

Bosch, Hieronymus 148

Boston 27, 322, 349

Botticelli, Sandro 95–8, 102; *La Derelitta* 95–6; *Primavera* 97–8, 102

Bradnam, Susan 13

Brandt, Allan 313

Brazil 175

Brecht, Bertolt 219

Bressan, Arthur 123, 126, 127

Bright Eyes 48

Briquet, Dr 58

Britain 9, 108, 179, 183, 193, 305, 314, 315, 317, 333, 334, 337–41, 351, 355

Bronski, Michael 129, 340

Brown, John 215, 218; Portfolio Two 5

Brunet-Weinmann, Monique 11, 205

Buchan, David 17; *plate* 1

Buckley, William F. 326

Buddies 123, 125–6, 127, 129, 130

Burton, Sir Richard 142–5

Bush, George 120, 284, 324, 342, 348

Butler, Sheila 215–16, 220; Portfolio Two 10

CAID (Community Acquired Immune Deficiency) 27, 47

Calgary 65, 210, 316

Callen, Michael 49, 50, 197, 200, 202

Canada 9, 78, 156, 174, 175, 180, 207, 229, 230, 244, 247, 249, 253, 294, 299, 300, 305, 309, 314, 333; British Columbia 316, 317; Manitoba 253; Yukon 253. *See also* Ontario; Quebec

Canadian AIDS Society 253

Canadian Charter of Rights and Freedoms 292, 295

Canadian Public Health Association 22, 310

Canadian University Students Overseas (CUSO) 12, 178

cancer 109, 147, 153–5, 224, 234, 255, 272–3, 275, 276; breast 349; gay 170, 258. *See also* Kaposi's sarcoma; leukemia

candidiasis 188–92
Cannadine, David 359–60, 362
Cant, George 108–9, 329, 355
capitalism 7, 92, 164, 183, 242–3, 262, 327
Catherine of Genoa, St 99–100
CBC (Canadian Broadcasting Corporation) 156, 169
CDC. *See* Centers for Disease Control
censorship: of AIDS representations 16, 84–5, 165, 166, 242, 252–3, 265, 309, 314–16, 351; of Gay History exhibit 343–4; of porn 134, 315
Centers for Disease Control (CDC) 13, 19, 27, 30, 36, 154, 185, 186, 187, 198, 261, 263, 312–13
Cézanne, Paul 75, 76
Chance of a Lifetime 36; 'Hank and Jerry' 123, 124, 125, 128, 130
Chapel Hill, NC 21, 206, 210
Charcot, Jean-Martin 56–60
chastity. *See* abstinence
Chicago 27
children 81, 100, 129, 143, 147, 175 181, 220, 224, 232, 254, 267, 269, 309, 310, 312; abuse of 298–9, 334; as 'innocent victims' 35, 229–30, 308; street kids 9, 173–4; with AIDS 25, 28, 156, 237, 280
cholera 4, 153
Christ 94, 105, 143, 262
Christian 131, 156, 230; fundamentalism 264, 268, 307, 310, 325; Grail myth 150, 158, 198; heterodoxy 100; moralization of AIDS 94–5, 108–9, 115–16, 119–20, 174, 179, 181, 197–8, 202, 229, 258–64, 276–7, 310–11; metaphysics, 330, 353; mysteries, 98–9, 104, 259, 362; sexual morality 142, 174–5, 179, 181, 194; teleology 172. *See also* abstinence; church; martyr; monogamy; moralism; Sebastian
ChromoZone 66
church 107–8, 110, 150, 203, 287, 295, 306, 318, 359–60; St James's, Piccadilly 109; St Mary's 110
Cinéaste, 116
civil rights and liberties 3, 5, 117, 251, 253–4, 299–300, 307, 342, 344
class 170, 172, 330, 345, 351, 362; and AIDS discrimination 42, 114, 257, 260, 324–35, 345
Clément, Catherine 55, 56
clones 139, 258
closet 267. *See also* coming out; gay identity
Coad, Wendy 215, 217; Portfolio Two 2
Coalition for Lesbian and Gay Rights 252
coming out 132, 223, 227, 232, 244, 258, 267, 346, 348, 354, 356. *See also* gay identity; gay liberation
Comité sida aide Montréal 150, 157
Communism 276
community-based groups 317–18, 339. *See also* AIDS service organizations
Conant, Marcus 24
condoms 9, 84, 116, 117, 128, 130, 131, 149, 150, 184, 209, 213, 270, 308–9, 310, 311, 313, 315, 318; 'Condoman' 182–3; 'El Preservativo' 183; hot rubbers 209; *plate* 59; Portfolio One 8–9. *See also* safer sex
Conkey, Kathleen 342
conservatives and conservatism 5, 9, 16, 19, 35, 94, 108, 113–15, 156, 180, 187, 193, 199, 205, 208, 231, 262–4, 276, 299–300, 306, 309, 317–18, 326, 358–9; on abortion, 308–9

constructivism, and disease 273–4
contraception, debates 308–9, 310, 314, 317–18
counterdiscourse 111, 114; AIDS education as 37, 175–6, 194, 202, 211, 314, 317–18, 357; gay identity as 352–4, 356; expressed in photography 33, 42; to developmentalism 172, 174–5; to heterosexism 138, 361; to mainstream AIDS discourse 5, 8, 29, 36, 55–6, 73, 112, 174–6, 201, 357, 361; to neo-puritanism 11, 99
Courbet, Gustave 75
COYOTE (Call Off Your Old Tired Ethics) 281
Criminal Code, Canadian 290
Crimp, Douglas 6–9, 13, 21, 51, 62, 116, 158, 159, 204, 206, 216, 257, 265, 273–4; 'AIDS: Cultural Analysis ...' 6, 21, 64, 158, 160, 204, 214, 271, 273, 285; *AIDS demo graphics* 21; 'How to Have Promiscuity ...' 50, 121, 270; *October* anthology 6–9, 13, 21, 46, 50, 141, 170, 206, 235, 265
crisis: as turning-point 29, 195, 363; history of term 195–6; interventions in 302–3; of authority 14–15, 281, 333; of bourgeois identity, 324–6, 327; of representation 70, 170, 187–8, 192–4, 203; of sexual identity 14, 57–61, 333, 341; postmodern 326. *See also* AIDS crisis
critical theory: applied to AIDS crisis 6, 8, 16, 62, 169–70, 202, 205–11, 237, 238; as shamanism 327–8; as stimulus for activism 4, 16, 202, 205–11. *See also* deconstruction; feminism; postmodernism
criticism. *See* critical theory
critics 188, 195, 199, 201, 360; as activists 201–11, 216. *See also* academics; artists; critical theory
Crossman, Clarence 13, 208, 242
Cruise, Tom 113
CRUSAID 108
cubism 70, 75–6
cultural activism: concept of 4, 9, 117, 141, 202–6, 265–6; history of 3–4, 54; testing of 9, 159, 202–11, 234, 241–53, 266, 268; versus aestheticism 15, 22, 66, 134, 135–6, 141, 265–6. *See also* AIDS activism; art; artist
cultural analysis 8, 136, 203, 216, 241, 249–50, 287–9, 321–8, 338. *See also* Crimp; critical theory; cultural activism
Curnoe, Greg 216, 220; Portfolio Two 11
Curtius, E.R. 151
cybernetics 321–2
cynicism 202, 321, 323–4

Dalglish, Peter 173
dandy(ism) 11; as activism 136–45
Danny 112, 126, 129
Davis, Christopher 267
Day, Susan 215, 218–19; Portfolio Two 6
DCAC Gallery 210
death 43, 83, 104, 119, 128, 141, 163, 190, 192, 207, 225–56, 269, 276, 350, 360, 362–3; and sex 11, 39, 86, 90, 92, 94, 128–9, 131, 147, 159, 178, 181, 189, 194, 209, 260, 266, 269–70, 305, 318, 323, 348, 363; and the Maiden 91; 'Architecture of' 17; by ignorance 84; dance of 147–9, 151, 164, 204, 205, 260, 267; equated with AIDS 40–1, 86, 146; gay versus straight 13, 258–64, 334, 354; medieval images of 11, 93–4, 108, 147–9, 151, 166, 180; of individual 146–7, 151–2, 154, 163–8, 223,

255–6, 268, 304, 308, 318, 355–6; of society 304, 318, 356; of species 146–7, 151–2, 154, 304, 356–7; of youth 104, 115, 148; representation of 17, 93, 139–40, 148, 151, 165–6, 200, 202, 209, 218–19, 233, 238–9, 241, 259–60; sacrificial 328; Triumph of 180; *plates* 1, 39, 41, 48; Portfolio One 2–4
Death in Venice 140
Decad 105, 106
deconstruction 8, 132, 134, 137, 182, 191–2, 201, 217, 314
Delaporte, François, 273
Demeter 99, 102
Denneny, Michael 68
dentists 188–92, 226, 233, 238, 248, 254
Denver 27
Denver Principles 7, 21, 48
Derelitta, La 94–5
dermatology 180, 184, 185, 188–92
Detroit 207
developmentalism 12, 169, 171–4, 178, 213
devil 80, 195; exorcism of 103, 104, 144, 198, 283; possession by 60, 198, 200, 261; virus as 104, 181, 197, 260–1, 264
dextran sulfate 5
Diana: Princess of Wales 96, 99, 100, 104, 106–9; Triformis (goddess) 99–100, 104, 107
Dickens, Charles 92, 229 232, 233, 257–8, 260, 264, 265
die-in 163, 207
Diocletian 101
discipline(s) 14; as knowledge systems 55, 81, 202, 220, 330, 333; in Foucault 7, 65, 81, 219, 357
discourse: academic/artistic 17–18, 114, 124, 138, 146, 163, 188–90, 332; analysis 7, 16, 46, 202, 203, 205, 273, 274, 313–14, 357; biomedical 23, 29, 31, 53–4, 56–7, 61, 138, 146, 170, 190, 195–6, 209, 274, 275, 278–80, 283, 325, 336, 337; erotic 116, 127, 376; legal/political 14, 117, 138, 169, 172, 176, 195–7, 201; lunatic 283; northern versus southern 172–5; of modernist art photography 39; of punitive fidelity 310; scientific 25–6, 146, 272, 274; sexist 264. *See also* AIDS discourse; counter-discourse
disease 152–5, 199; and desire 209, 216, 318, 357; and gay rights 350; and identity 336–7; and secrecy 227; as language 53–4, 87, 191, 201, 203, 205, 211, 234, 241, 273, 283, 305, 357; concept of 46, 53–4, 152, 195, 209, 276, 297, 305, 311; images of 23, 32, 57–8, 61, 72–3, 84, 90–1, 125, 143, 148, 151–2, 179–80, 184, 186–7, 191–2, 209, 272–5; sexually transmitted (STD) 183, 189, 309, 314, 337, 348; visible truth assigned to 57, 61, 114–15, 179–80, 254; Portfolio One 7; *See also* AIDS; cancer; plague; syphilis
disidentification 298–9, 300–2; of gays from straights 311, 339; rivers of 301, 303
doctors 109, 131, 141, 150, 153, 155, 156, 173, 185–92, 221, 226, 248, 254, 269–70, 336, 351; hubris of 199–201, 277–8, 311; power of 105, 182, 195, 197–8, 205, 233, 238, 277; *plate* 48
domino theory of contagion 311–12
Don't Die of Ignorance (campaign) 84, 193–4, 279; *plate* 51
Dreuilhe, Emmanuel 23, 103, 282–4
drugs: addictive 181, 269, 313, 361; experimental 5, 91, 153, 212, 225,

335, 336, 345; trials of 25, 28, 37, 85, 186, 187, 212–13, 318, 345, 357; War on 186, 203, 207, 248. *See also* AZT; dextran sulfate; IV drug users; pentamidine
Dugas, Gaetan 258
Durand, André 10, 89, 94–109; as numerologist 105, 106, 107; as theurgic artist 97–100, 108, 205; *Mystic Marriage*, 100, 107; *Votive Offering*, 10, 89, 94–109, 205; *plate* 39
Dyad, 106–7
Dyer, Richard 123
dying slave: motif in Fabo 70–4, 78, 82, 85, 86; of Michelangelo 70, 71, 75, 86; *plates* 25–7

Easter Seal Society 229, 230
Edwards, Owen 41
Elford, Jonathan 311
Elliot, Rose 107
Embassy Cultural House 12, 53, 66, 68, 69, 207–8, 215–21; *plate* 1
ephesis 106
epidemic: cultural responses to 4, 8, 27–9, 103, 107–8, 116, 118–19, 122, 124, 131–2, 150–2, 164, 179–84, 192, 202–3, 207, 209, 216, 220, 222, 228, 241, 249, 264–6, 268, 278, 281, 303–4, 334–9, 346–7, 350–2, 355–7, 360; history of 143, 272–3; medical/scientific research on, 27–9, 185, 274, 277–8; of bereavement 356; of meanings 274, 277, 355, 357, 363. *See also* AIDS; cholera; malaria
epidemiology 336–7
epistrophē (return) 106–7
Eros 90, 94, 98, 101, 105, 128–9, 209, 219, 267, 269–70, 314
erotophobia 17, 19, 84, 94, 101, 179, 181, 203, 209, 220, 268, 352
Esther 95
Etherington, James 210
Evans, Linda 35; *plate* 8
Eve 91, 179
eye: artist's 10, 79; critic's 188, 192; God's 106; initiate's 97–9, 106, 120, 188; of state surveillance 57, 78, 80, 81, 82, 202, 220–1; *plate* 31. *See also* gaze; power/knowledge; vision

Fabo, Andy 17, 21, 216, 220–1; against masterpiece notion 68–70, 82, 86; and Foucault 19, 65, 80, 81; biography 65–6, 79; *Body Under Duress*, 54, 74, 80, 83–4; bookworks of 10, 12, 54, 68–78, 205, 208, 220–1; *Catalogue of Accusations*, 68, 71, 78, 80, 82, 83, 85; *Conduct Sheet*, 68, 71, 74, 77, 78, 79, 80, 83; defies conventional representation 82, 85, 205; *dying slave* 68, 70, 74, 80, 85; *Encyclopedia of Experience* 220–1; exhibitions of 65–6; keynote address of 16–18, 83, 208, 288; self-portraits of 85–6; *Survival of the Delirious* 208; *The Wall* 66–7, 74, 75; *plates* 25–37; Portfolio Two 12
Fain, Nathan 31
Falwell, Jerry 360
familialism 262, 263, 264, 281, 310, 338, 353, 356; Portfolio One 6
family: coping with AIDS 175, 224, 233, 237, 244, 246, 248, 256, 259–61, 268, 299, 355; drama 112, 122–24, 226, 260–3; heterosexuality of the 353, 356; nuclear 123, 124, 147, 181, 226, 260, 305, 309–10; patriarchal 60, 108, 267, 305; power of 105, 155, 157, 220, 307, 309, 338; surrogate (chosen) 124, 128, 164, 225, 226–7, 256, 259, 306, 311, 315, 355; values 5,

19, 36, 148, 181, 201, 226–7, 229, 260, 264, 310, 314, 331, 338; violence 298–9. *See also* conservatives and conservatism; New Right
Family AIDS Caring Trust (FACT) 173; *plate* 46
Fatal Attraction 37
Federal AIDS Centre (Ottawa) 156
feminity 23, 56, 60, 74. *See also* gender; lesbian(s); women
feminism 5, 8, 10, 53–6, 59–60, 62, 63, 111, 123, 172, 217, 220, 307, 314, 353; Portfolio Two 1–2, 8
Ferro, Robert 268–9
Ficino, Marsilio 97, 105, 109
film 62; feminist 111–12; gay 8, 11, 37, 73, 112, 122–34, 316; lesbian 112; mainstream 37, 111–21, 123, 150, 267
Finger Lakes Trio 118
Finlayson, Catherine 210
Fire Island 117, 118–19
fisting 165
Fleck, Ludwik 25
Fleming, Marnie 208
Florence 98
fluids: bodily 19, 92, 198, 258, 321, 322, 323–6; contaminated 19–20, 70, 92, 198, 263–4, 322, 324, 325; night sweats 261, 269; semen 312; symposiastic 18–20; tears 122, 124, 141, 224, 256, 259; urine 325, 348; wisdom as 20; *plate* 36. *See also* blood
Food and Drug Administration 37
Forest City Gallery 66
Foster, Dr Geoffrey 173
Foucauldianism 21, 56, 108, 112, 115, 169, 173, 192–3, 204–6, 216, 274. *See also* Foucault
Foucault, Michel: *Archaeology of Knowledge* 75, 146; *Birth of the Clinic* 88, 306; death from AIDS 7; *Discipline and Punish* 81, 88, 306, 319; 'Film and Popular Memory' 329, 364; 'Friendship' 364; *History of Sexuality* 306, 319, 366; 'Nietzsche, Genealogy, Practice' 74; on bodies 65, 75–6, 80, 216, 326; on death 356–7; *Order of Things* 75, 88; on sexuality 173, 330, 333; *Power/Knowledge* 319; Quilt panel for 356; scepticism 8, 19, 169; social philosophy 7, 56–7, 75–6, 80, 146, 204–6, 219, 258, 306–7, 321, 326, 357, 362–3; 'Social Triumph of the Sexual Will' 364
France 339
Francis, Don 198
Friedlander, Julia 343
Friends of Photography 210
Freud and Freudianism 57, 60–1, 111, 184, 220, 262, 330, 352
Freytag, Gustav 196, 200
fund-raising 229, 317, 343, 349, 358; and AIDS art 38, 72, 118, 157–9, 163, 266, 267–8, 351
Funnel, The 65

Gagnon, Monika 10, 219
Gallo, Robert 31, 199–201, 257, 263, 265, 277, 282, 283
Garnet Press 66
Gauguin, Paul 71; *plate* 30
gay bars 36, 128, 165, 356
gay-bashing 345
gay communities 14, 31, 33, 36, 46, 65, 114, 117, 122, 124, 130, 165, 222, 235, 243, 249, 260, 261, 311, 327, 329, 334, 335–6, 339, 342–4, 351, 354, 356, 361; disunity among, 347; gays and lesbians united in 345, 350, 351; invisibility of 335–6, 340
gay culture 352, 354–6, 361
gay identity: and memory 359–63;

as counterdiscourse 352; before AIDS 331, 362–3; denial of 351; equated with safer sex 341; fatalistic 353; formation of 219, 331, 334, 352, 359; impact of AIDS activism on 340, 351–2, 354, 359–60, 362; in Britain 337–8; not homosexuality 337–8, 354, 362; politics of 329, 332, 337, 351; problematics of representing 65, 112–16, 140, 258–9, 335–6; radicalization of 14, 112, 250, 332, 334, 347–8, 350, 360–1; rebirth of 10, 119, 334, 360, 362; re-homosexualized 354; sexual re-affirmation of 36, 79, 125, 126–7, 354, 358, 362; socio-political character of 332, 350–1; subsumed by AIDS 36, 86, 163–8, 234–5, 241, 244, 261, 333–4, 335–6, 341, 346, 348
gay liberation: against racism and sexism 348–9, 351; erotics 8, 10, 112, 126–7, 131, 209, 307, 314, 333, 345, 352, 362; impact of AIDS on 36, 87, 112, 118, 131, 134, 148, 165, 187, 223, 249, 250, 307, 341, 348, 349–52, 354–5; leadership of 348; pre-AIDS 4–5, 73, 112, 123, 126–7, 131, 339–40, 358, 361–2; strategic and tactical aims of 345, 350–2, 354, 363; values of 36, 130, 134, 138, 140, 174, 212, 250, 256, 332, 334, 346, 349, 352, 354, 356, 362
gay lifestyle 116, 119, 227, 260–1, 266, 279, 352
gay love 66, 125–7, 167, 221, 227, 256, 268, 311, 334, 361; spiritualized 78, 82, 83, 225, 259, 339; *plates* 31–2, 37, 52
gay men
- as activists 56, 66, 69, 77, 87, 112, 118–19, 136, 138, 141, 187–8, 212, 223, 241–53, 308, 317–18, 329, 336, 339, 342–3, 347–52, 360; *plate* 17
- as 'high-risk' group 16, 25, 29, 30, 55, 86, 120, 188–9, 198, 231, 248, 267, 276, 279–80, 309, 310, 335–6, 343, 356
- discrimination against 4, 13, 36, 65, 177, 222–3, 248–53, 259, 314, 315, 327, 332, 339, 343, 345
- history of 67–9, 73, 114, 123, 126, 306, 340, 342–3, 352–4, 361–3
- representation of 11, 35–6, 39, 65, 69, 73–4, 77, 79, 79–86, 114–21, 122, 140–5, 188–2, 194, 222–7, 256, 258–61, 266–9, 311, 340, 342; *plates* 16–18
- self-representation of 124–31, 135–45, 163–8, 205, 222–27, 238, 242–7, 255–6, 311; *plates* 12–14
- stereotyping of 67, 82, 116, 143, 222–7, 232, 241–2, 279–80, 311, 333, 353

See also homosexual; homosexuality
Gay Men's Health Crisis (GMHC) 27, 32, 33, 36, 44, 48–9, 50, 116, 123, 346, 349, 358; *plates* 13–15, 25, 33, 37
gay plague 27, 30, 91, 191, 244, 260, 266, 269, 281, 313, 337, 341
gay politics 332–3, 339–44, 355, 358–9; activism versus assimilationism in 346–52, 360. *See also* AIDS politics; Foucauldianism
gay pride 350, 360, 361–2; events 342–3, 361
gay rights: 348–9, 351; inseparable from AIDS activism 350, 355, 358–9. *See also* AIDS activism; gay liberation; gay politics
gay sensibility 11, 137–45, 361; camp 132, 136, 140, 163, 258, 268; drag 340; in popular culture 123, 134, 163–8; *plate* 18

gay studies 6; conference at Yale 122; students 341
gay women. *See* lesbian(s)
gaze: film spectator's 113–20; magical 107; medical 7, 56–7, 59–61, 76, 84, 174, 185–6, 205, 218; non-medical 8, 93; patriarchal 63; technocratic 221, 304, 325; *plates* 31, 47
Geleynse, Wyn 217
gender 53, 54, 58, 61, 76, 111, 171, 176, 216, 293, 307, 314, 330, 331, 345; and AIDS discrimination 42, 293; reversal 59, 74, 353; *plate* 3
general public 35, 111–12, 207, 231, 237, 266, 269, 274, 277; myth of 3, 16, 86, 112, 170–1, 193–4; threatened by AIDS 3, 16, 22, 31, 32, 33, 69, 84, 86, 116, 173, 203, 209, 231, 264, 278–9, 310, 337, 353; threatened by gays 353; versus private 164–6, 230–1, 241, 250
genocide 186, 241, 244, 341, 356, 358. *See also* Holocaust
George, St 101
Germany 14, 132, 149; terrorism in 111
Germany Year Zero 114
Get It On (campaign) 194; *plates* 52–3
Gevisser, Mark 341
Gibson, William 322
Gilman, Sander 72, 74, 76, 88, 143, 148, 152, 160
Girard, René 323
Glasgow 360
Gleizes and Metzinger 75, 76
Glück, Robert 334, 335, 336
GMHC. *See* Gay Men's Health Crisis
God 80, 81, 105, 106, 108, 109, 169, 241, 258, 263, 280, 304
Goldstein, Richard 135
Golub, Leon 207, 215, 219; Portfolio Two 7
Gomez, Jewelle L. 348
Gone with the Wind 124, 184
gonorrhea 309
Gordon, John 13, 22, 102, 202, 208, 222–7, 228–30, 232–4, 236–9, 242–47, 250, 252, 253
Gordon, Linda 308–9, 310, 314, 317–18
government: as institution constructing AIDS 28–9, 31, 35, 55, 78, 85, 108, 111, 171–4, 193, 211–13, 305–18; opposed to gays 334; oppression of body 216, 219 220; response to crisis 249, 266, 268, 295–6, 299–300, 314–18, 326, 336, 349, 358–60
Graces, the 98, 99, 107
Grand Bend 241–7
Gran Fury 21, 118, 136, 139, 360, 361
Green Monkey 13, 139, 141–4, 171, 200, 257, 263, 265
Greyson, John 11, 13, 130, 132, 135–45
GRID (Gay-Related Immune Deficiency) 27, 46, 152
Grover, Jan Zita 10, 18, 66, 87, 206, 207, 231, 233, 235, 279
Grundmann, Roy 116
guilt: disease and 311–12, 317; *plate* 9. *See also* Christian; moralism; victim
Gusfield, Joseph 307

Haitians 4, 307, 308, 312–13
Halifax 316
Haman 95
Hardy, William 206
Harris, Daniel 11
Hassan, Jamelie 12, 18, 69, 207, 217
Hay, Louise 362
healing 163, 176; artistic 103–9,

135, 220, 266, 282–3; mystical 218; political 197, 266, 282–3; sexual 125, 130–1. *See also* drugs; magic; medicine; talismans
health 195, 273, 337, 362; and development 171–6; as sobriety 362; images of 23, 49, 108, 180, 195, 197, 230. *See also* public health
Health and Welfare Canada 181
heart disease 153–4
Hecate 99, 100, 101
Heckler, Margaret 31, 258
Helms Amendment 29, 36, 315, 334, 358
Helms, Jesse 36, 120, 201, 358–9
hemophilia and hemophiliacs 28, 35, 152, 250, 251, 311
hepatitis B 152, 154, 183, 261, 347
herpes 183, 307, 347
heterosexism 9, 11, 40, 55, 67, 74, 116, 118, 193, 233, 264
heterosexual(s) 16, 28, 30, 33, 34, 37, 63, 72, 75, 84, 113, 117, 127, 149, 156, 171, 183, 194, 198–9, 231, 241, 251, 257, 268–70, 280, 309, 310, 311, 312, 330–3, 337, 340, 346, 351, 358; as 'innocent victims' 35, 115, 258, 261–4, 281; *plates* 10–11, 42, 53; Portfolio One 10–11
heterosexuality 23, 54, 92, 142, 251, 269–70, 280–1, 330; hegemony of 342; versus homosexuality 331, 353; as ideology 331–2, 336–7, 352–4, 359
high-risk groups. *See* risk groups
Hiroshima 303
Hiroshima Mon Amour 147
Hispanics 25, 29, 114, 118, 313, 317, 351
HIV (Human Immunodeficiency Virus)
– antibody testing or status 28–9, 31, 35–7, 212, 224, 226, 248, 253–4, 255, 269, 290–3, 313, 335, 341, 346, 347, 351
– as cause of AIDS 26, 28, 241, 280, 312
– discovery of 28, 31, 102, 155, 199–200, 277, 280, 285–6, 304, 310
– infection 14, 35, 55, 61, 63, 84, 92, 153, 182, 184, 190, 221, 222, 232, 250, 264, 279–80; *plate* 3
– naming of 28, 31, 47, 211
– physical impact of 3, 170, 182, 255, 262, 280
– representations of 17, 24, 31, 61, 63, 92, 180, 181–2, 186, 189, 199–201, 258, 264, 274, 276, 280, 284, 322, 341; *plate* 4
– socio-cultural impact of 3, 55, 87, 102, 104, 152, 196, 209, 211, 226–7, 231, 250, 264, 298–9, 303–4, 333–9, 348, 363
– transmission of 36, 28, 170, 172, 173, 174, 183, 202, 213, 224, 234, 239, 270, 278–80, 290, 298, 299, 301, 312, 334, 351, 352
– victory over 102, 103, 104, 149, 197, 241, 284
See also AIDS
Hoffman, William 123, 128
Holocaust: AIDS as 95–6, 117, 131, 137, 186–7, 241, 244, 262–3, 341, 343, 347, 360
homoeroticism 314, 334. *See also* Eros; gay love; sex
Homophile Association of London Ontario (HALO) 243
homophobia 55, 62, 83, 119, 120, 170, 193, 203, 223, 227, 243, 248, 250–1, 259, 267, 270, 280, 281, 337, 339, 342, 346, 348, 358–9; internalized 46, 117, 143, 223, 227, 241, 258, 261, 348; rationalizations for 352–4; *plate* 57. *See*

also Helms Amendment; heterosexism
homosexual: concept of the 14, 31, 46, 55, 61, 126, 139, 198, 251, 293, 311, 312, 318, 330–1, 333, 337–8, 340, 362, 363; desire 331–2, 346, 352–3, 363; liberal 342; lifestyle 30, 116, 340–1; male 4, 10, 25, 74, 169, 227, 241, 279–81, 307, 308, 346, 347, 351. *See also* gay men; homosexuality; lesbian(s)
homosexuality 74, 92, 114, 117, 165, 171, 223, 227, 281, 305, 315, 332; and communism 276; and death-fear 354; criminalized 62, 84, 293, 315, 334; desexualized 340; equated with AIDS 30–1, 61, 86, 114, 171, 223, 232, 276, 312; exotic 26, 142, 165, 223, 308, 312; explanations for 233, 331, 352–3; medical concept of 54, 55, 60, 331
Horton and Aggleton 25–6, 30; *plate* 2
hospice 38; *plate* 16
hospital 57–8, 82, 114–15, 125, 131, 140, 143, 147–8, 169, 248, 250–1, 254, 262, 263–4, 266, 267, 311, 316; Hôtel-Dieu (Montreal) 156; Mama Yemo (Kinshasa) 190; Middlesex (London, England) 96; of the Mysteries 94, 101, 107, 108; Salpêtrière (Paris) 57, 59; University (London, Ontario) 15, 19, 206; Victoria (London, Ontario) 226, 233
Houston 26; Center for Immunological Disorders 317
HTLV-III. *See* HIV
Hudson, Rock 24, 28, 29, 33, 35, 49, 130, 142, 148, 198, 308; *plate* 8
human condition, AIDS as 41–2, 237–8, 262–3
Human Immunodeficiency Virus. *See* HIV
human rights 3, 291, 292–3, 294–5, 299–300, 302–3, 306, 333
human T-cell lymphotropic virus (HTLV-III). *See* HIV
Huysmans, Joris-Karl 136
hyper-reality 91, 107, 262
hysteria 53; etymology 58; female 54, 56–8; grande hystérie 57, 59; male 54, 58–9; *plates* 21–4

imaging therapy 109
immigrants, discrimination against 4, 177, 316
immigration 42, 212, 290, 299–300
immune system 91, 148, 150, 170, 186, 197–8, 202, 225, 231, 274–6, 280, 284, 326; *plates* 3–4, 58
immunology as discourse 333
imperialism 170, 180, 217, 218
impotence, societal 295–6, 311–12
Indianapolis 27
individualism 148, 362
Inevitable Love 123, 124, 128, 130
infantilization: of homosexuals 352–3; of PWAs 232–3, 237, 259, 269
inferiorization 5, 10, 56, 63, 114, 170, 175, 202, 218, 219, 220, 241, 326–7
innocence 311–12. *See also* Christian; moralism; victim
Institut Unzeit, Das 66
insurance industry 28, 37, 207, 227, 254
intravenous drug abusers (addicts). *See* IV drug users
Ischar, Doug 137
isolation: of PWA 72–3, 300; ritual 301–2, 303. *See also* AIDS representation; marginalization
IV drug users 28, 30, 115, 131, 152, 157, 212, 231, 248, 276, 312,

361–2; images of 149, 181, 279, 280, 281, 307, 308, 316, 360

jack-off parties 352
Jackson, Bruce 323
Jack the Ripper 76
Jamaica 174; *plate* 47
Janson, H.W. 71
Jaret, Peter 197–8, 200
Jarman, Derek 73
Jocelyn, Tim 66, 72, 83
Jolicoeur, Nicole 56
Jones, Cleve, 355
Jones, James 311
Jordan, 180; Portfolio One 3
Journal of the American Medical Association (JAMA) 24, 28, 33
Journal of the Canadian Medical Association 152–3
Jungianism 219

Kampala 182
Kaposi's Foundation 27, 33
Kaposi's sarcoma (KS) 30, 62, 125, 127, 143, 153, 184, 255, 261; lesions as spectacle 17, 23, 32, 255, 258, 266–7, 360; medical images of 24, 31, 182, 186
Kaufman, David 68
Kaunda, Kenneth 186, 187
Kelly, Mary 56
Kenya 186
Kinahan, David 13, 18, 208, 236–9
King's College (UWO) 223, 228
Kinshasa 190, 301
Kirby, Lynne 59
Kirk and Madsen 340
kissing 35, 118, 124, 130, 143
Kleiman, Dena 335
Klute 111
Knott, Norman 181
knowledge systems. *See* discipline(s)
Koch, Ed 258, 342–4
Kolovakos, Gregory 341–2
Krafft-Ebing, Richard von 329–30, 331, 333
Kramer, Larry 133, 198, 262, 341, 342, 344, 346, 347
Kroker, Arthur 14, 132, 188, 262, 321–8
KS. *See* Kaposi's sarcoma
Kuropat, Rosemary 342, 349
Kybaratas, Stash 126

Lacanian theory 111, 326
Lancet 24
Laplanche and Pontalis 330
Lapointe, Norman 156
Larouche Initiative 28, 29, 37
La Tour, Georges de 93
La Tourette, Gilles 59, 60
LAV. *See* HIV
law 56, 194, 195, 242, 276, 287–8, 315, 331, 332; against gays 333–4, 340, 345; AIDS-specific 290–3, 299–300, 316, 318, 346; aims of 292–3; and lawmakers 293–4, 315; and PWAs 252, 293, 296, 346; and science, 296–7, 315; and symbolism 297, 298, 307, 315; and wishful thinking 302–3; as art-form 14, 16, 287–8, 304; reform 340; setting precedents 302–3; relativism of 288–9. *See also* AIDS legislation
leather 9, 34, 36, 128, 143, 340, 356
Left, the 120, 134, 169, 197, 216, 308, 341, 347–8, 350. *See also* radicals and radicalism
Leibowitch, Jacques 30
Leigh, Carol 281
Lepois, Charles 58
leprosy and lepers 39, 143, 261–2
Lesbian and Gay Health Foundation 37
lesbian(s) 330, 339, 340; activists 56, 138–9, 249, 259, 336, 345,

347, 353, 360; archives 44–5; artists 137; black 348; constituency 231, 242, 243, 309, 342, 343, 345, 346, 351–2, 359, 361, 363; filmmaking 112; images 78; relationships 212, 306, 353, 356; rights 251, 348, 351; students 341; studies 122; with gay men 345, 349, 351, 355, 356, 359, 363
lesions. *See* Kaposi's sarcoma
Let the Record Show ... (installation) 13, 207, 217, 266, 361
leukemia 153
leukoplakia, hairy 188–92, 201, 204
Levine, Carol 318
Lévis-Strauss, Claude 58
Lewis, C.S. 98
Lianna 112
Liberace 148
liberals and liberalism 4–5, 16, 18, 21–2, 113, 116, 117, 120, 148, 169, 172, 173, 178, 230, 264, 299–300, 306, 342, 348, 358
Life 35, 89, 90, 92, 94, 95, 96, 99, 101, 205, 267–8; *plate* 38
Lippi, Filippino 95
lithomancy 102, 103, 225
living with AIDS (theme). *See* AIDS
Londe, Albert 60
London, England 3, 9, 100, 206, 210, 345, 356
London Free Press 13, 222–8, 232, 234, 236–9, 246, 247, 255–6; *plates* 55–6
London Life, sponsor of Visual AIDS 179, 210; *plate* 40
London Lighthouse 210
London, Ontario 17, 68, 193, 222–7, 256; as local focus of volume 9–10; cultural activism in 12, 13, 21, 159, 177–9, 194, 206–11, 215–21, 243–53, 288; discrimination in 248–9, 250
London Regional Art and Historical Museums 177, 207, 208
Longtime Companion 11, 111–21
Los Angeles 26, 136–7, 267, 327; Artists' Space (LACE) 136–7
Lovett, Joe 32
Luna 99–100; lunaria 99
Lusaka 9, 178
lymphadenopathy 30, 261, 266
lymphadenopathy-associated virus (LAV). *See* HIV
lymphocytes 103, 197, 277, 283

MacLaine, Shirley 131, 362
magic: against AIDS 15, 89, 225, 283, 338; healing 96–7, 99–100, 102, 103, 104, 105, 109, 119–20, 225, 283
Magnan, Victor 60
Magdalen, Mary 93–4
Main, Stewart 123, 129
malaria 4
Mandate 79; *plate* 33
Manifeste de Montréal, Le 7, 187, 211–13
Mann, Jonathan 279
Mansfield, Glenn 36; *plate* 12
Mantegna, Andrea 93
maple leaf, as motif in Fabo 78, 85
Mapplethorpe, Robert 17; Portfolio Two 1
marginalization 5, 54, 112, 170, 174, 178, 204, 215, 249; and exclusion 55, 137, 140, 143, 166, 173, 279, 328, 344, 351, 358; as subject for art 67, 77, 112, 114, 217–19, 276, 324, 334; Portfolio Two 2
Marianne and Julianne 111
marker events 301
marriage: heterosexual 312, 346, 353, 355; same-sex 345–6. *See also* familialism; monogamy; moralism

Marshall, Stuart 48
martyr 219, 229; athlete as 230–1; PWA as 93, 96, 100, 104, 107–8, 129, 168, 235, 258–61, 268, 269, 363. *See also* Sebastian
Marx, Karl 327
masculinity 74, 75, 79, 138; crisis of 59–61; oppressively heterosexual 55, 59, 113, 138, 353
Massa, Robert 349–50
Masters, Brian 103, 110
Masters and Johnson 29, 198–9, 200, 257, 278–81, 282, 283
masturbation 79, 127; as safer-sex practice 36, 125, 126, 130, 315, 352
Maupin, Armistead 268–9
Maurice 124, 130
Mayes, Sharon 269–70
McCabe, Colin 113
McCarthyism 93, 276, 280, 325; Body 321, 325–6
media 13, 16, 25–53, 55, 61, 63, 73, 83–7, 89–91, 100, 101, 104, 119, 141, 187, 193, 200, 201, 203, 205, 206, 221, 222–7, 229, 231, 247, 252, 262, 264, 307, 310, 312, 321, 337–8, 340, 361; British 6, 107, 311, 335; gay 23, 27–31, 34, 124; mainstream 4–6, 8, 13, 24, 32–4, 222–8, 230–1, 239, 265, 344; sensationalism 17, 23, 24, 32, 61, 90, 125, 126, 137, 165, 198, 326, 338. *See also* press; television
Medici, Lorenzo de' 97
medicine 83, 102, 155, 195, 199, 238, 249, 298, 331, 335–7; as discourse constructing AIDS 15, 27–30, 55–6, 87, 146–8, 152, 159, 175, 182, 186–92, 197, 265, 276, 315, 326, 350; as political practice 53–4, 76, 115, 258, 265, 266, 275, 281, 283, 287, 336, 357; as religious cult 100, 101; genito-urinary 337; panic 326; Western versus Eastern 218; Portfolio One 7
melodrama 11, 92, 120, 122–34
memento mori (theme) 11, 17, 93, 149, 180, 189, 190, 192
memorials 8, 11, 159, 355, 360
memory: and mourning 66, 80, 82, 83; collective 15, 126, 149; popular 329, 359–63
men: fallible victims 16; hysteria patients 10, 58–60; lawmakers 293–4; saintly athletes 230–1; sex objects 124, 128, 140, 144–5, 268, 330, 331, 351; soldiers 10, 59, 309; super 182–3; Third World 175, 180–4; white heterosexual 16, 63, 293, 351; who have sex with men 351–2; Portfolio One 2, 4–8, 10–11. *See also* gay men; gender; masculinity
Mercer Union 66
Mercury, with Caduceus 98
Metz, Christian 113
Mexico 183, 269; Portfolio One 9
Miami 26, 143
Michals, Duane 39; *plate* 19
Michelangelo 70, 71, 73, 75, 78, 86; *plates* 25–8, 32, 54
Middle Ages: return to 147–51, 204, 259, 261–2, 304, 326–7; *plates* 41–3. *See also* death; periodization; renaissance
military metaphors (for AIDS) 13, 14, 17, 22, 23, 103, 137, 138, 147, 166, 169, 183, 186, 187, 188, 191 197–8, 199, 201, 209, 224, 272–84, 326; civil war 360; First World War 359–60; Gulf War 284; medieval 149; nuclear 147, 150, 153, 303; Second World War 262; terrorism 274, 277–8, 358; *plates* 3, 4, 42, 58; Portfolio One 9
Millais, John Everett 96

millennium 297: fin-de-millénium 321, 322, 323, 325, 326, 347; millenarianism 151, 160. *See also* Age of AIDS; AIDS apocalypse; periodization
Miller, James 66, 147, 149, 157, 158, 159, 160, 216, 217; *plate* 54
Milton, John 190
misogyny 261, 353
modernism 70, 76–7, 176
Mohr, Richard 192
MOMA. *See* Museum of Modern Art
Monad 105, 106, 107
monarchy 108, 151, 205, 268
Monette, Paul 263, 267
monogamy 12, 37, 115–16, 171, 183–4, 263–4, 281, 310, 312, 314, 315, 338, 355; cocooning 352; serial 339. *See also* moralism
Montagnier, Luc 31, 155, 279–80, 282, 283
Montreal 3, 11, 12, 147, 153, 154, 156, 157–9, 185–92, 200, 210, 351–2
moralism 19, 91–3, 107, 115–16, 119, 150, 152, 165–6, 168, 169, 171, 173–5, 179–81, 189, 194, 199, 203, 205, 209, 224, 228, 230, 257–65, 272, 276, 280–1, 304, 307, 310–12, 314, 317, 326–7, 333, 338, 348, 353, 362
Morbidity and Mortality Weekly Report 94, 263, 267
Mordecai 95
Morin, Edgar 147
Morrison, Ken 159
mourning 66, 83, 122, 124, 126; loss and 334–5, 355, 360; rites 11, 15, 39, 119–20, 128, 131, 141, 163–8, 225, 227, 260, 327, 355, 360
Mulroney, Brian 348
Mulvey, Laura 113
Museum of Modern Art (MOMA) 39, 62, 63
mysticism 106–9, 119–20, 181, 218, 225, 259, 262, 283; *plate* 39; Portfolio One 5

NAMES Project. *See* Quilt
Nashe, Thomas 93, 189, 191, 192, 194, 202
National Association of PWAs 37, 44, 48
National Cancer Institute 31
National Enquirer 26, 258
National Gay and Lesbian Health Conference 349
National Gay Rights Advocates 350
National Geographic 197, 275–7; *plates* 3, 58
National Institutes of Health 37, 199
nationalism 330, 338, 360
native peoples: in Australia 182–3; in Canada 180–1, 294; Portfolio One 4–6, 8
Natural History Museum 143
nature: amoral 304; erotic 269–70; homosexuality against 353; tragic 199–200, 277–8, 323
Nature 24, 25
Navy Blue 128
Nazis. *See* Holocaust
necrophilia 90, 142
Neoplatonism 71, 75, 86, 96–8, 99, 105–7, 109
Neumann, Franz 324–5
New England Journal of Medicine 24
New Historicism 206
New Museum of Contemporary Art 13, 207, 217, 266, 360
New Right 5, 19, 22, 27, 36, 197, 202, 276, 281, 307, 308
Newsweek 26, 36; *plates* 9–11
New York 3, 9, 13, 21, 26, 27, 28, 29, 30, 32, 33, 36, 39, 40, 62, 66, 108, 114, 117, 119, 143, 157, 158,

159, 186, 207, 217, 266, 267, 335, 342, 344, 345, 356, 360
New York Native 47–8, 342–4
New York Post 341; *plate* 17
New York Times 26, 33, 153, 334–5
New Zealand 123, 124
Nicholas, St 80
Nietzsche, Friedrich 326–7
nihilism 327
Nixon, Nicholas 39–41, 51, 62; *plate* 20
non-government organizations (NGOs) 171, 173, 351, 358
No Sad Songs 124
novel 257; of Cultural Activism 265–9; of Social Criticism 257–5
numerology, as healing magic 105, 106
nurses 250–1

obituaries 11, 112, 163–8; *plate* 45
object-choice 330–2, 345, 353
O'Brien, Paddy 208
occult, the 97–107; forces of sympathetic cosmos 104. *See also* magic; Neoplatonism; theurgy
October 43 (anthology). *See* Crimp
O'Malley, Jeff 12, 18
Omni 279–80
Ontario 241–2, 252–4
Ontario Charter of Human Rights 13, 242, 244, 247, 251–4
Ontario Human Rights Commission 242, 247, 249
Oppenheim and Thompsen 59
opportunistic infections 313. *See also* psoriasis; thrush
Oral AIDS Epidemiology Project 188, 190
oral sex. *See* sex
Orpheus 80, 83–5; *plates* 35, 44
Other, the 56, 61, 115, 170, 173, 217, 220, 223, 301, 317, 356; killable 323–4; Self and 311–12
Ottawa 316
Ouerd, Michele 58
OutRage 5
Outrageous Too 127

paedophilia 142; equated with homosexuality 353
pain: and disidentification 300–1, 323; and law 298–9, 300, 302. *See also* AIDS tragedy; body
painting 10, 65–110, 129, 157, 168, 180, 192, 205, 217–21; problematics of portraiture 66–7, 70, 77, 85, 166, 168, 217–18, 288–9; *plates* 25–37, 39, 43, 44, 48; Portfolio Two 1–5, 7–12
Pandora 91
panic 321–4, 326–8. *See also* AIDS phobia; postmodernism
panopticon 81, 306, 325
Papua New Guinea 183; Portfolio One 10
Paris 57, 200
Paris Match 32
Parting Glances 123, 124, 127, 129, 130
Päs, Gerard 215, 218, 228–30; Portfolio Two 4
Passing Strangers 126
Pasteur Institute 32, 155, 200
Patient Zero (myth) 198, 258
patriarchy 15, 56, 63, 111, 123, 217, 219, 263, 305, 318
Patton, Brian 13, 18, 208
Patton, Cindy 36, 46, 49, 50, 84, 88, 134, 235, 276, 285, 320, 329, 350, 363, 366
PCP. *See* Pneumocystis carinii pneumonia
Pelagianism 260
penis 76, 79, 84, 182, 184, 269–70, 322
pentamidine 29, 37, 266

people of colour. *See* blacks; Hispanics
People Weekly 251; *plates* 5, 7
periodization 15, 19, 25–30, 86, 123, 137, 257, 308; 'before-and-after' 19, 34, 87, 126, 129, 152, 179, 181, 198–9, 303–4, 362; *plate* 48; Portfolio One 1–2. *See also* Age of AIDS; AIDS apocalypse; millennium
Persephone 99
Personal Best 112
person with AIDS. *See* PWA
Peter Pan 120
phallocentrism 79
phallus 76, 78; *plate* 36; Portfolio One 12; Portfolio Two 1
pharmaceutical industry, as activist target 21, 187, 350, 359
philia 78; *plates* 31–2
Photo (Paris) 32
photography 23–64, 77, 89–92, 185, 192, 217, 267; concerned/documentary 40–3, 62–3, 89–91, 173, 191, 197, 237–9, 243; didactic 42–4, 90, 94; exhibitions 8, 10, 39–42, 62–3, 360; of hysterics 57–8, 60; of PWAs 10, 11, 13, 23, 31–43, 61–3, 89–91, 93, 99, 143, 163, 164, 188, 191, 205, 222, 233, 234, 237–9, 360; photographer as subject of art 39–41; use in prevention campaigns 19, 43; *plates* 3, 5–10, 16–24, 55–6
Picasso: *Demoiselles* 71, 74, 76–7, 79, 86; *Guernica* 204; *Las Meninas* 96; *plate* 29
Pien, Ed 215, 217–18; Portfolio Two 3
pink triangle 77, 187, 241, 360
plague 192, 204, 211, 264; anxiety 20, 189, 231; bubonic (Black Death) 72, 93–4, 140, 143, 149, 205; fantasies 10, 16, 94, 102, 103, 104, 117, 140, 144, 150, 153, 180, 199–200, 202, 260–4, 270, 277
Plato 106, 205, 263; *Symposium* 18, 20, 188
pleasure: and gay identity 329, 333, 352, 358; and power/knowledge 306. *See also* Eros; safer sex; sex
PLWA (Person Living With AIDS). *See* PWA
Pneumocystis carinii pneumonia (PCP) 29, 30, 31, 91, 115, 143, 261
Poe, Edgar Allan 72
Poland 178, 184; Portfolio One 12
Policing Desire. See Watney
polio, 228–9, 231, 234
politics. *See* AIDS politics; gay politics; power structures
Poole, Nancy 207, 208
pornography 159, 194, 217, 312, 315, 334, 338; as film genre 123, 126–8; as safer-sex aid 316, 334; industry 133–4, 142; medical 126, 185, 188–9
posters 16–18, 77, 138; AIDS prevention 8, 9, 11, 12, 19, 22, 118–19, 147–9, 174–5, 177–84, 193–4, 201, 205, 209–11, 351; protest 180–1, 186–7, 360. *See also* Visual AIDS
postmodernism 5, 17, 91, 132, 138, 205, 262, 274, 277, 321–8
poststructuralism 4–5, 14
power/knowledge 56–7, 61–2, 81–2, 169–70, 193, 205, 220, 278, 306–8, 342
power structures 7–8, 54–6, 104, 105, 108, 115, 176, 216, 217, 220, 312, 341–2, 350, 356, 362
Praunheim, Rosa von 112, 131–2
pre-Raphaelite art, 96
Presidential Commission on HIV Epidemic 29, 349
press: AIDS coverage in 27–38, 72, 107–8, 198, 277, 334–7, 347–8,

350, 357; gay 11, 27–9, 33, 163–8, 308, 329, 339, 361; magazines 8, 26, 32, 89–92, 100, 242, 251, 315–16, 361; newspapers 8, 13, 26–9, 175, 222–35, 236–9, 293, 329, 335; tabloids 8, 24, 26, 92, 101, 198. *See also* media
Preston, John 354, 356
Pride Institute 361–2
Primavera. See Botticelli
prisons 220, 306; AIDS and 57–8, 65, 71, 79, 212, 224, 248; HIV-antibody testing in 37, 316
procession (pro-odos), 106–7
Progeria Longaevus, 150–2; *plate* 43
Prohibition 307
Project Inform 29
promiscuity 37, 115, 171, 199, 267, 281, 310, 312, 315, 338, 341
prostitutes: female 4, 35, 74–7, 93–4, 156, 175, 187, 231, 258, 281, 301, 309, 312; male 173–4; *plates* 9, 49
psoriasis 261–2
psychiatry 331, 332
psychoanalysis 332; and activism 359; Freudian 111, 113, 220; post-Freudian 8, 14, 111, 113, 233, 352
psychology 14, 109, 226–7, 259, 300–2; of sexuality 331
public. *See* general public; public health
public health 16, 43, 96, 117, 119, 156, 171–4, 178, 205, 244, 278–9, 290, 297, 299, 309, 313, 316, 317, 350; discourse 4, 12, 19, 208, 221, 333. *See also* general public; government; medicine
Public Studio One 66
Purdy, Richard 11, 150–2; *plate* 43
PWA (person with AIDS) 13, 69, 83, 137, 154, 177, 191, 231, 232–4, 248, 250, 266, 278, 282, 317–18, 346, 359; disposal of 17, 89–90, 163–4, 166–7, 355; identity of 357–8; images of 10, 16, 23–44, 61–3, 72, 85, 89–92, 94, 95, 101, 107–9, 114, 118–19, 124–32, 137, 163–8, 188–92, 204, 205, 208, 218, 222–7, 228–35, 241–7, 258–60, 268–70, 355–7; invisibility of 313; life expectancy of 24–5, 87, 119, 224–5, 313; not victim 48, 62, 85, 91, 95, 101, 103, 108–9, 154, 155, 175, 187, 197, 202, 224–5, 234–5, 241, 247, 254, 268–9, 282–3, 355–6, 357–8; rights of 211–13, 226, 247, 251–4, 290, 292–3, 294–5, 316–18, 349–50; scapegoat 323–4, 326–7, 328; *plates* 5–11, 15–20
PWA Coalition 7, 28, 38, 197, 203
Pythagoreanism 106–7

Quadlund, Michael 316
quarantine 35, 148, 186, 212, 290, 291, 301, 316, 318, 319; of hysterics 56; of PWAs in California proposed 28–9, 50
Quebec 154, 156–9, 253, 258
Queensland 317
queer, as counterdiscursive identity 353
Quilt (The NAMES Project) 11, 29, 45, 159, 163, 355–6, 360, 361

race and racism 40, 55, 114, 121, 170, 180, 193, 197, 217–18, 313, 330, 345, 348, 362
radicals and radicalism 3, 5, 11, 14, 15, 16, 18, 21–2, 84, 111–12, 118, 141, 187–8, 194, 197, 203–4, 207, 211, 346, 360
radio 43, 164, 207
railway spine and brain 59
Ramsauer, Kenneth 32, 34; *plate* 6
Raphael 71, 77, 78, 80, 81, 86; *plate* 29

Ray, Gypsy 38; *plate* 16
Reagan, Ronald 31, 37, 117, 186, 231, 275, 310, 316, 324, 342, 348, 349
realism 75–6, 329; gay 342; reactionary 11, 81–2, 112–14, 118, 119–21, 238–9, 264–5, 311, 342
Recross Knight 100
Redon, Odilon 83
Reed, Paul 266–7
Régnard, Paul 60; *plate* 22
Reich, Dahlia 13, 222–7, 228, 232, 233, 236–9, 243, 255–6; *plates* 55–6
religion. *See* Christian; church; moralism
Renaissance 72, 85–6, 93, 94–7, 100, 106, 148, 189, 191, 192, 195, 197, 205; as resistance movement 159–60; ecphrastic rivalry in 7; versus resistance movement 10, 11, 108–9, 135, 141
Réne, Norman 11, 112, 113
representation 25–6, 53–4, 56, 73, 75, 76, 86, 115, 148, 159, 160, 170, 194; as empowerment 32, 62, 77, 84–5, 97, 102, 104, 137, 174, 187, 217–18, 235, 282–4, 317; as re-creation and disposal 17, 82, 97; problematics of 67–8, 70, 73, 80–2, 113–15, 178, 192–4, 234–5, 272–84; *plate* 34. *See also* AIDS representation; crisis
Representing AIDS (conference) 15–19, 53, 68, 83, 134, 178, 206, 208, 242, 288, 318; criticized 54, 138; reviewed 21–2; *plate* 1
repression 58, 123, 202
Resnais, Alain 147
resurrection 119–20, 166; of cosmos 104; of Gary Walsh 259; of Sunnye Sherman 97, 99, 102
retrovirus. *See* HIV; immune system
Rhodes, Richard 67
Richer, Paul 60
Right, the. *See* conservatives and conservatism; New Right
risk: legal concept 294–5; living with 295–6
risk groups 31; discrimination against 4, 16, 22, 121, 209, 276, 308, 312; 'high' and 'low' 22, 35, 37, 173, 279–80, 351. *See also* blacks; gay men; Haitians; immigrants; IV drug users; prostitutes; PWAs; women
Rist, Darrell Yates 342–50, 352, 359
Rivera, Geraldo 33
Rosenberg, Charles E. 152–3
Rosett, Jane 38–9; *plates* 17–18
Rosler, Martha 63
Rossellini, Roberto 114
Rossetti, Dante Gabriel 96
Rowe, Bill 226–7
royal touch 100, 104
Rubin, Gayle 311–12
rupture 11, 63, 86, 151–2, 181; of representational strategies 66, 146–60, 314
Ruse, Michael 21
Russo, Vito 343

sado-masochism (S/M) 143, 165, 219, 312, 324, 327, 334
safer sex: and gay identity 341–2, 347, 352, 354, 357–8; calendar 36; cartoon 9; comics 36, 182; eroticizing 84, 116, 117, 120, 125–6, 144, 209, 352, 362; films 125–6, 128, 130–1, 133; information 116, 178, 190, 193, 202, 203, 213, 309, 314, 315, 317, 318, 341; manuals 50, 116; politics of 15, 36, 329; practices 36, 84, 116, 130, 144, 268, 282, 313, 352, 358; publications 29, 33, 36, 201; Socratic dialectic as 20; taboos against 314, 352, 358; theorized and in-

vented by gay activists 36–7, 84, 116–17, 352, 354; *plates* 12–14
Salpêtrière 57, 59, 60; *plates* 22–4
Sanders, Marie 219
San Francisco 3, 9, 10, 26, 27, 29, 30, 32, 33, 41, 43, 50–1, 119, 126, 144, 163–8, 169, 188, 190, 191, 206, 210, 258–64, 270, 335; the Castro 11, 199, 258, 260, 268, 269, 356, 351
San Francisco AIDS Foundation 33, 36, 38, 45
Sappho 144
satellite dish, motif in Fabo 84, 220–1; *plates* 35–6
Schatz, Ben 350–2
Schweitzer, John A. 157, 158, 159; Galerie 149, 157–8, 160, 210; *plates* 40–1
science: as discourse 57, 146, 152, 159, 173, 174, 178, 188–9, 265, 273, 274, 315, 330; authority of 9, 26, 105, 154–5, 158, 173, 188–90, 201, 209, 274–5, 277–9, 283, 296–7, 330, 336, 350
Science 24, 25
Scientific American 199–200, 277; *plate* 4
Scott, Mary 54, 210, 215, 217; Portfolio Two 1
Sebastian, St 10, 70, 71, 73, 93, 94, 101, 268; *plates* 25–8, 30
Sebastiane 73
Segal, Lynne 55
Selene 99–100
Self 330; and Other 311–12
Senegal 179–80; Portfolio One 2
sex 19, 89–90, 130, 159, 165, 175, 179, 189, 194, 209, 248, 260, 266, 281, 305, 307, 309, 314, 337, 357, 362; anal 116, 117, 130, 165, 312, 313, 315, 315, 337; anal-oral 188–92; and family 308–11; blamed for AIDS 358; cynical 321–2; deviant 115, 142–3, 169, 171, 268, 280, 306, 333; equated with AIDS 181; gay 36, 79, 116, 117, 125, 130–1, 142, 165, 258, 260, 308, 312, 338, 340, 352, 354, 358; genital-oral 116, 130, 189; panic 14, 132; premarital 338; procreative 308–9, 312, 353; represented in art 5, 79–83, 142–3, 178, 181, 183, 216, 269–70, 321; sacrificial 321–8; toys 312; unsafe 299, 310, 318, 347; vaginal 313, 337; *plates* 12–14, 59–60; Portfolio One 10–12; Portfolio Two 1, 9. *See also* safer sex; sexuality
sexism 40, 121, 197, 269, 348. *See also* heterosexism; homophobia
sexology 329–31
sexual acts, discourse of 333, 336, 337
sexual diversity, and gay identity 332, 338
sexuality 33, 54, 56–9, 61, 62, 74, 86, 176, 181, 251–2, 309, 313, 314, 332–3, 336–7, 342, 362; as discourse 14, 124, 173, 306–7, 318, 321–8, 330, 333–4, 336, 359; female 349; gay 36, 73–4, 84, 124–5, 127, 128, 251–2, 332, 340, 345, 353; invention of 331; rigid categories of 345. *See also* heterosexuality; homosexuality
sexually transmitted disease (STD). *See* disease; gonorrhea; syphilis
sexual politics 330–2, 348, 359; of Foucault 333, 357. *See also* AIDS politics; gay liberation
Shanti 38
Sheehan, Nick 124
shell shock 59–60
Sherman, Ina 92; as Demeter 102
Sherman, Sonya (Sunnye) 89–109, 205; daughter of Murray 92, 102; *plates* 38–9

Sherwood, Bill 123
Shilts, Randy 13, 48, 198, 257–65, 268, 342, 348; *And the Band Played On* 46, 257–65
Showalter, Elaine 56, 59, 61
Sibyl, the 78
SIDACTION 186; *plate* 50
SIDART 159
silence equals death (theme) 21, 77, 144, 170, 187, 191, 194, 207, 221, 222–3, 227, 235, 263, 266, 270, 308, 314, 317, 326, 360
Silin, Jonathan 318
sin 311–13, 333, 353. *See also* Christian; God; moralism; plague; victim
Sisters of Perpetual Indulgence 258, 261
Sisyphus 82
slim disease 182
Sloterdij, Pietr 323
Socrates 15, 18–20
Sokolowski, Thomas 41, 51
Solomon, Rosalind 39–41, 51, 62
Somerville, Margaret 14, 19, 21
Sontag, Susan 39, 46, 51, 138, 160, 272–6, 282, 285, 297
sotadic zones 142
soul 71, 80, 81–3, 98, 102, 202, 218, 259, 263, 267, 330
specularity, dominant 61–3, 113–15, 120
Spence, Jean 217
Spenser, Edmund 100
Spero, Nancy 54, 207, 215, 218; Portfolio Two 8
spiritus: astral 105; 'discretio spirituum' 259
Sri Lanka 184; Portfolio One 11
Star 26
Star Wars (Strategic Defense Initiative) 37, 275
State. *See* government; monarchy; power structures
STD (sexually transmitted disease). *See* disease; gonorrhea; syphilis
Stockholm 356
straights. *See* heterosexual(s)
Street Kids International 173
structuralism 4
Sun (Toronto) 72
Sunday People (UK) 32
Survivors 173
Switzerland 150, 177, 210
symposium: etymology of 19; versus anti-symposiastic spirit 18–20
syndrome 84–5, 111, 181, 194, 196, 203, 228, 307, 337; as system 112–13, 118–21, 157; 'do something' 296. *See also* AIDS; discourse; disease
syphilis 39, 72, 74, 76, 143, 152, 183, 309

tabloids. *See* press
talismans 97, 100, 102, 103, 105–6, 108, 109, 182–3, 220, 283
technology: and sex 321–2; as virus 322
television: AIDS movies 122, 130, 311; commercials 91–2, 156, 260, 262, 310, 351; coverage of AIDS crisis 8, 32, 33, 35–6, 43, 48, 49, 100, 140, 144, 166, 169, 192, 197, 261, 350, 356; 'Dynasty' 35, 49; Gulf War coverage 284; 'Morton Downey' 327; 'Star Trek' 143; 'The Journal' 169; '20/20' 32, 33, 34. *See also* media; press; radio
testing: anonymous 213, 251; ethics of 37, 212, 251, 254, 290, 295, 299–300, 313, 316, 348; mandatory 290, 292–3, 295, 316, 348; *plate* 15. *See also* HIV; law; quarantine
Testing the Limits 136
Tetrad 107
text: body as 55–63, 219; film as

progressive 114–15, 117, 119–20; film as subversive 114
Thanatos, and Eros 90, 94, 209, 267. *See also* AIDS allegory; death; sex
The ADS Epidemic 130
The Advocate 361
The AIDS Support Organization (TASO) 175
theatre, as cultural activist site 122, 133
The Body & Society (exhibition) 12, 13, 53–4, 66, 68, 207, 215–21; Portfolio Two 1–12
The Handmaid's Tale 114
The Jungle Boy 132
The Nation 341, 345, 347
The Navigator 150
The Normal Heart 133
therapy: industry 361–2; PWAs and 225, 226, 227, 259, 269, 282–3
theurgy 97–8, 100, 103, 105–6, 109
Third World 3, 12, 169–76, 178–84, 217, 313. *See also* Africa; developmentalism
thrush 189, 191, 261
Tidmus, Michael 137
Time 26, 180, 284
Timmy: Easter Seal 13, 228–30; PWA as 13, 228–9
Toronto 3, 9, 10, 11, 17, 65, 72, 144, 186, 207, 223, 224, 225, 229, 242, 256
transfusion, AIDS 28, 35, 258, 260, 308, 311–12
Treichler, Paula 29–30, 46, 47, 49, 53, 63, 274, 285, 286; *plate* 4
triad: of Dianas 99; of Graces 98, 99, 102, 107; princess-priestess-PWA 99–102, 107
Trinity, the 99
Trotta, Margarethe von 111
T-shirts: activist 118, 187, 346; erotic 70; homophobic 13, 241–7, 250, 252; *plate* 57
tuberculosis 148, 272
Turner, Bryan 53, 216, 276, 285
twelve-step movement 361–2

Uganda, 175, 182; Portfolio One 7
Ulrichs, Karl 331, 334
Una, 100
United States 9, 14, 23–51, 93, 96, 111–21, 168, 180, 186, 198, 260, 264, 276, 279–80, 284, 290, 305, 309, 311, 313, 314, 333, 334, 355, 360–1; California 259, 269, 321, 322, 325, 339–42, 346, 348, 351, 352, 358; Colorado 316; Illinois 316; Minnesota 316; Texas 317
university: as site of AIDS activism 4–5, 8, 202–11; Concordia 11, 14; hierarchy 8; Laval 156; McGill 14; of California 188; of Calgary 65; of Montreal 156; of North Carolina 206, 210; of Western Ontario 10, 11, 12, 13, 15, 53, 68, 159, 177, 193–4, 206, 207, 216, 223, 228, 241, 318; of Windsor 14, 318; Rice 168; Rutgers 206
unnaturalness, homosexuality as 353
Urinal 132
urn: funeral 89, 91, 92, 93, 96, 101, 163; as death aestheticized 17–18; *plates* 1, 38
USA Today 26

vagina 78, 179, 312, 322, 337
Vance, Carole S. 330
vanitas mundi (theme) 93, 148
Venus 98–9, 102, 269
Veronica, St 143
victim 147, 170, 195, 196, 202, 219, 228, 268, 272, 302, 321, 323–4; guilty 34, 61, 126, 310, 311; innocent 34, 62, 93, 168, 229, 308, 311; sacrificial 323, 326, 328;

plates 9, 10. *See also* AIDS victim; children; moralism
Vidal, Gore 342, 348
video 49, 122–3, 126, 208; as activist documentary 8, 11, 132, 137; as educational tool 9, 36–7, 128, 130, 132, 173–4; games 284; music 130, 137
Village Voice 135
Virgin, the 77, 80, 89, 98; in Majesty 99
virginity 98–102. *See also* abstinence; monogamy; moralism
vision 192; intellectual 109; physical 109, 322; spiritual 103, 104, 106, 109; virtual 322. *See also* eye; gaze; power/knowledge; specularity; voyeurism
Visual AID (San Francisco charity) 211
Visual AIDS (New York arts group) 159
Visual AIDS (poster exhibition) 147, 149, 160, 177–84, 206–11; *plates* 40–2, 47–8, 52–3, 59–60; Portfolio One 1–12
Votive Offering. See Durand
voyeurism 61, 63 185, 258

Waddell, Tom 50–1
Walsh, Gary 258–61, 268
War on AIDS. *See* military metaphors
Washington, DC 27, 29, 91, 92, 210
Watney, Simon 6, 9, 14–15, 47, 61, 72, 74, 83, 170, 187, 192–3, 206, 216, 265, 310–11; 'AIDS and Photography' 366; 'Homosexual Body' 364; *Policing Desire* 6, 9, 20, 47, 48, 170, 214, 234, 310–11, 315, 320, 332, 364, 465; 'Rhetoric of AIDS' *plate* 6; 'Safer Sex' 365, 366; 'Spectacle of AIDS' 6, 55, 61, 63, 64; *Taking Liberties* 365; 'Visual AIDS' 211, 214
Waugh, Thomas 11
Weeks, Jeffrey 330, 345, 362
Weeks, Ned 71
Weinmann, Heinz 147
Wells, Peter 123, 129
White, David 10, 18, 65–88, 187, 194, 205, 206, 220
White, Edmund 68, 141
White, Ryan 251; *plates* 5, 10
WHO. *See* World Health Organization
Wilson, Ruth 12, 22, 178–9
Wind, Edgar 97
WOG (Wrath-of-God) 27, 47, 258, 304
Wolf, Susan 318
Women 123, 175, 177, 309, 330, 331, 334; and AIDS 30, 40, 91–2, 227, 312, 317; artists 137, 143; bodies of 54–7, 76, 213, 219, 262, 308; 'fallen' 16, 76, 90–1, 94, 102, 263–4, 308, 309, 312; images of 19, 54–61, 63, 74, 77, 89, 93–6, 98–9, 100, 101, 111–12, 114, 131, 178–9, 217, 218–19, 262, 267, 269–70, 309; in liberation movements 4, 111, 148, 213, 246, 306, 308–9, 314; patients 10, 54–61, 91, 262, 349; PWAs 4, 89, 91, 99, 156, 175, 176, 212, 260–2, 269–70, 281, 311; rights of 306, 308; *plates* 8–11, 16, 21, 31, 38–9, 42, 49; Portfolio One 1, 6, 7, 10–11; Portfolio Two 2, 6, 8. *See also* feminism; lesbian(s); prostitutes
workplace: AIDS and the 43–4, 248, 251, 254, 256
world: as symbolic order 284, 314, 350; dual AIDS 186–8, 192, 194, 205, 350; real 3, 5, 185, 186, 196, 274, 349; turned upside down 103, 151, 186–7, 283; virus as 186–7; *plates* 2, 50

World Health Organization (WHO) 9, 12, 120, 171, 279, 300

xenophobia 330; and AIDS discrimination 16, 27, 180, 300–2

Yates, Frances 97

Zaire 190, 191, 301
Zambia 9, 174, 178; Portfolio One 1
Zimbabwe 173

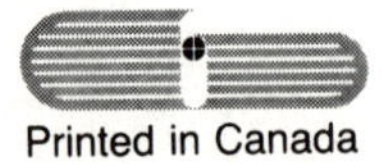
Printed in Canada

PRICE
PRICE
1 23456 78900 5